Prostheses in Antiquity

Today, a prosthesis is an artificial device that replaces a missing body part, generally designed and assembled according to the individual's appearance and functional needs with a view to being both as unobtrusive and as useful as possible. In classical antiquity, however, this was not necessarily the case. The ancient literary and documentary evidence for prostheses and prosthesis use is contradictory, and the bioarchaeological and archaeological evidence is enigmatic, but discretion and utility were not necessarily priorities. So, when, how and why did individuals utilise them? This volume, the first to explore prostheses and prosthesis use in classical antiquity, seeks to answer these questions, and will be of interest to academics and students with specialist interests in classical archaeology, ancient history and history, especially those engaged in studies of healing, medical and surgical practices, or impairment and disability in past societies.

Jane Draycott is Lord Kelvin Adam Smith Research Fellow in Ancient Science and Technology at the University of Glasgow, UK. Previously she was Lecturer in Classics at the University of Wales Trinity Saint David, Associate Teacher in Roman Archaeology at the University of Sheffield, all in the UK, and 2011–2012 Rome Fellow at the British School at Rome, Italy.

Medicine and the Body in Antiquity

Series editor: Patricia Baker, University of Kent, UK

Advisory board:
Lesley A. Dean-Jones, University of Texas at Austin, USA
Rebecca Gowland, University of Durham, UK
Jessica Hughes, Open University, UK
Ralph Rosen, University of Pennsylvania, USA
Kelli Rudolph, University of Kent, UK

Medicine and the Body in Antiquity is a series which aims to foster interdisciplinary research that broadens our understanding of past beliefs about the body and its care. The intention of the series is to use evidence drawn from diverse sources (textual, archaeological, epigraphic) in an interpretative manner to gain insights into the medical practices and beliefs of the ancient Mediterranean. The series approaches medical history from a broad thematic perspective that allows for collaboration between specialists from a wide range of disciplines outside ancient history and archaeology such as art history, religious studies, medicine, the natural sciences and music. The series will also aim to bring research on ancient medicine to the attention of scholars concerned with later periods. Ultimately this series provides a forum for scholars from a wide range of disciplines to explore ideas about the body and medicine beyond the confines of current scholarship.

Available:

Tertullian and the Unborn Child: Christian and Pagan Attitudes in Historical Perspective – Julian Barr

Bodies of Evidence: Ancient Anatomical Votives Past, Present, and Future – Jane Draycott and Emma-Jayne Graham

Hippocratic Oratory: The Poetics of Early Greek Medical Prose – James Cross

Forthcoming:

Becoming a Woman and Mother in Greco-Roman Egypt: Women's Bodies, Society, and Domestic Space – Ada Nifosi

Cultural Systems of Classification: Sickness, Health, and Local Epistemologies – Ulrike Steinert

Empathy and Compassion in the Medicine and Literature of Greece and Rome – Amber J. Porter

Music Therapy in Ancient Greece – Antoinetta Provenza

Retail Therapy: Selling Pharmaka, Buying Health in Ancient Greece and Rome – Laurence Totelin

Roman Homes, Gardens, and Domestic Medical Practice – Jane Draycott

https://www.routledge.com/classicalstudies/series/MBA

Prostheses in Antiquity

Edited by Jane Draycott

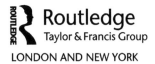

Routledge
Taylor & Francis Group

LONDON AND NEW YORK

First published 2019 by Routledge

2 Park Square, Milton Park, Abingdon, Oxon, OX14 4RN
605 Third Avenue, New York, NY 10017

Routledge is an imprint of the Taylor & Francis Group, an informa business

First issued in paperback 2020

British Library Cataloguing-in-Publication Data
A catalogue record for this book is available from the British Library

Library of Congress Cataloging-in-Publication Data
Names: Draycott, Jane (Jane Louise), editor.
Title: Prostheses in antiquity / edited by Jane Draycott.
Description: Abingdon, Oxon ; New York, NY : Routledge, 2018. |
Series: Medicine and the body in antiquity | Includes bibliographical
references and index.
Identifiers: LCCN 2017038466 (print) | LCCN 2017038988 (ebook) |
ISBN 9781351232388 (Web PDF) | ISBN 9781351232371 (ePub) |
ISBN 9781351232364 (Mobi/Kindle) | ISBN 9781472488091
(hardback : alk. paper) | ISBN 9781351232395 (ebook)
Subjects: | MESH: Prostheses and Implants—history | History, Ancient
Classification: LCC RD130 (ebook) | LCC RD130 (print) | NLM QT
11.1 | DDC 617.9/56—dc23
LC record available at https://lccn.loc.gov/2017038466

ISBN: 978-1-4724-8809-1 (hbk)
ISBN: 978-0-367-73360-5 (pbk)

Typeset in Bembo
by Florence Production Ltd, Stoodleigh, Devon

For Kyle Erickson, in recognition of and gratitude for everything that you did and continue to do for me

Contents

Figures

Tables

Abbreviations

AHR – *American Historical Review*
AJA – *American Journal of Archaeology*
AJP – *American Journal of Philology*
AJ – *Archaeological Journal*
ANRW – *Aufstieg und Niedergang der Römischen welt. Rise and Decline of the Roman World*
CAJ – *Cambridge Archaeological Journal*
CCRH – *Les Cahiers du Centre de recherches historiques*
CIL – *Corpus Inscriptionum Latinarum*
CJ – *Classical Journal*
CQ – *Classical Quarterly*
CW – *Classical World*
G&R – *Greece and Rome*
GRBS – *Greek, Roman and Byzantine Studies*
HSCP – *Harvard Studies in Classical Philology*
IA – *Internet Archaeology*
IG – *Inscriptiones Graecae*
ILS – *Inscriptiones Latinae Selectae*
IJO – *International Journal of Osteoarchaeology*
JEA – *Journal of Egyptian Archaeology*
JHS – *Journal of Hellenic Studies*
JRA – *Journal of Roman Archaeology*
JRS – *Journal of Roman Studies*
JRSM – *Journal of the Royal Society of Medicine*
LIMC – *Lexicon Iconographicum Mythologiae Classicae*
OJA – *Oxford Journal of Archaeology*
PBSR – *Papers of the British School at Rome*
PPS – *Proceedings of the Prehistoric Society*
REG – *Revue des études grecques*
SHM – *Social History of Medicine*
SJA – *Stanford Journal of Archaeology*
TAPA – *Transactions of the American Philological Association*

All papyri are abbreviated according to the conventions of the *Checklist of Greek, Latin, Demotic and Coptic Papyri, Ostraca and Tablets*, available at https://library.duke.edu/rubenstein/scriptorium/papyrus/texts/clist.html (accessed January 2018).

Contributors

Ellen Adams is Senior Lecturer in Classical Art and Archaeology at King's College London, UK. She has published extensively on Minoan Crete, including a book entitled *Cultural Identity in Minoan Crete: Social Dynamics in the Neopalatial Period* (Cambridge, 2017). For some years, she has been investigating the field of Disability Studies, in a project entitled 'The Forgotten Other: Disability Studies and the Classical Body'. Papers produced in this area include: 'Fragmentation and the Body's Boundaries: reassessing the Body in Parts', in J. Draycott and E.-J. Graham (edd.) *Bodies of Evidence: Ancient Anatomical Votives Past, Present and Future*. She has also learned British Sign Language to an advanced level, and has a keen interest in signed art tours and the relationship between visual culture and visual language.

Marshall Joseph Becker is Professor Emeritus of Anthropology at West Chester University, USA, and a Distinguished Member of the American Anthropological Association. He has authored numerous publications in the fields of forensic anthropology, ancient cremation, Maya archaeology, Native American archaeology and ethnohistory, and the analysis of human skeletal material from Iron Age and later sites in Italy.

Michaela Binder is a bioarchaeologist and is currently Research Associate at the Austrian Archaeological Institute, Vienna, Austria.

Jane Draycott is Lord Kelvin Adam Smith Research Fellow in Ancient Science and Technology at the University of Glasgow, UK. Previously she was Lecturer in Classics at the University of Wales Trinity Saint David, Associate Teacher in Roman Archaeology at the University of Sheffield, all in the UK, and 2011–2012 Rome Fellow at the British School at Rome, Italy. Her research focuses on the history and archaeology of medicine in classical antiquity, and her publications include *Bodies of Evidence: Ancient Anatomical Votives Past, Present and Future* with Emma-Jayne Graham (2017) and *Approaches to Healing in Roman Egypt* (2012).

Josef Eitler is an independent archaeologist in Vienna, Austria. His research focuses particularly on Late Antiquity and Early Christianity, as well as on transition processes at the beginning of the Early Medieval Period. Currently he is head of the Austrian Science Fund project 'Cult Continuity at the Summit of Hemmaberg' at the Landesmuseum Kärnten.

Jacky Finch is now an Independent Researcher after spending five years as a Visiting Scientist at the University of Manchester, UK. The research presented in her paper was undertaken at the KNH Centre for Biomedical and Forensic Egyptology at the University of Manchester, UK between 2006 and 2009. It formed part of the PhD awarded in 2009 and continues to attract attention worldwide.

Lennart Lehmhaus is Harry Starr Fellow in Judaica at the Harvard University Centre for Jewish Studies, USA. He is also a postdoctoral research associate within the Collaborative Research Center SFB 980 'Episteme in Motion' on transfer of knowledge at Freie Universität Berlin. As a member of the project A03 (on Encyclopaedic medical episteme in Late Antiquity), he inquires into Talmudic medical discourses, their Jewish epistemologies and encyclopaedic dimensions, with a comparative eye on Graeco-Roman and (Ancient) Near Eastern cultures. His dissertation and first book on Seder Eliyahu Zutah combines a first-time annotated German translation and bilingual edition with a thorough study of the innovative literary, discursive and socio-cultural dimensions of this work. He has published several articles on rabbinic Judaism and midrashic traditions in a multi-cultural context, and on Jewish literature and knowledge. His research interests comprise ancient Jewish cultures and literatures; knowledge and science in the ancient world; literary theory, intertextuality and socio-cultural readings of texts; and trajectories of Jewish traditions into contemporary Jewish and Israeli culture.

Jean MacIntosh Turfa is a Consulting Scholar in the Mediterranean Section of the University of Pennsylvania Museum, USA, and teaches and researches in Etruscan archaeology and ancient religious cults. She is editor of *The Etruscan World*, and, with Stephanie L. Budin, *Women in Antiquity* (2013 and 2016), and author of *Divining the Etruscan World* (2012) and, with Marshall J. Becker, *The Etruscans and the History of Dentistry: The Golden Smile Through the Ages* (2017).

Anne-Sophie Noel is currently a scholar-in-residence and adjunct assistant professor at American University (Washington, DC, USA) as well as an associate researcher at HiSoMA (Lyon, France). She is a cultural historian of ancient Greece, specialising in the performance and reception of Greek drama. For the academic years 2015–2017, she was a Junior fellow of Harvard's Center for Hellenic Studies, where she continued work on her book manuscript that combines her interest in ancient drama and object studies, *Things that Move: Objects and Feelings in Ancient Greece*. She has published widely on Greek tragedy; her forthcoming publications include projects on a cognitive approach to the interactions between verbal and visual inputs in ancient performance, the ancient Greek worship of objects, and female affective relationships with daily-life instruments. She is also involved in a French collaborative translation and commentary of Pollux' *Onomasticon* book IV (section on theatre).

Katherine D. van Schaik is a research affiliate of the Harvard Department of the Classics, a postdoctoral fellow in Harvard's Program in Science, Religion, and Culture, and a medical resident at Harvard Medical School's teaching hospitals. She completed her PhD in Ancient History at the Harvard Department of the Classics, USA, and her MD training at Harvard Medical School. Katherine's research in ancient history and in modern medical education investigates changes in definitions of disease over time, medical training and knowledge transmission, and medical decision-making in Greco-Roman antiquity and in contemporary settings. A particular focus of her work is the development and evolution of disease classification methods and treatment algorithms from the period of the Hippocratic physicians to Galen. She has published in the *Journal of the American Medical Association, Academic Radiology, PLoS ONE* and the *American Journal of Physical Anthropology,* and has contributed to edited volumes focusing on ancient medicine, including the *Studies in Ancient Medicine* series.

Acknowledgements

The core of this book stems from a conference entitled 'Prostheses in Antiquity' organised by the editor and hosted by the University of Wales Trinity Saint David on the Lampeter campus on 30th June 2015. I would like to thank all the staff and students of UWTSD who provided administrative and technical support in the lead-up to the conference and on the day itself.

I would also like to express my gratitude to the Wellcome Trust, which funded the entirety of the conference through the Small Grant scheme (small grant reference number 108557/Z/15/Z), and the Classical Association, which funded five bursaries for postgraduate students. Without this generous financial support, the conference would not, could not, have taken place.

Special thanks are due to Kyle Erickson, who was supportive of my research into prostheses in antiquity from its inception, to Emma-Jayne Graham, who was a thoughtful, critical and exacting reader of early drafts of each chapter, to the anonymous reviewers engaged by Routledge for their feedback on the initial manuscript, and finally to Patty Baker, not just in her capacity as editor of Routledge's Medicine and the Body in Antiquity series, but as a mentor and a source of inspiration in my ongoing efforts in the field of the history and archaeology of medicine in antiquity.

Jane Draycott

Introduction

Jane Draycott

Lydian Pelops, with whom mighty Earthholder Poseidon fell in love, after Clotho pulled him from the pure cauldron, distinguished by his shoulder gleaming with ivory . . .[1]

The earliest mention of a prosthesis in Graeco-Roman literature can be found in Pindar's retelling of the myth of Pelops in the first *Olympian Ode* (*circa* 522–433 BCE).[2] While the fine details of the myth vary from source to source, ancient authors are generally in agreement regarding the fact that his father Tantalus wished to make a suitable offering to the gods of the Olympian pantheon, so killed his son, cut him up and cooked him in a stew which he served to them.[3] All the gods except for Demeter declined the stew; she was distracted by the loss of her daughter Persephone following her abduction by Hades so ate the portion she was offered, a portion which contained Pelops' left shoulder. Upon discovering what Tantalus had done, the gods reassembled and resurrected Pelops, and replaced his missing shoulder with an ivory prosthesis.

Even though Pelops' prosthesis is mythological rather than historical, it offers us a suitable starting point for an examination of prostheses in classical antiquity, broadly defined.[4] Many of the aspects of ancient prostheses, prosthesis use and prosthesis users that will be explored over the course of this volume are present here. The myth of Pelops demonstrates an individual losing a body part and replacing it with an artificial substitute; ancient authors emphasise that his incomplete body is subsequently rendered complete through this action.[5] It demonstrates a particular emphasis being placed upon the material from which the prosthesis is manufactured, the exotic and luxurious imported substance ivory; ever after, this ivory shoulder serves to distinguish its user; it gleams, it shines, it glows.[6] It demonstrates that subsequently the prosthesis, in conjunction with his prowess as an equestrian, is what he is famous for and reference to it serves almost as a heroic epithet.[7] Ancient paintings of Pelops include the prosthesis and make a feature of it.[8] Intriguingly, Pelops' prosthesis is also an object in its own right; it has a life and story of its own separate from him. After Pelops' death, the prosthesis was exhibited in a sanctuary at

Elis; the rest of his bones were interred at the temple of Artemis Cordax some distance from Olympia.[9] It was the subject of a prophecy regarding how the Greeks could win the Trojan War.[10] After the fall of Troy, on its way back to Elis, it was lost at sea.[11] However, many years later it was recovered by the fisherman Damarmenos, and he took it to the Oracle at Delphi to find out whose bone it was and what he should do with it.[12] The Oracle told him to give the bone to the Eleian embassy, the members of which were also at Delphi seeking help with a plague that was ravaging Elis, and they rewarded him by naming him and his family guardians of the bone.[13] Much later, authors exaggerated its connection with the fall of Troy by claiming that it was turned into the Palladium.[14] And yet, for all the attention paid to the prosthesis, one dissenting voice questions the relevance of it, and the extent to which we should focus our attention on it at all. Dio Chrysostom (*circa* 40–115 CE) in his eighth oration *On Virtue* bemoans the fact that 'as if there were any use in a man having a golden or ivory hand or eyes of diamond or malachite; but the kind of soul he had men did not notice'.[15]

Context: history, culture, society

What, exactly, *is* a prosthesis? In the twenty-first century, a prosthesis is a device that replaces a missing body part, usually designed and assembled according to the individual's appearance and functional needs, as unobtrusive and as useful as possible so as to maximise the chances of their acceptance of it.[16] The missing body part can be missing due to a congenital or an acquired impairment, although in the case of the former scenario it could be argued that the individual is not, in fact, impaired as they have never known any different.[17] Studies have shown that if an individual both mentally and physically accepts their prosthesis and is satisfied with it, they will be more likely to use it.[18] Users are more inclined to accept a prosthesis that is aesthetically pleasing to them and consequently considerable effort is expended on the part of the prosthetist to match skin tone, hair colour etc., or to design and create something unusual and truly unique if that is what the user desires.[19] Users are also more inclined to accept a prosthesis that makes their life easier than one that makes their life harder.[20] Thus it is necessary to consider each contemporary prosthesis as having a dual role, one aspect of this being its form and another being its function, although these aspects can also overlap. The nature of these forms and functions varies from prosthesis to prosthesis. An extremity prosthesis such as a finger, hand or arm not only resembles the missing finger, hand or arm but can also restore some but not all of its functionality. A facial prosthesis – or cosmesis, as it is sometimes designated – such as an eye or a nose resembles the missing eye or nose and while it does not restore the lost sense of sight or smell, it does enable the user to 'pass' if that is what they wish to do.[21]

The English term 'prosthesis', which is used today to refer to an artificial device that replaces or augments a missing or impaired part of the body, is a compound of the Greek terms πρός ('on the side of') and θέσις ('setting' or 'placing'). It entered the English language in 1533, used in a grammatical capacity to designate the addition of a syllable to the beginning of a word, but it was not until 1704 that it was used in a medical capacity to refer to an artificial device that replaces or augments a missing or impaired part of the body, and only in the middle of the nineteenth century that it came to mean this almost exclusively.[22] It is not a term that was readily utilised by ancient authors, at least not quite in the way we use it today. When the word πρόσθεσις ('application') is used in Greek literature, it indicates the application of an object for a specific purpose, as in the application of a medicinal remedy such as a pessary or a piece of medical equipment such as a cupping vessel.[23] No ancient Greek or Latin medical treatise mentions prostheses, however; clearly the application of a prosthesis to the body for the purpose of replacing a missing part was not considered a medical remedy. The nearest any ancient Greek or Latin medical writer gets to this is recommending that gold wire be utilised to fix loose teeth in place; there is, however, no mention of the possibility of utilising a dental prosthesis to replace these loose teeth if the gold wire is unable to secure them and they are lost.[24]

Perhaps the closest an ancient author comes to our modern understanding of prostheses is Philostratus (*circa* early third century CE) when he discusses the application of false hair in a love letter to an anonymous woman:

> The woman who beautifies herself seeks to supply what is lacking; she fears the detection of her deficiency. The woman whose beauty is natural needs nothing adventitious, for she is self-sufficient to the point of utter perfection. Eyes underlined with kohl, false hair (κόμης προσθέσεις), painted cheeks, tinted lips, all the enhancements known to the beautifier's art, and all the deceptive bloom achieved by rouge have been invented for the correction of defects; the unadorned is the truly beautiful.[25]

Here, Philostratus is part of a long tradition of male Greek and Roman authors that excoriate women for seeking to augment and amplify their natural beauty with artificial substances.[26] While the use of items such as creams or face packs to preserve one's natural beauty was, in the eyes of the male authors writing on the subject at least, permissible, the use of items such as cosmetics to embellish one's natural beauty and in so doing make it unnatural was not.[27] And yet there is a considerable amount of archaeological evidence to suggest that women utilised cosmetics anyway, and that in addition to cosmetics they also utilised not only 'false' hair, but also 'false' teeth, that is to say prosthetic hair and prosthetic teeth.[28] On the one hand, prosthetic hair and prosthetic teeth come in for a considerable amount of criticism from Roman authors such as Martial (*circa* 38 CE – *circa* 104 CE) and Juvenal (*circa* late first century CE – *circa* mid second century CE), particularly when they are being worn by elderly women in an attempt to disguise baldness and tooth loss.[29] On the other hand, the Jewish Talmud (*circa* third century CE) advises furnishing a woman with a prosthetic tooth in order to make her more attractive and in doing so facilitate marriage.[30] Clearly the Roman and the Jewish understandings of what were essentially the same objects that were in use at broadly the same time and often in the same places, or at least the ways that these objects were discussed in works of literature written by male authors, varied considerably. Is there any indication that other types of prostheses or other types of prosthesis users came in for similar criticism regarding their inherent falsity? On the one hand, the Roman general Marcus Sergius Silus, while serving as praetor in 197 BCE, was forced to defend himself against peers who believed that the loss of his right hand during the Second Punic War (218–201 BCE) and his replacement of it with an iron prosthesis was grounds for excluding him from religious rites.[31] On the other hand, Tabaketenmut (either the 22nd or 23rd Dynasty, *circa* 950–710 BCE), the daughter of a priest and so potentially herself a priestess, may only have been able to take part in religious rites *because* she replaced her missing toe with a wooden prosthesis.[32]

Whereas in the twenty-first century we tend to refer to prostheses using the noun 'prosthesis' or the adjective 'prosthetic', whatever the type of prosthesis under discussion, when extremity prostheses are referred to in ancient literature, they are described using the combination of the substitute body part and the substance from which it is made. Thus, Pelops has a shoulder of ivory (ὦμος ἐλεφάντου or *umerus eburno*), Pythagoras has a thigh of gold (μηρός χρυσοῦν), Hegesistratus has a foot of wood (πούς ξυλίνου), Marcus Sergius Silus has a hand of iron (*manus ferream*), Statyllius has the hair belonging to another (ἀλλότριος πλόκαμος).[33] This begs the question: is the ancient practice of referring to prostheses in this way indicative of a particular way of thinking about them, of conceptualising them? And does this tell us something about the relationship between the human body and technology in classical antiquity?[34] Did the use of technology to create humanoid objects such as statues and automata, and equipment such as weapons, armour and shoes perhaps inspire artisans and craftsmen to create prostheses?[35] From the earliest works of classical literature and art, individuals with physical impairments are described and depicted as taking advantage of a range of different types of assistive technology such as staffs, sticks, canes, crutches, walking frames and prostheses.[36] Certainly, classical prostheses were objects that were highly individualised, just as specially commissioned statues, automata, weapons, armour and shoes were.[37] As we can see from the images painted on the Berlin Foundry Cup (see Figure I.1), an ancient metal workshop produced items ranging from statues to armour, all individually crafted.[38]

This ancient metal workshop is also depicted manufacturing votive offerings, and a notable feature of ancient ritual practice in classical antiquity is the offering of anatomical votives, that is votive offerings in the form of parts of either the external or internal body.[39] It has been suggested that anatomical votives were used to represent the fragmentation or disaggregation of the dedicant's ailing body, with the healing process conceived of as the reintegration of the fragmented parts leading to the reconstitution of the dedicant's body.[40]

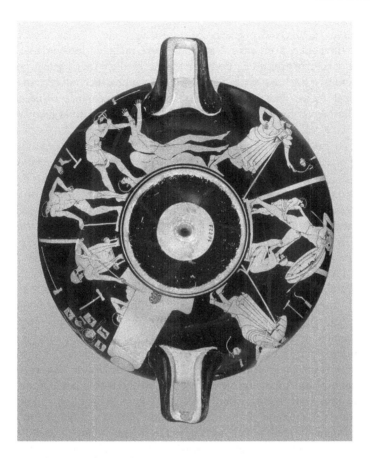

Figure I.1 Berlin 'Foundry Cup', *circa* 490–480 BCE, inv. F2294. Image courtesy of © Antikensammlung der Staatlichen Museen zu Berlin.

Anatomical votives have been described as 'a kind of "non-amputation" underscoring the integrity of the absent, cured dedicant'.[41] Conversely, an actual amputation served to salvage the body at the expense of the body part in question, restoring a degree of bodily integrity by curing the body of an injury or an infection but leaving it absent a previously present part.[42] Were prostheses viewed as a means of reintegrating fragmented parts and reconstituting the body?[43] There is literary and documentary evidence for there having been something of an overlap between prostheses and anatomical votives in classical antiquity; a papyrus dating from 118 CE describes a 'maker of artificial limbs' as manning a healing shrine on a private estate in the Hermopolite nome of Roman Egypt, while a number of poems included in the *Greek Anthology* record individuals who were coming to the end of their working lives dedicating the tools of their trades to the gods, and among them is an example of a devotee to Aphrodite dedicating his prosthetic hair.[44] While this was clearly not the case with all ancient prostheses – many of the surviving examples have survived precisely because they were *not* separated from the body of their user, even after death, and were included in their user's burial, either as a part of the user's body or as one of their user's grave goods – it was obviously the case with some, and the appearance of certain types of anatomical votives likely corresponded with the appearance of certain types of prostheses (see Figure I.2, a collection of anatomical votives recovered from the sanctuary of Asklepios at Corinth).

How far can utilising contemporary prostheses, prosthesis use and prosthesis users as points of comparison assist us in our attempt to understand ancient prostheses, prosthesis use and prosthesis users? It is important to remember that not only is our contemporary understanding of impairment and disability not necessarily applicable to ancient societies, but also that our contemporary understanding of prostheses, prosthesis use and prosthesis users might not necessarily be either. See for example the case of an extremity prosthesis recovered from a grave in Turfan, China, dating to approximately 300–200 BCE.[45] The deceased, a man between the ages of 50 and 65, suffered from a severe case of tuberculosis that froze his left knee and rendered walking unaided impossible.[46] Since traditional Chinese law utilised mutilation punishment (*xing*) for a range of transgressions, impaired individuals experienced a considerable amount of stigmatisation, and this might explain why, rather than undergo surgical amputation of the left leg and replace the missing limb with a prosthesis, the deceased chose to utilise a prosthesis in conjunction with his impaired limb for many years.[47] This prosthesis was made from leather, sheep or goat horn and the hoof of a horse or an Asiatic ass, and comprised a plate that was fastened to the thigh by leather straps and tapered into a peg-leg (see Figure I.3).[48] No attempt was made to carve the peg-leg to resemble a human limb; on the contrary, the peg-leg terminated in a hoof, and ultimately this may have rendered the prosthesis easier to use. Other finds recovered during archaeological excavation of the site have indicated that the local

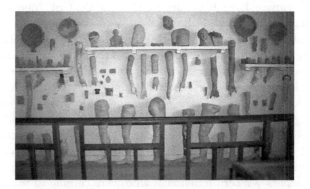

Figure I.2 Collection of anatomical votives recovered from the sanctuary of Asklepios at Corinth. Image courtesy of A. L. Lesk.

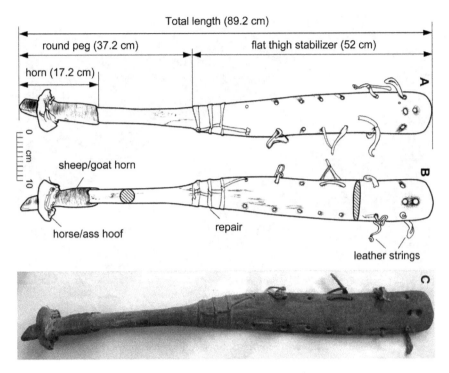

Figure I.3 Chinese prosthetic leg excavated from a grave in Turfan, *circa* 300 BCE. Image courtesy of the Deutsches Archäologisches Institut.

population were relatively poor, and the goods recovered from the deceased individual's grave do not indicate that he was in any way unusual as far as wealth or social status were concerned.[49]

Let us compare the 'Turfan Limb' with the famous 'Capua Limb', a Roman prosthetic leg recovered from a tomb in Capua dating to approximately 300 BCE that was, prior to the discovery of the 'Turfan Limb', the oldest known functional prosthetic limb in the world.[50] The 'Capua Limb' was made from wood, iron and bronze, and comprised a wooden core covered in bronze sheeting worn in conjunction with a leather and bronze belt to hold it in place and, assuming that the prosthesis could be securely fastened at the thigh and the waist, facilitate a limited amount of movement in conjunction with a staff, stick or crutch (see Figure I.4, a copy of the original which was destroyed in an air raid during the Second World War).[51] Other finds recovered from the tomb were a bronze urn and some locally produced red-figure pottery. Judging by the materials used in the limb's construction, it was likely worn by a high-status individual, or at the very least, a wealthy one, perhaps a veteran of the Second Samnite War (327–304 BCE) or even a retired gladiator.[52] Capua is noted in ancient literature as a city of considerable wealth and luxury and

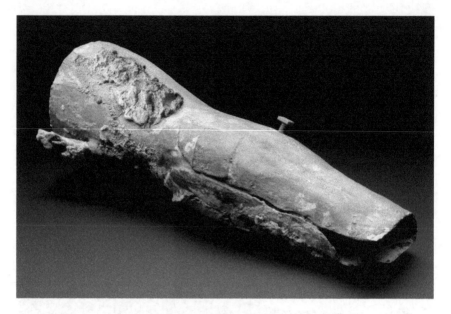

Figure I.4 Copy of Roman prosthetic leg, *circa* 1910, inv. A646752; the original
was excavated from a grave in Capua, *circa* 300 BCE. Image courtesy of
© Science Museum/Science & Society Picture Library.

particularly feted for its bronze.[53] In his discussion of the 'Capua Limb',
Lawrence Bliquez has proposed the following:

> From a cosmetic point of view, the owner of the leg must have cut some-
> thing of a fashionable figure. His artificial limb was designed with an eye
> to the real thing, and the glint of the bright Italian sun on the then deep
> gold of his leg's bronze covering must have made a splendid impression.[54]

This leads us to another aspect of ancient prostheses, prosthesis use and
prosthesis users that it is necessary to take into account: since each ancient
prosthesis was entirely unique and designed and manufactured in isolation by
the user, one craftsman (for example a carpenter), or a team of craftsmen (for
example a carpenter, a metal-worker, and a leather-worker), ancient prostheses
can, perhaps, give us an insight into ancient cultures and societies and their
users' places within those, in addition to telling us something about the
individuals themselves. Whether the prosthesis is cosmetic or functional or a
combination of both, how far are the substance from which it is made and
the way in which it is made (for example design, craftsmanship etc.) intended
to serve an additional purpose related to conspicuous consumption to either
demonstrate or enhance the status and prestige of its wearer?[55] The owner of

the 'Turfan Limb' was seemingly determined not to allow his impairment to become a disability and result in him being stigmatised in a society where impairments were viewed as highly undesirable at best, punishment for major transgressions at worst. As a member of a relatively poor community with no access to prestige materials such as gold, silver, bronze, iron, etc., he utilised materials that were in plentiful supply in his agrarian and pastoral society, the animal products of leather, horn and even a hoof to create his prosthesis. While the form that his prosthesis took can be seen as entirely practical, a means of stabilising him as he moved around, it is also possible that his choice of an animalistic rather than humanoid limb was influenced by his Subeixi culture's interaction with the Pazyryk culture of the Scythian communities in the nearby Altai Mountains.[56] The owner of the 'Capua Limb' did not necessarily have to worry about stigmatisation due to his impairment, since, whether a veteran or a gladiator or neither, he was an impaired individual in a society with a long history of warfare and was likely surrounded by others who had received equally debilitating injuries.[57] It is also clear from the materials utilised in the creation of his prosthesis that he was an individual of means. While the owner of the 'Turfan Limb' may have had to resort to creating his own prosthesis, the owner of the 'Capua Limb' certainly outsourced the creation of his to one or more craftsmen. While, like the 'Turfan Limb', the form that the wooden core of the 'Capua Limb' took is entirely practical, the bronze sheeting has the appearance of a military greave, potentially an indicator of the (former) occupation of the user or perhaps the specialisation of the craftsman responsible for the metal components.[58]

So we have two extremity prostheses produced in neighbouring ancient civilisations at roughly the same time, yet despite servicing broadly the same aim (the replacement of an impaired or missing lower limb), the prostheses themselves are entirely different in design and construction, the prosthesis use would have been entirely different, and the prosthesis users themselves came from not only different societies but also different (in fact, entirely opposite) sections of their respective societies. That there has long been a relationship between wealth and class and the extent of an individual's disability (as opposed to their impairment) has been readily acknowledged by historians in discussions of the lived experience of impairment and disability in past societies.[59] Thus, we should not be surprised to see that this relationship extends to prostheses, prosthesis use and prosthesis users too.[60] However, wealth and status do not automatically guarantee an impaired individual a technologically advanced prosthesis and minimal resultant disability: Lucian (*circa* mid second century CE) tells of a rich man who lost both of his feet to frostbite and replaced them with wooden prostheses that he covered with expensive shoes, but these prostheses were cosmetic rather than functional and he still required the assistance of slaves to move around.[61] Indeed, perhaps those wealthy and powerful enough to requisition the labour of others, whether free or slave, had little need of functional prostheses at all.[62]

This volume focuses primarily on prostheses as material objects and considers their role (or roles) in the cultures and societies of classical antiquity.[63] If a prosthesis is a 'tool' that a person intentionally uses for his or her own purposes, we can only progress in our attempt to understand prostheses, prosthesis users and prosthesis use in antiquity if we consider prostheses as social objects with a complex set of meanings in the daily lives of people in the ancient world.[64] Social contexts produce cultural practices which produce distinctive biological bodies.[65] The people of the ancient cultural contexts that feature in this volume – the Greeks, the Etruscans, the Romans, the Egyptians, the Jews and the Franks – had very different aesthetic standards to the people of the contemporary, predominantly Western cultural contexts that will be reading this book. However, common to all of them is that a degree of bodily difference or disparity was taken for granted, yet how an individual presented his or her difference or disparity in public indicated both their social and economic background, and their aspirations regarding both. While it is clear that the inhabitants of classical antiquity experienced a variety – indeed, a 'sliding scale' – of physical and mental impairments, the ancient literary, documentary and archaeological evidence for prostheses is not as comprehensive as we might expect or even hope.[66] In point of fact, a number of suggested representations have in recent years been comprehensively debunked, while others remain ambiguous (see, for example, the image on the cover of this volume, a depiction of a prosthesis user that has been dated to both the Roman period and the twelfth century). Compare, for example, the Moche (a people dating to the Early Intermediate Period of Prehispanic Peru, *circa* 100–800 CE) and the considerable amount of evidence for limb loss and prosthesis use in their society (see Figure I.5).[67] To date, four skeletons definitively attesting amputation of one or both feet and almost 100 artistic representations of prosthesis users have been identified in the Peruvian archaeological record.[68] While it has been suggested that these amputations should be interpreted as having been punitive as opposed to surgical because many of the amputees and prosthesis users also display what appears to be intentional mutilation of facial features including the nose and lips, more recently an argument has been made for ritual mutilation.[69] Consequently, depending upon the reason for the mutilation, it could be seen and interpreted as a marker of either low or high status. Whatever the context of prosthesis, prosthesis use and prosthesis users in that society, it is indisputable that all three featured prominently in it.

Thus, we should consider the evidence that we do have for prostheses and prosthesis use in classical antiquity extremely carefully and comprehensively. The logical inference is that prostheses were rarely used; as mentioned above, they are certainly not in the place where we, with our twenty-first century perspective, would expect them to be, in the extensive Greek and Latin medical literature that survives from classical antiquity. While in the twenty-first century we see prostheses of all types as medical, it is debateable whether

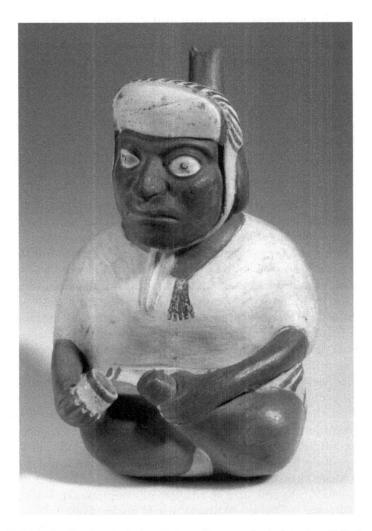

Figure I.5 Moche figurine depicting a man with a prosthetic foot, inv. B4919. Image courtesy of © Division of Anthropology, American Museum of Natural History, New York.

most, if any, ancient prostheses were viewed in this way. As far as the ancient Greek *iatros* (male) or *iatrinē* (female), or Roman *medicus* (male) or *medica* (female) was concerned, medical treatment for an amputated limb went no further than the amputation itself once the stump had begun to heal. Thus, because the prostheses of classical antiquity were not considered thera-peutic, they were not included in ancient medical literature, and we must look elsewhere for information regarding their role in classical culture and society.

Context: impairment, disability and disability studies

Today, the World Health Organisation uses disability as an umbrella term that covers impairments, activity limitations and participation restrictions:

> An impairment is a problem in body function or structure; an activity limitation is a difficulty encountered by an individual in executing a task or action; while a participation restriction is a problem experienced by an individual in involvement in life situations. Disability is thus not just a health problem. It is a complex phenomenon, reflecting the interaction between features of a person's body and features of the society in which he or she lives.[70]

This distinction between the term 'impairment' and the term 'disability' has proved useful for the development of the academic discipline of Disability Studies, which aims to offer a critical perspective with which to think differently about the way that disability is constructed, created and related to everyday life.[71] It has identified a series of models through which to approach disability both in the contemporary world and in the past. The Medical Model of disability involves a gaze which views disability as a personal limitation arising from an impairment (whether congenital or acquired) and consequently the individual's problem, and emphasises the necessity of medical intervention to fix or cure that problem.[72] In contrast, the Social Model of disability involves a gaze that views disability not as a personal or individual problem but as a societal structural issue, recognising that an individual might have a congenital or acquired physical or mental impairment but that it is society's response to this impairment that renders that individual disabled.[73] Yet the Social Model has been criticised for either ignoring or being unable to deal with a number of aspects of the realities of impairment.[74] An alternative model, the Interactional Model, has been proposed since impairment is a fact and without it a society would have nothing with which to base its preconceptions in relation to the individual on and the individual would not be disabled.[75]

Starting with Martha Lynn Edwards (later Martha Lynn Rose), ancient historians have begun to utilise disability theory in their examinations of impairment and disability in the past.[76] Simultaneously, ancient historians and archaeologists have suggested ways in which Disability Studies can benefit from incorporating approaches from their disciplines.[77] It is important to acknowledge that in classical antiquity a congenital or acquired impairment did not automatically result in disability; there was not, in fact, any recognition of disability or 'disabled' as a category or classification of person at all.[78] Martha Lynn Edwards has proposed what she has termed the Community Model, and sees the impaired as having been thoroughly integrated into ancient society; hence the difficulty in uncovering any literary, documentary or archaeological evidence that is specifically about them and their experiences.[79] Sara Newman has expanded upon this and proposed the Civic Model, in which representations of disability were associated with concepts of citizenship and belonging.[80] For our purposes, it is necessary to consider how a prosthesis user would have been viewed in classical antiquity. Would a prosthesis user have been considered impaired? Would a prosthesis user have been considered disabled? To date, prostheses, prosthesis use and prostheses users have rarely featured in discussions of impairment and disability in classical antiquity.[81]

Context: scholarship

Prostheses seem to have been utilised either during life or after death in a variety of civilisations for thousands of years, but while the earliest surviving prosthesis, an artificial eye recovered from a grave at Cingle del Mas Nou i Cava Fosca in Spain, has been dated to *circa* 5000 BCE, and the earliest literary reference, an account of Vishpala, a female warrior with an iron leg, in the *Rigveda*, has been dated to *circa* 1500–1200 BCE, it is not until the Graeco-Roman period that both archaeological and literary evidence begins to proliferate, making both diachronic and synchronic studies possible.[82]

To date, however, only one substantial piece of academic research has been devoted solely to prostheses in Graeco-Roman antiquity: Lawrence Bliquez's 'Prosthetics in Antiquity: Greek, Etruscan, and Roman Prosthetics' in *Aufstieg und Niedergang der Römischen Welt* 37.3, published in 1996.[83] Bliquez chose to focus on Greece and Italy at the expense of other areas of the ancient Mediterranean, and to concentrate his attention on 'those devices attached to the human body which had some practical as well as cosmetic purpose', thus including dental and extremity prostheses while excluding other types of mobility aids, wigs, bodily padding, etc.[84] While impairment and disability in classical antiquity have been increasingly studied over the last decade, prostheses, prosthesis users and prosthesis use have been overlooked, even in the most recent and comprehensive study, Christian Laes' edited volume *Disability in Antiquity*.[85] This can perhaps be accounted for by the fact that the subject falls somewhere between medical history and disability history, between ancient history and archaeology.

General surveys of the history of surgery, amputation and prosthetic medicine from antiquity to the present have been undertaken, but not by academics for an academic audience.[86] The subject of impairment and disability in antiquity should in theory touch upon the issue of prostheses, but scholarship has so far not covered it in any kind of depth, whether the subject is approached from the perspective of ancient literature, history or archaeology.[87] Additionally, despite some consideration of care-giving in the past, the role of other human beings, whether free or slave, in relation to the use (or lack of use) of prostheses has not been considered.[88] Specific types of prostheses (for example dental appliances and artificial eyes) have succeeded in garnering attention from scholars.[89] Likewise, famous prostheses, newly discovered prostheses and historically significant individuals known to have used prostheses have been showcased in articles for both specialist and general audiences, while skeletons displaying evidence of amputation have been published individually as curiosities, collectively according to type of amputation, and as part of cemetery populations in archaeological reports.[90] Additionally, some attention has been paid to items that, while not prostheses, served as mobility aids.[91]

The core of this collection lies in the papers presented at the Wellcome Trust and Classical Association–funded 'Prostheses in Antiquity' workshop held at the University of Wales Trinity Saint David (30th June 2015), during which a group of international scholars working on the social, cultural and historical contexts of health and disease from the disciplines of Classics, Ancient History, Archaeology, Bioarchaeology, Egyptology and Biblical Studies in universities and museums were invited to discuss how ancient prostheses should be defined and evidence for their usage interpreted.[92] The fact that the study of prostheses in antiquity is an emerging area of enquiry in a range of academic disciplines is attested by the fact that a high proportion of the speakers were early career researchers, and that previously unpublished archaeological discoveries and the findings of experimental archaeological investigations were presented. Contributions revealed the depth and vitality of current studies of health and disease in antiquity but also the extent to which their dissemination has tended to remain confined by the traditional disciplinary and language boundaries of academia. Consequently, critical new works (particularly archaeological discoveries) have not always reached the wider audience that they deserve, frequently being presented as amusing curiosities in publications aimed at medical practitioners such as *The Lancet*.[93] This volume responds to this, presenting innovative and varied research which reveals the extent to which the study of prostheses is at once a vibrant, dynamic and stimulating field of enquiry, and has the potential to have far-reaching implications for the study of the history of health and well-being, impairment and disability, and understandings of the body, as well as for the medical sciences. It does not attempt to provide a catalogue or even a typology of ancient prostheses (the approach taken by Bliquez), but rather exploits the interpretive potential of situating prostheses in their historical, cultural and social contexts.

The papers which comprise this volume represent the current work of a range of scholars, some leaders in their field, most early career researchers, dedicated to the study of health and well-being in antiquity. Some were presented at the UWTSD conference (subsequently expanded and written up into formal chapters) whilst others have been commissioned as a means of addressing lacunae in the initial coverage of the subject. The volume is not intended as an historical account of the development of prostheses in the classical world, or as a repository for typological studies of different types of prosthesis, although the chapters that deal with specific types of prosthesis do include information on these subjects.[94] Rather, it is intended to provide a primary point of reference for any scholar working in the fields of history of medicine or body-related subjects who wishes to engage with the multiplicity of approaches and potential interpretations that might be applied to this important but often undervalued category of evidence. Importantly, it also seeks to bring to the attention of the wider archaeological, historical and classicist community a range of material that is known but poorly understood outside of specialist publications, whether in the humanities or the sciences.

Contents

In the volume's opening chapter, Jacky Finch recounts her experiences undertaking experimental archaeological reconstructions of two prosthetic great toes recovered from Egypt and enlisting amputees to test the reconstructions in laboratory trials. Since first-hand accounts of what it was like to live with an impairment or disability in classical antiquity are exceedingly rare to start with, it is not a surprise that we should be lacking a first-hand account of a prosthesis user in classical antiquity.[95] Concerns have been raised about the extent to which impaired and disabled individuals have participated in scholarly inquiry related to impairment and disability in past societies, but here they are placed at the heart of the investigation and their personal experiences used to better inform our contemporary understanding of these two artefacts.[96] The technical sophistication and possible functionality of ancient prostheses have often been questioned with negative conclusions drawn but here Finch offers conclusive proof that it was entirely possible for ancient prostheses to have a degree of functionality and so serve practical as well as cosmetic purposes, in addition to providing useful guidance for any future scholars seeking to undertake experimental archaeological reconstruction of prostheses from the past.[97] Since one of the prostheses that she investigates here was originally recovered attached to a mummy of an individual whose identity is known and whose personal circumstances are somewhat recoverable, she is also able to contextualise the prosthesis, the prosthesis user and the prosthesis use, something that is not possible for any of the other prostheses that survive from antiquity.

The next two chapters examine the two types of prosthesis that are most frequently attested in ancient literary, documentary, archaeological and bioarchaeological evidence: teeth and hair. These types of prosthesis have often been overlooked or dismissed as having been simply a fashion accessory, but both chapters argue that they were far from insignificant in ancient Etruscan, Italian and Roman culture and society. These types of prosthesis are also the ones that are most frequently described in negative terms as being 'false' and 'purchased', and whose users (primarily women but also, on occasion, men who were deemed effeminate) are criticised for using them. First, Jean MacIntosh Turfa and Marshall Becker present a comprehensive inventory of all known ancient Etruscan and Italian dental appliances, and contextualise them in relation to the conceptions of gender, beauty, class, wealth and status held by individuals within Etruscan and Italian societies. While dental appliances are known to have been utilised contemporaneously in the neighbouring societies of Greece and Rome, the Etruscan and Italian dental appliances are entirely different in design and execution. Unlike the wiring recommended by the Hippocratic treatise *On Joints* (*circa* mid fifth century BCE) and Celsus' *On Medicine* (*circa* early first century CE) as a means of fixing loose teeth in place, and unlike the extremity prostheses presented by Finch, the dental appliances presented here were not functional in the sense of helping the individuals who wore them to eat; on the contrary, they rendered that process much more difficult. Additionally, they did not seek to replace a body part that had already been lost; on the contrary, teeth were voluntarily removed to accommodate them. Their functionality seems to have laid in the information that they communicated about their wearers' status in their society. Second, Jane Draycott explores the role of the wig and the hair piece in imperial Rome. Unlike other types of ancient prosthesis, including the dental appliances presented by Turfa and Becker, an ancient wig or hair piece was most commonly made from body parts either voluntarily or involuntarily harvested from someone else, frequently a lower status individual such as a slave.[98] She assesses the significance and potential ramifications of a high status Roman utilising someone else's hair as a substitute for their own and explores the reasons behind the popularity of certain types of hair, most notably the red or blonde hair harvested from Germanic prisoners of war and slaves. More than any other type of prosthesis discussed in this volume, wigs and hair pieces seem to have been simultaneously desirable and undesirable: to some, they were markers of status, wealth, elegance, fashion, beauty and sex appeal; to others, they were dishonest, immoral and potentially even contaminated.

How to attempt to understand a civilisation's prostheses without being able to access any extant examples of them? Lennart Lehmhaus investigates the role that prostheses played in Late Antique Jewish culture and society by examining discussions of them in Talmudic literature, surmising that they were a means of bypassing certain types of bodily dysfunction. The possibility that Jewish prosthesis users were prohibited from using their prostheses at certain times indicates that in Jewish communities at least prostheses were viewed as tools – and fairly labour-intensive ones at that – as opposed to parts of the body. Perhaps because of this, they seem to have been viewed relatively positively, as a means by which impaired individuals could participate more fully in society and accomplish things that might otherwise be beyond their reach, such as contracting a suitable marriage. Alternatively, how to attempt to understand a civilisation's prostheses without being able to study any extant discussions of them? Josef Eitler and Michaela Binder present the findings of a recent excavation at the Late Antique pilgrimage centre of Hemmaberg in Carinthia, which unexpectedly revealed the grave of a man whose left foot had been amputated and replaced with a prosthesis that, while not suitable for putting weight on and walking, served to hold in place a compress absorbing pus, offering an indication of the ways in which prostheses could be personalised according to the medical needs of their user in addition to the societal. Since considerable archaeological excavation has taken place at Hemmaberg over a period of some years, enough is known about the site and its inhabitants to attempt a preliminary contextualisation of the prosthesis user and his place within this small community.

The final three chapters in the volume move away from prostheses proper, each one expanding the scope of the discussion of prostheses, prosthesis use and prosthesis users in new and unexpected ways. Katherine van Schaik considers what happens when body parts are not lost but rather become useless because of irreversible nerve injury. Surveying the literary, documentary and archaeological evidence for the diagnosis and treatment of paralysis from a range of Mediterranean civilisations, and assessing the significance of care-givers, she reminds us that the role of carers – human prostheses, if you will – is frequently overlooked or elided when the lives of the impaired and disabled in classical antiquity are discussed.[99] In view of this, it is important to note that, no matter how functional ancient extremity prostheses such as the examples recovered from the archaeological record and discussed by Finch and Eitler and Binder were, carers – whether family members, friends, servants or slaves – still supplemented and perhaps even complemented them, playing a significant part in the daily lives of prosthesis users and their prosthesis use. Consequently, it was possible for ancient impaired individuals to adapt to their new life circumstances. Then, Anne-Sophie Noel approaches the fundamental ambiguity of prostheses in ancient thought, exploring whether people's use of prostheses in Athenian society during the fifth century BCE inspired tragedians to incorporate the prosthetic experience into their works through their depictions of significant relationships between certain individuals and their possessions.[100] She argues that certain theatrical objects were transformed by usage into living things, acquiring not just movement but also, on occasion, emotions and even speech. This leads her to question the extent to which prostheses were considered to have agency independent of their user, whether they were thought of as inert and passive devices used to replace a missing body part, or things infused with nonhuman agency as they interacted with the body in a dynamic way. Finally, Ellen Adams brings the volume to a close by noting that since prostheses are often expected to fulfil the function of a missing physical part, the distinction between them and aids in general becomes blurred. She engages critically with the terminology utilised in contemporary discussions of prostheses and aids, and suggests that just as notions of impairment and disability are culturally specific, so are notions of prostheses and aids, and understanding this can assist in clarifying the framework through which we approach them in the ancient world in future studies.

One last thing to bear in mind when exploring prostheses and prosthesis use in antiquity is that however primitive or advanced – depending upon your perspective – we consider the prostheses of the Graeco-Roman world to be, they served their purposes while remaining the height of technological sophistication until Ambroise Paré's advances in the sixteenth century.[101] Consequently, it is our hope that this volume proves useful not just to those whose research interests focus on the ancient world, but also to those who work on later periods.

Notes

1 Pindar, *Olympian Ode* 1.24–28 (trans. W. H. Race): Λυδοῦ Πέλοπος ἀποικίᾳ· τοῦ μεγασθενὴς ἐράσσατο Γαιάοχος Ποσειδάν, ἐπεί νιν καθαροῦ λέβητος ἔξελε Κλωθώ, ἐλέφαντι φαίδιμον ὦμον κεκαδμένον. For commentary, see Gerber, 1982, pp. 55–59. On Pindar's version of the myth, see Griffith, 2000.

2 Ironically, Pindar's account relates then refutes that Pelops' ivory shoulder was a prosthesis yet retains this as a key feature of the myth, arguing that he was born with it as a sort of birthmark rather than acquired it later in life. According to Paley, 1868, p. 3 n. 2, since the name Pelops means 'dark faced', this could be seen to refer to a pale shoulder that is revealed when clothing is removed. According to Gerber, 1982, p. 58, since the ivory shoulder is one of the most consistent and conspicuous features of the myth, it was probably considered to be a mark of beauty. For further discussion of this, see Noel, this volume. This is not, however, the earliest mention of prostheses in world literature: that honour belongs to the iron leg of Vishpala, referred to in the *Rig Veda* (*circa* 1500–1200 BCE), see 1.118.8; Vishpala is mentioned in several other places in the Rig Veda, see 1.112.10, 1.117.11 and 10.39.8. For similarities between the Greek of Pindar and the Sanskrit of the *Rig Veda*, see Watkins, 2002.

3 Lycophron, *Alexandra* 149; Ovid, *Metamorphoses* 6.405; Seneca, *Thyestes* 145; Pseudo-Apollodorus, *Library* 2.1–3; Pseudo-Hyginus, *Fables* 83; Eugentius, *Mythologies* 2.15.

4 There have been some attempts to rationalise the myth and situate it within the trajectory of the development of orthopaedics, see for example Donati *et al.*, 2009 on the myth's place in the history of bone-grafting which argues that ivory is tolerated quite well by the human body.

5 Ovid, *Metamorphoses* 6.405; Pseudo-Hyginus, *Fables* 83.

6 Pindar, *Olympian Ode* 1.37; Tibullus, *Elegies* 1.63–64; Philostratus the Elder, *Imagines* 1.30.7–11. According to Lorimer, 1936, pp. 32–33, the gods utilise ivory because, when suddenly called upon to provide a spare part, they can only produce one made from their own substance. According to Kenna, 1961, p. 100 n. 10, this could be an allusion to a seal stone worn either around the neck or on the upper arm that, due to being made from a tusk, resembled a shoulder blade. For discussion of the origin of the elephant or possibly hippopotamus ivory utilised in Bronze Age Greece, the time that Pindar was writing about, see Hayward, 1990.

7 Vergil, *Georgics* 3.7.

8 Philostratus the Elder, *Imagines* 1.30.25. For Pelops in classical art, see the *LIMC*, *s.v.* 'Pelops'.

9 Shoulder-blade at Elis: Pliny the Elder, *Natural History* 28.6.34; Pausanias, *Description of Greece* 5.13.4–6. Bones at Olympia: Pausanias, *Description of Greece* 6.22.1. According to Mayor, 2000, p. 105, the shoulder-blade could in actuality have been a mammoth scapula, since Olympia is sited on the Aleiphos River and the surrounding valleys contain dense concentrations of Pleistocene mammal fossils.

10 Pseudo-Apollodorus, *Library* 5.10–11; Parke, 1933.

11 Pausanias, *Description of Greece* 5.13.4.

12 Pausanias, *Description of Greece* 5.13.5. According to Mayor, 2000, p. 106, Damarmenos could have recovered some sort of prehistoric mammal bone, since the shallow seas around Euboea were once Neogene valleys that were populated by animals now extinct. There are other accounts of ancient fishermen recovering large bones from the sea that they then dedicated to the gods, see *Greek Anthology* 6.222, 6.223.

13 Pausanias, *Description of Greece* 5.13.6.

14 Clement, *Exhortation to the Greeks* 4.

15 Dio Chrysostom, *Eighth Oration: On Virtue* 28.

16 Murray, 2005. A presentation on the prosthetic service today was given at the 'Prostheses in Antiquity' workshop by Ian Massey, a prosthetist based at the Cardiff Artificial Limb and Appliance Centre.

17 On the relationship between parts of the body and the whole body, and the extent to which the body can be fragmented or considered fragmented, see Adams, 2017; on the issue of whether individuals born with a condition such as deafness are, in fact, impaired or disabled, see Adams, this volume.

18 The reasons why individuals abandon their prostheses are complex, and are as much to do with the individuals themselves (for example, age, sex, gender, ethnicity, level of education etc.) as the prostheses, but studies have made the importance of comfort and functionality in successful prosthesis use clear, see for example Murray and Fox, 2002; Pezzin *et al.*, 2004; Biddiss and Chau, 2009.

19 See for example the work of Sophie Oliveira Barata at the Alternative Limb Project, http://www.thealternativelimbproject.com/ (accessed January 2018), where 'alternative' prostheses are designed and constructed in consultation with the client and their prosthetist according to the client's specific tastes and preferences. See also the work of Limbitless Solutions, https://limbitless-solutions.org/ (accessed January 2018), where 3D-printed bionic prostheses are made for children at affordable cost. Particularly interesting is the company's use of the actor Robert Downey Jr in character as the Marvel superhero Tony Stark/Iron Man to present a 3D-printed prosthesis to a young boy with a partially developed right arm in a promotional short film. This stunt was subsequently critiqued by Smith, 2016.

20 Studies have shown that the sooner after the amputation the prosthesis is fitted, the more likely the user is to accept the prosthesis and use it successfully, see Pezzin *et al.*, 2004.

21 A recent study has shown that facial prosthesis users tend to prefer implanted prostheses over adhesive prostheses; the users of the latter type feel more self-conscious, see Wondergem *et al.*, 2016. As far as the functionality of facial prostheses is concerned, in recent years, scientists have had some success in developing a prosthetic retina that has partially restored the sight in mice, see Nirenberg and Pandarinath, 2012.

22 Wills, 1995, p. 218; Davis, 2013, p. 68.

23 Pessary: Hippocrates, *The Affections of Women* 1.11, and *On the Nature of Women* 11; ladder: Thucydides, *History of the Peloponnesian War* 4.135, see also Polybius, *Roman Histories* 5.60.7; cupping vessel: Aristotle, *Rhetoric* 1405b3.

24 See Hippocrates, *On Joints* 33.9–10; Celsus, *On Medicine* 6.12.1; this process is discussed in more detail in Turfa and Becker, this volume.

25 Philostratus, *Letters* 22 (trans. A. R. Benner and F. H. Forbes): Ἡ καλλωπιζομένη γυνὴ θεραπεύει τὸ ἐλλιπὲς φοβουμένη φωραθῆναι ὃ οὐκ ἔχει·χή φύσει καλὴ οὐδενὸς δεῖται τῶν ἐπικτήτων ὡς προσαρκοῦσα ἑαυτῇ πρὸς πᾶν τὸ ὁλόκληρον. ὀφθαλμῶν δὲ ὑπογραφαὶ καὶ κόμης προσθέσεις καὶ ζωγραφίαι παρειῶν καὶ χειλέων βαφαὶ καὶ εἴ τι κομμωτικῆς φάρμακον καὶ εἴ τι ἐκ φυκίου δολερὸν ἄνθος, ἐπανόρθωσις τοῦ ἐνδεοῦς εὑρέθη·ὑπὸ δὲ ἀκόσμητον ἀληθῶς καλόν. On real, false and artificial hair in antiquity, see Draycott, 2017; on prosthetic hair, see Draycott, this volume.

26 The Roman idea (and ideal) of female natural beauty is expressed most frequently in elegiac poetry, see for example Lilja, 1965, pp. 119–132; Richlin, 1992, pp. 44–46; Wyke, 2002, pp. 152–153; Olson, 2009; Olson, 2012, pp. 58–59.

27 See Gibson, 2003 for discussion of this tradition.

28 On prosthetic hair, see Draycott, this volume. On prosthetic teeth, see Turfa and Becker, this volume.

29 See for example Horace, *Satires* 1.8.47–50; Martial, *Epigrams* 1.72, 2.41, 5.43, 9.38, 12.23, 14.56; Lucian, *Professor of Public Speaking* 24; Lucillius, *Greek Anthology* 11.310; Macedonius, *Greek Anthology* 11.374.

30 See the Palestinian Talmud, in tractate Nedarim 9; 41c, and the Babylonian Talmud, Nedarim 66b. For discussion of the way that prostheses are treated in the Talmud, see Lehmhaus, this volume. See also Turfa and Becker, this volume.

31 Pliny the Elder, *Natural History* 7.29. For discussion of this, see Beagon, 2002; Van Lommel, 2015, p. 111, p. 115.

32 See Finch, this volume. The mummy of the priest of Mut Ankhefenmut (21st Dynasty, *circa* 1085–950 BCE) likewise shows a missing toe that has been replaced with a prosthesis, this one made of ceramic rather than wood, but unlike Tabaketenmut's prosthesis, Ankhefenmut's was not worn in life, only in death, see Brier *et al.*, 2015 for discussion.

33 Interestingly, the first well-known modern prosthesis user, Gottfried von Berlichinger, a German knight who lost his right hand at the siege of Landshut at the age of 25, was likewise referred to in this way, as '*Götz mit der eisernen Hand*' ('Götz with the iron hand'). During the Second World War, the 17 SS Panzer Grenadier Division was named after him and used an iron hand as its emblem.

34 The relationship between the impaired and disabled body and technology in the contemporary world is increasingly controversial, see Mitchell and Snyder, 1997, pp. 7–8.

35 Despite the recent proliferation of scholarship on ancient science and technology, these works have contained relatively little discussion of the use of technology for medical purposes; see for example the brief acknowledgement that machines were used for surgical traction in a broader discussion of machines in Greek and Roman technology, Wilson, 2008, pp. 345–346. To date, examinations of the use of technology for medical purposes in antiquity have concentrated predominantly on medical instruments, such as most recently Bliquez, 2014, with discussion of machines deliberately excluded, p. x.

36 See for example Hephaistos' appearance in Book 18 of the *Iliad*, where he is presented as using a staff to move around but has also created a set of automata in the form of golden maidens to assist him, *Iliad* 18.410–422. For discussion of this, see Kalligeropoulos and Vasileiadou, 2008; Paipetis, 2010, pp. 107–111.

37 Acton, 2014, p. 135.

38 Mattusch, 1980. For discussion of the links between weapons and armour and prostheses, see Noel, this volume.

39 For the most recent discussion of ancient anatomical votives, see Draycott and Graham, 2017; Hughes, 2017.

40 Hughes, 2008; this argument is expanded in Hughes, 2017, pp. 25–61.

41 Rynearson, 2003, p. 10.

42 See Aelius Aristides, *Sacred Tales* 48.27 for the god Asklepios requesting that he amputate a body part to ensure the safety of the whole.

43 A paper that focused on the relationship between prostheses and anatomical votives in antiquity was presented at the 'Prostheses in Antiquity' workshop by Alyce-Rose Cannon but she was unfortunately unable to contribute to this volume.

44 The papyrus is *P.Giss.* 20; also known as *W.Chr.* 94 and *P.Giss.Apoll.*11: http://papyri.info/ddbdp/p.giss.apoll;;11 (accessed January 2018). Translation and discussion of the papyrus regarding this aspect of it can be found in Draycott, 2014. The epigram is *Greek Anthology* 6.254. Discussion of the dedication of all types of hair can be found in Draycott, 2017.

45 Li *et al.*, 2012.

46 See Li *et al.*, 2012, pp. 338–339 for discussion of the skeleton and palaeopathology.

47 See Milburn, 2017 for discussion of impairment and disability in ancient China.

48 See Li *et al.*, 2012, p. 339 for discussion of the technical aspects of the prosthesis.

49 See Li *et al.*, 2012, p. 336 for discussion of the archaeological context.

50 See Bourguignon and Henzen, 1885; Sudhoff, 1917; von Brun, 1926 for the announcement of the discovery and early discussion and analysis of it.

51 See Bliquez, 1996, pp. 2669–2671 for discussion of the prosthesis' functionality.

52 Despite the fact that the sex of the skeleton is not explicitly stated in any of the reports of the find, it has consistently been assumed to be a male skeleton, see Bliquez, 1996, p. 2667 n.47. The perceived cost of a prosthesis plays a role in contemporary prosthesis adoption and successful use; users are more likely to adopt and use a prosthesis they perceive to be expensive, see Roeschlein and Domholdt, 1989. For further discussion of the issue of conspicuous consumption in relation to dental prostheses, see Turfa and Becker, this volume, and Lehmhaus, this volume; for discussion of this in relation to hair prostheses, see Draycott, this volume.

53 On Capua as a place of wealth and luxury, see Athenaeus, *Learned Banqueters* 13.528b; Florus, *Epitome* 1.11.6–8. On Capua's bronze industry, see Pliny the Elder, *Natural History* 34.39; see also Cato the Elder, *On Agriculture* 135.2.

54 Bliquez, 1996, p. 2671.

55 For the role that certain types of prosthesis played in demonstrating social status through their material, see Turfa and Becker, this volume, Draycott, this volume, Lehmhaus, this volume. For conspicuous consumption in relation to prostheses in later historical periods, see Kwass, 2006; Warne, 2009.

56 On stigmatisation, see Goffman, 1963 reissued 1990.

57 See Van Lommel, 2015 for discussion of the variability of attitudes towards wounded veterans in the Roman Republic and Empire.

58 Bliquez, 1996, p. 2672.

59 For a case study focusing on an individual in Egypt during the Roman period, see Draycott, 2015.

60 Ott *et al.*, 2002; Warne, 2009; Neumann, 2010; Jones, 2017. Even today, the cost of different types of prostheses varies considerably, and consequently what is available to different types of prosthesis user varies considerably; for example, in the United Kingdom, the National Health Service provides prostheses to anyone who needs them, but former and current service men and women who lost a limb as a result of an injury sustained while in military service can access funding through the Veterans' Prosthetics Panel (VPP) that is not available to either civilians or former or current service men and women who lost a limb while in military service but not as a result of an injury sustained in that military service: https://www.england.nhs.uk/commissioning/armed-forces/veterans-prosthetics/ (accessed January 2018). The Alternative Limb Project's 'realistic' limbs start at around £700 while its 'alternative' limbs start at around £1,000: http://www. thealternativelimbproject.com/about/the-alternative-limb-project/ (accessed January 2018). Limbitless Solutions believes that 'no family should have to pay for their child to receive an arm', and 3D prints its prostheses to minimise their cost: https://limbitless-solutions.org/about-us/ (accessed January 2018).

61 Lucian, *The Ignorant Book Collector* 6; for discussion of the role that other people play in assisting those with mobility impairments, see van Schaik, this volume.

62 For slaves as prostheses, see Blake, 2013 and 2016.

63 According to Vivian Sobchack, herself a prosthesis user, there are two ways of looking at prostheses: literally and figuratively, see Sobchack, 2006, p. 18. For an example of the latter, see Mitchell, 2002.

64 Ott, 2002, p. 16. New Materialism and Material Engagement theory frequently approach the subject of prostheses in material culture, see for example Knappett, 2005, pp. 11–34. See also Brown, 2003; Murray, 2005; Bennett, 2010. On relationships between humans and non-human things in regard to theatrical props, see Noel, this volume.

65 Sofaer, 2006.

66 Graham, 2013, p. 249.

67 Verano *et al.*, 2000; Więckowski, 2016.

68   Verano *et al.*, 2000, p. 182 states that more than fifty per cent of these representations show individuals missing both feet, twenty-six per cent show individuals missing one foot, while the remainder show individuals missing entire arms, lower arms, or hands.

69   Punitive mutilation: Urteaga-Ballon, 1991. Ritual mutilation: Arsenault, 1993.

70   http://www.who.int/topics/disabilities/en/ (accessed January 2018).

71   Cameron, 2013a, p. xvi.

72   See Cameron, 2013b, pp. 98–101 for a concise overview.

73   See Cameron, 2013c, pp. 137–140 for a concise overview.

74   See Oliver, 2004 for analysis and discussion.

75   See Riddle, 2013; Grue, 2015, pp. 47–50.

76   Rose, 2003 reissued 2013.

77   Southwell-Wright, 2013.

78   There were many different types of impairment; see for example Samama, 2017 for collation of the Greek terminology utilised to refer to different types of congenital and acquired impairment.

79   Edwards, 1997.

80   Newman, 2013, p. 12.

81   They have, however, been discussed in relation to impairment and disability in later historical periods, notably the American Civil War (1861–1865), the First World War (1914–1918) and the Second World War (1939–1945), see Ott *et al.*, 2002. Here, nascent prosthetics industries have been viewed as seeking to restore wholeness to divided countries by restoring wholeness to soldiers who had sacrificed parts of their bodies, and, through the manufacture of realistic looking prostheses, obfuscating the fact that conflict had ever occurred in the first place, see Davis, 2013, pp. 69–70.

82   On the artificial eye from Spain, see Enoch, 2009. On the iron leg of Vishpala, see *Rig Veda* 5.1.116; there is some debate over whether Vishpala was a woman or a horse, see O'Flaherty, 1981, p. 183, p. 185. For an enigmatic artificial tooth dating from the Neolithic period, an incisor carved from a seashell that may have been intended to be worn in life or after death, see Irish *et al.*, 2004.

83   Bliquez, 1996; this was preceded and inspired by a shorter piece for a general audience, Bliquez, 1983.

84   Bliquez, 1996, p. 2641.

85   Garland, 1995 reissued 2010; Rose, 2003 reissued 2013; Breitwieser, 2012; Laes, Goodey and Rose, 2013; Laes, 2014; Krötzl, Mustakallio and Kuuliala, 2015; Laes, 2017.

86   See for example Phillips, 1990; Kirkup, 2007.

87   See for example Ohry and Dolev, 1982; Garland, 1995 and 2010; Abrams, 1998; Salazar, 2002; Rose, 2003 and 2013; Kelley, 2007; Avalos *et al.*, 2007; Fishbane, 2008; Breitwieser, 2012; Laes, Goodey and Rose, 2013; Laes, 2014; Krötzl, Mustakallio and Kuuliala, 2015; Laes, 2017.

88   Tilley, 2015; Tilley and Schenk, 2017; Powell *et al.*, 2017.

89   Becker and Turfa, 2017; Becker has also published many articles on the subject of Etruscan dental appliances; Martin, 2015.

90   On famous prostheses, newly discovered prostheses, and historically significant prosthesis users, see for example Reeves, 1999; Nerlich *et al.*, 2000; Seguin *et al.*, 2014; Beagon, 2002. On skeletons, see for example Verano *et al.*, 2000; Dupras *et al.*, 2010; Stukert and Kricun, 2011.

91   See for example Loebl, 1997; Armstrong, 2014.

92   Wellcome Trust small grant reference number 108557/Z/15/Z.

93   See for example Nerlich *et al.*, 2000; Finch, 2011.

94   For the former, see Draycott, in preparation; for the latter, see Turfa and Becker, 2017.

95 See Draycott, 2015 for discussion of a rare example of the former.
96 Cross, 2007, p. 179, p. 18; Hubert, 2000, p. 2; Mitchell and Snyder, 1997, p. 2. For another recent successful example of this approach to impairment and disability history, albeit one focussed on mental rather than physical impairment and disability, see the Wellcome Trust–funded project 'All the King's Fools', http://www.allthekingsfools.co.uk/site/ (accessed January 2018); an interim report on this project is provided in Lipscombe, 2011.
97 See for example Rose, 2003 reissued 2013, p. 26.
98 There is one example of an ancient dental prosthesis that utilises a tooth harvested from an animal, see Turfa and Becker, this volume, dental appliance No. 12 from Tarquina.
99 For a description of slaves as 'articulate tools' (*instrumentum vocale*), see Varro, *On Agriculture* 1.17.1. What has been designated the 'bioarchaeology of care' is of increasing importance for studies of impairment and disability in the past, see Tilley, 2015; Tilley and Schrenk, 2017; Powell *et al.*, 2017.
100 See also Mueller, 2016.
101 Thurston, 2007.

Bibliography

Abrams, J. Z. (1998) *Judaism and Disability: Portrayals in Ancient Texts from the Tanach through the Bavli*. Washington, DC: Gallaudet University Press.

Acton, P. (2014) *Poiesis: Manufacturing in Classical Athens*. Oxford: Oxford University Press.

Adams, E. (2017) 'Fragmentation and the Body's Boundaries: Reassessing the Body in Parts', in Draycott, J. and Graham, E.-J. (edd.) *Bodies of Evidence: Anatomical Votives Past, Present and Future*. Abingdon: Routledge, pp. 193–213.

Armstrong, K. (2014) 'Possibly the First Wheeled Walking Aid', personal communication.

Arsenault, D. (1993) 'El personaje del pie amputado en la cultura Mochica del Peru: un ensayo sobre la arqueologia del poder', *Latin American Antiquity* 4, pp. 225–245.

Avalos, H., Melcher, S. and Schipper, J. (edd.) (2007) *This Abled Body: Rethinking Disabilities in Biblical Studies*. Atlanta, GA: Society of Biblical Literature.

Beagon, M. (2002) 'Beyond Comparison: M. Sergius Silus, Fortunae Victor', in Clark, G. and Rajak, T. (edd.) *Philosophy and Power in the Graeco-Roman World. Essays in Honour of Miriam Griffin*. Oxford: Oxford University Press, pp. 111–132.

Becker, M. J. and Turfa, J. M. (2017) *The Golden Smile: Etruscan Dental Appliances*. London: Routledge.

Bennett, J. (2010) *Vibrant Matter: A Political Ecology of Things*. Durham, NC: Duke University Press.

Biddiss, E. A. and Chau, T. T. (2009) 'Upper Limb Prosthesis Use and Abandonment: A Survey of the Last 25 Years', *Prosthetics and Orthotics International* 31.3, pp. 236–257.

Blake, S. (2012) 'Now You See Them: Slaves and Other Objects as Elements of the Roman Master', *Helios* 39.2, pp. 193–211.

Blake, S. (2016) 'In Manus: Pliny's Letters and the Arts of Mastery', in Keith, A. and Edmondson, J. (edd.) *Roman Literary Cultures: Domestic Politics, Revolutionary Poetics, Civic Spectacle*. Toronto: University of Toronto Press, pp. 89–101.

Bliquez, L. J. (1983) 'Classical Prosthetics', *Archaeology* September/October, pp. 25–29.

Bliquez, L. J. (1996) 'Prosthetics in Classical Antiquity: Greek, Etruscan, and Roman Prosthetics', in *ANRW* II 37.3, pp. 2640–2676.

Bliquez, L. J. (2014) *The Tools of Asclepius: Surgical Instruments in Greek and Roman Times*. Leiden: Brill.

Bourguignon, A. and Henzen, G. (1885) 'Scavi di Santa Maria di Capua', *Bullettino dell'Instituto di Correspondenza Archeologica* 7/8, p. 169.

Breitwieser, R. (ed.) (2012) *Behinderungen und Beeinträchtigungen/Disability and Impairment in Antiquity*. Oxford: Archaeopress.

Brier, B., Vinh, P., Schuster, M., Mayforth, H. and Chapin, E. J. (2015) 'A Radiologic Study of an Ancient Egyptian Mummy with a Prosthetic Toe', *The Anatomical Record* 298.6, pp. 1047–1058.

Brown, B. (2003) *A Sense of Things: The Object of Matter in American Literature*. Chicago, IL and London: University of Chicago Press.

Cameron, C. (2013a) 'Introduction', in Cameron, C. (ed.) *Disability Studies: A Student's Guide*. London: Sage, pp. xv–xvii.

Cameron, C. (2013b) 'The Medical Model', in Cameron, C. (ed.) *Disability Studies: A Student's Guide*. London: Sage, pp. 98–101.

Cameron, C. (2013c) 'The Social Model', in Cameron, C. (ed.) *Disability Studies: A Student's Guide*. London: Sage, pp. 137–140.

Cross, M. (2007) 'Accessing the Inaccessible: Disability and Archaeology', in Insoll, T. (ed.) *The Archaeology of Identities: A Reader*. Abingdon: Routledge, pp. 179–194.

Davis, L. (2013) *The End of Normal: Identity in a Biocultural Era*. Ann Arbor, MI: University of Michigan Press.

Donati, D., Zolezzi, C., Tomba, P. and Viganò, A. (2009) 'Bone Grafting: Historical and Conceptual Review, with an Old Manuscript by Vittorio Putti', *Acta Orthopaedica* 78.1, pp. 19–25.

Draycott, J. (2014) 'Who is Performing What, and For Whom? The Dedication, Construction and Maintenance of a Healing Shrine in Roman Egypt', in Gemi-Iordanou, E., Gordon, S., Matthew, R., McInnes, E. and Pettitt, R. (edd.) *Medicine, Healing, Performance: Interdisciplinary Approaches to Medicine and Material Culture*. Oxford and Philadelphia: Oxbow, pp. 42–54.

Draycott, J. (2015) 'The Lived Experience of Disability in Antiquity: A Case Study from Roman Egypt', *G&R* 62.2, pp. 189–205.

Draycott, J. (2017) 'Hair Today, Gone Tomorrow: The Use of Real, False and Artificial Hair as Votive Offerings', in Draycott, J. and Graham, E.-J. (edd.) *Bodies of Evidence: Ancient Anatomical Votives Past, Present and Future*. Abingdon: Routledge, pp. 77–94.

Draycott, J. (in preparation) *In the Footsteps of Hegesistratus: Prostheses, Prosthesis Use and Prosthesis Users in Classical Antiquity*.

Draycott, J. and Graham, E.-J. (edd.) (2017) *Bodies of Evidence: Ancient Anatomical Votives Past, Present and Future*. Abingdon: Routledge.

Dupras, T. L., Williams, L. J., De Meyer, M., Peeters, C., Depraetere, D., Vanthuyne, B. and Willems, H. (2010) 'Evidence of Amputation as Medical Treatment in Ancient Egypt', *IJO* 20, pp. 405–423.

Edwards, M. L. (1997) 'Constructions of Physical Disability in the Ancient Greek World: The Community Concept', in Mitchell, D. and Snyder, S. (edd.) *The Body and Physical Difference: Discourses of Disability*. Ann Arbor, MI: University of Michigan Press, pp. 35–50.

Enoch, J. M. (2009) 'A Mesolithic (Middle Stone Age!) Spanish Artificial Eye: Please Realize This Technology is circa 7000 Years Old!', *Hindsight: Journal of Optometry History* 40.2, pp. 47–62.

Finch, J. (2011) 'The Ancient Origins of Prosthetic Medicine', *The Lancet* 37.9765, pp. 548–549.

Fishbane, S. (ed.) (2008) *Deviancy in Early Rabbinic Literature: A Collection of Socio-Anthropological Essays*. Leiden: Brill.

Garland, R. (1995, 2010) *The Eye of the Beholder: Deformity and Disability in the Graeco-Roman World*. London: Bristol Classical Press.

Gerber, D. E. (1982) *Pindar's Olympian One: A Commentary*. Toronto, Buffalo, NY and London: University of Toronto Press.

Gibson, R. (2003) *Ovid* Ars Amatoria *Book 3*. Cambridge: Cambridge University Press.

Goffman, E. (1963 reissued 1990) *Stigma: Notes on the Management of Spoiled Identity*. London: Penguin.

Graham, E.-J. (2013) 'Disparate Lives or Disparate Deaths? Post-mortem Treatment of the Body and the Articulation of Difference', in Laes, C., Goodey, C. and Rose, M. (edd.) *Disabilities in Roman Antiquity: Disparate Bodies* a Capite ad Calcem. Leiden: Brill, pp. 249–274.

Griffith, R. D. (2000) 'Pelops and the Speal-bone (Pindar "Olympian" 1.27)', *Hermathena* 168, pp. 21–24.

Grue, J. (2015) *Disability and Discourse Analysis*. London and New York, NY: Routledge.

Hayward, L. G. (1990) 'The Origin of the Raw Elephant Ivory used in Greece and the Aegean during the Late Bronze Age', *Antiquity* 64.242, pp. 103–109.

Hubert, J. (2000) 'Introduction: The Complexity of Boundedness and Inclusion', in Hubert, J. (ed.) *Madness, Disability and Social Exclusion: The Archaeology and Anthropology of 'Difference'*. Abingdon: Routledge, pp. 1–8.

Hughes, J. (2008) 'Fragmentation as Metaphor in the Classical Healing Sanctuary', *SHM* 21.2, pp. 217–236.

Hughes, J. (2017) *Votive Body Parts in Ancient Greek and Roman Religion*. Cambridge: Cambridge University Press.

Irish, J. D., Bobrowski, P., Kobusiewicz, M., Kabaciski, J. and Schild, R. (2004) 'An Artificial Human Tooth from the Neolithic Cemetery at Gebel Ramlah, Egypt', *Dental Anthropology* 17.1, pp. 28–31.

Jones, C. L. (ed.) (2017) *Rethinking Modern Prostheses in Anglo-American Commodity Cultures, 1820–1939*. Manchester: Manchester University Press.

Kalligeropoulos, D. and Vasileiadou, S. (2008) 'The Homeric Automata and their Implementation', in Paipetis, S. (ed.) *Science and Technology in the Homeric Epics*. Dordrecht, Heidelberg, London and New York, NY: Springer, pp. 77–84.

Kelley, N. (2007) 'Deformity and Disability in Greece and Rome', in Avalos, H., Melcher, S. and Schipper, J. (edd.) *This Abled Body: Rethinking Disabilities in Biblical Studies*. Atlanta, GA: Society of Biblical Literature, pp. 31–45.

Kenna, V. E. G. (1961) 'The Return of Orestes', *JHS* 61, pp. 99–104.

Kirkup, J. (2007) *A History of Limb Amputation*. London: Springer.

Knappett, C. (2005) *Thinking through Material Culture: An Interdisciplinary Perspective*. Philadelphia, PA: University of Pennsylvania Press.

Krötzl, C., Mustakallio, M. and Kuuliala, J. (2015) *Infirmity in Antiquity and the Middle Ages: Social and Cultural Approaches to Health, Weakness and Care*. Farnham: Ashgate.

Kwass, M. (2006) 'Big Hair: A Wig History of Consumption in Eighteenth-Century France', *AHR* 111.3, pp. 631–659.

Laes, C. (2014) *Bepurkt? Gehandicapten in het Romeinse rijk*. Leuven: Davisfonds.

Laes, C. (ed.) (2017) *Disability in Antiquity*. London: Routledge.

Laes, C., Goodey, C., and Rose, M. (edd.) (2013) *Disabilities in Roman Antiquity: Disparate Bodies* a Capite ad Calcem. Leiden: Brill.

Li, X., Wagner, M., Wu, X., Tarasov, P., Zhang, Y., Schmidt, A., Goslar, T., and Gresky, J. (2013) 'Archaeological and Palaeopathological Study on the Third/Second Century BC Grave from Turfan, China: Individual Health History and Regional Implications', *Quaternary International* 290–291, pp. 335–343.

Lilja, S. (1965) *The Roman Elegists' Attitude to Women.* New York, NY: Garland.

Lipscombe, S. (2011) 'All the King's Fools', *History Today* 61.8, available online at http://www.historytoday.com/suzannah-lipscomb/all-king's-fools (accessed January 2018).

Loebl, W. Y. (1997) 'Staffs as Walking Aids in Ancient Egypt and Palestine', *JRSM* 90.8, pp. 450–454.

Lorimer, H. L. (1936) 'Gold and Ivory in Greek Mythology', in Bailey, C., Bowra, C. M., Barber, E. A., Denniston, J. D. and Page, D. L. (edd.) *Greek Poetry and Life: Essays Presented to Gilbert Murray on his Seventieth Birthday, January 2, 1936.* Oxford: Clarendon Press, pp. 14–33.

Martin, J.-P. (2015) *Ocularistes et yeux artificiels: de l'Antiquité au XXe siècle.* Paris: L'Harmattan.

Mattusch, C. (1980) 'The Berlin Foundry Cup: The Casting of Greek Bronze Statuary in the Early Fifth Century BC', *AJA* 84, pp. 435–444.

Mayor, A. (2000) *The First Fossil Hunters : Paleontology in Greek and Roman Times.* Princeton, NJ: Princeton University Press.

Milburn, O. (2017) 'Disability in Ancient China', in Laes, C. (ed.) *Disability in Antiquity.* London: Routledge, pp. 106–118.

Mitchell, D. (2002) 'Narrative Prosthesis and the Materiality of Metaphor', in Snyder, S. L., Brueggemann, B. J. and Garland-Thomson, R. (edd.) *Disability Studies: Enabling the Humanities.* New York: The Modern Language Association of America, pp. 15–30.

Mitchell, D. and Snyder, S. (1997) 'Introduction: Disability Studies and the Double Bind of Representation', in Mitchell, D. and Snyder, S. (edd.) *The Body and Physical Difference: Discourses of Disability.* Ann Arbor, MI: University of Michigan Press, pp. 1–31.

Mueller, M. (2016) *Objects as Actors: Props and the Poetics of Performance in Greek Tragedy.* Chicago, IL and London: University of Chicago Press.

Murray, C. D. (2005) 'The Social Meanings of Prosthesis Use', *Journal of Health Psychology* 10.3, pp. 425–441.

Murray, C. D. and Fox, J. (2002) 'Body Image and Prosthesis Satisfaction in the Lower Limb Amputee', *Disability and Rehabilitation* 24.17, pp. 925–931.

Nerlich, A. G., Zink, A., Szeimies, U. and Hagedorn, H. G. (2000) 'Ancient Egyptian Prosthesis of the Big Toe', *The Lancet* 356.9248.23–30, pp. 2176–2179.

Neumann, B. (2010) 'Being Prosthetic in the First World War and Weimar Germany', *Body & Society* 16.3, pp. 93–126.

Newman, S. (2013) *Writing Disability: A Critical History.* Boulder, CO and London: First Forum Press.

Nirenberg, S. and Pandarinath, C. (2012) 'Retinal Prosthetic Strategy with the Capacity to Restore Normal Vision', *Proceedings of the National Academy of Sciences of the United States of America* 109.37, 15012–15017.

O'Flaherty, W. D. (1981) *The Rig Veda: An Anthology: One Hundred and Eight Hymns, Selected, Translated and Annotated.* London: Penguin.

Ohry, A. and Dolev, E. (1982) 'Disabilities and Handicapped People in the Bible', *Koroth* 8.5–6, pp. 63–67.

Oliver, M. (2004) 'If I Had a Hammer: The Social Model in Action', in Swain, J., French, S., Barnes, C. and Thomas, C. (edd.) *Disabling Barriers – Enabling Environments*. London: Sage, pp. 7–12.

Olson, K. (2009) 'Cosmetics in Roman Antiquity: Substance, Remedy, Poison', *CW* 102.3, pp. 209–310.

Olson, K. (2012) *Dress and the Roman Woman: Self-Representation and Society*. Abingdon: Routledge.

Ott, K. (2002) 'The Sum of its Parts: An Introduction into Modern Histories of Prosthetics', in Ott, K., Serlin, D. and Mihm, S. (edd.) *Artificial Parts, Practical Lives: Modern Histories of Prosthetics*. New York, NY and London: New York University Press, pp. 1–42.

Ott, K., Serlin, D. and Mihm, S. (edd.) (2002) *Artificial Parts, Practical Lives: Modern Histories of Prosthetics*. New York, NY and London: New York University Press.

Paipetis, S. A. (2010) *The Unknown Technology of Homer*. Dordrecht, Heidelberg, London and New York, NY: Springer.

Paley, F. A. (1968) *The Odes of Pindar*. Cambridge: Deighton, Bell and Co.

Pezzin, L. E., Dillingham, T. R., MacKenzie, E. J., Ephraim, P. and Rossbach, P. (2004) 'Use and Satisfaction with Prosthetic Limb Devices and Related Services', *Archives of Physical Medicine and Rehabilitation* 85.5, pp. 723–729.

Phillips, G. (1990) *Best Foot Forward: Chas. A. Blatchford and Sons (Artificial Limb Specialists) 1890–1990*. Aylesbury: Granta.

Powell, L., Southwell-Wright, W., and Gowland, R. (edd.) *Care in the Past: Archaeological and Interdisciplinary Perspectives*. Oxford: Oxbow.

Reeves, N. (1999) 'New Light on Ancient Prosthetic Medicine', in Davies, V. W. (ed.) *Studies in Egyptian Antiquities. A Tribute to T.G.H. James*. London: British Museum Press, pp. 73–77.

Richlin, A. (1992) 'Making up a Woman: The Face of Roman Gender', in Doniger, W. and Eiberg Schwartz, H. (edd.) *Off with her Head!: The Denial of Women's Identity in Myth, Religion and Culture*. Berkeley, CA: University of California Press, pp. 185–213.

Riddle, C. A. (2013) 'The Ontology of Impairment: Rethinking how we Define Disability', in Wappett, M. and Arndt, K. (edd.) *Emerging Perspectives on Disability Studies*. New York, NY: Palgrave Macmillan, pp. 23–39.

Roeschlein, R. A. and Domholdt, E. (1989) 'Factors Related to Successful Upper Extremity Prosthesis Use', *Prosthetics and Orthotics International* 13.1, pp. 14–18.

Rose, M. (2003, 2013) *The Staff of Oedipus: Transforming Disability in Ancient Greece*. Ann Arbor, MI: University of Michigan Press.

Rynearson, N. (2003) 'Constructing and Deconstructing the Body in the Cult of Asklepios', *SJA* 2, available online at http://web.stanford.edu/dept/archaeology/journal/newdraft/2003_Journal/rynearson/paper.pdf (accessed January 2018).

Salazar, C. (2000) *The Treatment of War Wounds in Graeco-Roman Antiquity*. Leiden: Brill.

Samama, E. (2017) The Greek Vocabulary of Disabilities', in Laes, C. (ed.) *Disability in Antiquity*. London: Routledge, pp.121–138.

Seguin, G., d'Incau, E., Murail, P. and Maureille, B. (2014) 'The Earliest Dental Prosthesis in Celtic Gaul? The Case of an Iron Age Burial at La Chêne, France', *Antiquity* 88, pp. 488–500.

Smith, S. (2016) '"Limbitless Solutions": The Prosthetic Arm, Iron Man and the Science Fiction of Technoscience', *Science Fiction and Medical Humanities* 42, 259–264.

Sobchack, V. (2006) 'A Leg to Stand on: Prosthetics, Metaphor, and Materiality', in Smith, M. and Morra, J. (edd.) *The Prosthetic Impulse: From a Posthuman Present to a Biocultural Future*. Cambridge, MA: MIT Press, pp. 17–41.

Sofaer, J. R. (2006) *The Body as Material Culture: A Theoretical Archaeology*. Cambridge: Cambridge University Press.

Southwell-Wright, W. (2013) 'What can Archaeology Offer Disability Studies?', in Wappett, M. and Arndt, K. (edd.) *Emerging Perspectives on Disability Studies*. New York, NY: Palgrave Macmillan, pp. 67–95.

Stuckert, C. M. and Kricun, M. E. (2011) 'Bilateral Food Amputation from the Romano-British Cemetery of Lankhills, Winchester, UK', *Journal of Paleopathology* 1, pp. 111–116.

Sudhoff, K. (1917) 'Der Stelzfuß aus Capua', *Mitteilungen zur Geschichte der Medizin und Naturwissenschaften* 76/77, pp. 291–293.

Thurston, A. J. (2007) 'Paré and Prosthetics: The Early History of Artificial Limbs', *ANZ Journal of Surgery* 77.12, pp. 1114–1119.

Tilley, L. (2015) *Theory and Practice in the Bioarchaeology of Care*. New York, NY: Springer.

Tilley. L. and Schenk, A. A. (edd.) (2017) *New Developments in the Bioarchaeology of Care*. New York, NY: Springer.

Urteaga-Ballon O. (1991) 'Medical Ceramic Representation of Nasal Leishmaniasis and Surgical Amputation in Ancient Peruvian Civilization', in Ortner, D. J. and Aufderheide, A. C. Jr. (edd.) *Human Paleopathology: Current Syntheses and Future Options*. Washington, DC: Smithsonian Institution Press, pp. 95–101.

Van Lommel, K. (2015) 'Heroes and Outcasts: Ambiguous Attitudes towards Impaired and Disfigured Roman Veterans', *CW* 109.1, pp. 91–117.

Verano, J. W., Anderson, L. S., and Franco, R. (2000) 'Foot Amputation by the Moche of Peru: Osteological Evidence and Archaeological Context', *IJO* 10.3, pp. 177–188.

von Brun, W. V. (1926) 'Der Stelzfuß von Capua und die antiken Prothesen', *Archiv für Geschichte der Medizin* 18.4, pp. 351–360.

Warne, V. (2009) '"To Invest a Cripple with Peculiar Interest": Artificial Legs and Upper-Class Amputees at Mid-Century', *Victorian Review* 35.2, pp. 83–100.

Watkins, C. (2002) 'Pindar's Rigveda', *Journal of the American Oriental Society* 122.2, p. 432.

Więckowski, W. (2016) 'A Case of Foot Amputation from the Wari Imperial Tomb at Castillo de Huarmey, Peru', *IJO* 26, pp. 1058–1066.

Wills, D. (1995) *Prosthesis*. Stanford, CA: Stanford University Press.

Wilson, A. I. (2008) 'Machines in Greek and Roman Technology', in Oleson, J. P. (ed.) *The Oxford Handbook of Engineering and Technology in the Classical World*. Oxford: Oxford University Press, 337–392.

Wondergem, M., Lieben, G., Brouman, S., van den Brekel, M. W. F. and Lohouis, P. J. F. M. (2016) 'Patients' Satisfaction with Facial Prostheses', *British Journal of Oral and Maxillofacial Surgery* 54.4, 394–399.

Wyke, M. (2002) *The Roman Mistress: Ancient and Modern Representations*. Oxford: Oxford University Press.

1   The complex aspects of experimental archaeology: the design of working models of two ancient Egyptian great toe prostheses

Jacky Finch

Introduction

Processes required when studying any ancient object are sadly often limited to desk-bound research. This may be due to constraints imposed externally on the researcher, such as time, money and resources. However, it may indicate an unwillingness to explore a whole range of practical skills that can only be available by enquiring if others in a totally unrelated field could assist in the project. To fully understand the very essence of any artefact a more practical approach should always be considered. However, as a consequence this requires skills that may go far beyond those that are demonstrated by the researcher. Seeking out the required expertise and allowing those with the skills and interest to become part of the project naturally alters the direction in which the research is taken. This in due course extends the time frame required and increases the demands on resources. In turn, this also has an impact on the financial demands. With this approach, however, comes also the gradual realisation that a more satisfying understanding of the cultural and social significance of the object emerges.

The quote below is a most fitting résumé of how such a multipronged approach can be of value. It refers to the reconstruction of an ancient Egyptian New Kingdom loom. This project undertaken by Barry Kemp and Gillian Vogelsang-Eastwood was to clarify how the wonderfully fine linen found at the royal site of Amarna could have been woven. Loom fragments and remnants of ancient linen along with copies of wall scenes showing weavers in action were consulted:

> The obvious drawback of attempting within a short space of time to deploy skills which originally would have taken part of a lifetime to acquire can, to some extent, be alleviated by involving people with experience of a related technology. And even if experimental replication does not follow exactly the pattern of the ancient model, the search for working solutions clarifies to some degree what was and what was not

feasible and can bring in the contribution of people possessed of skills and specialist knowledge whose critique of scholarly interpretations proceeds from an altogether different point of view.[1]

The project described in this paper involved assessing the functionality of two ancient Egyptian great toe prostheses. Luckily both artefacts were relatively complete and accessible in their respective holding institutions. Thanks must go to the Supreme Council of Antiquities in Egypt, Dr Wafaa el-Saddik, the Director of the Egyptian Museum, Cairo and Dr J. H. Taylor at the British Museum, London who were incredibly generous in making the artefacts available along with their accompanying documentation. It became obvious at the outset that due to the rarity of the artefacts working replicas would have to be constructed. Experts from many and varied fields had therefore to be co-opted. Specialists in orthotic and prosthetic design and testing, in rehabilitation medicine, wood analysis and wood carving and those with a knowledge of ropes and knots, all gave generously of their time and expertise. It was most gratifying to receive so many enquiries from potential volunteers and I especially applaud the patience and good humour of the two individuals who eventually became involved in the trials.

Historical perspective: surviving for eternity

Death to the ancient Egyptians was an unavoidable fate, but it was not seen as absolute destruction, nor the discontinuity of life nor the isolation of the individual. Life would continue, immortality achieved and a peaceful eternity in a land identical to their beloved Egypt would be attained. In order to achieve this, they would build a home for their body (a tomb, a coffin or a sarcophagus) and they would ensure every aspect of their being would be catered for or recognised in the Afterlife.

The Egyptians perceived the individual to be a composite of physical and non-physical elements or manifestations. Recognition of the deceased's bodily form was part of the Egyptian consciousness from as early as the Old Kingdom (2686–2160 BCE) with preservation of the body, especially the heart, paramount. Completeness would ensure that the physical body would be able to house two important aspects of the individual, the *ka* and the *ba*. The *ka* and *ba* were seen as non-physical elements of the individual. The *ka*, seen as the twin or double of a person, connected with the life force of the individual which needed a physical body in which to reside after death. This was achieved through mummification, the *ka* being fed from offerings left at the tomb. The *ba* on the other hand represented the spirit of the individual, and in the form of a bird was able to leave the body to move freely beyond the tomb. The *ba* was able to speak, drink and feed. Two other essential manifestations of the individual were the shadow and the name. Only by the survival and union of all these aspects would immortality be assured and resurrection as a blessed spirit be achieved.[2]

Many funerary texts allude to the importance of a complete body.[3] Artificial restoration or reconstruction of missing body parts by the ancient Egyptian embalmers was thus viewed as a form of religious ritual, guaranteeing completeness of the body. This ensured that there was a fitting house in which the *ka* could reside and to which the *ba* could return. Reports from mummy 'unrollings' and from radiographic imaging provide ample evidence for a huge range of restorative practices. These range from moulding the external features of the body with linen and plaster (evident in the Old Kingdom 2686–2160 BCE, and to some extent during the Roman Period 30 BCE–395 CE), the use of subcutaneous packing of the body using sand, mud, linen or sawdust to plump out the body after desiccation with drying agents, the inclusion of false eyes using a wide range of materials plus the addition of false ears, noses, nipples, vertebrae and genitals. Many incomplete bodies were also supplied with false upper and lower limbs made from plant stems, linen, mud and resin. All these examples are non-functional additions applied *post mortem*.[4]

From the rather crudely fashioned restorations recorded in the above list there are three examples designed to replace the right great or big toe. One has been visualised within the wrappings of a female mummy dated 1069–945 BCE.[5] A cartonnage (a linen and animal glue composite) example is in the British Museum collection and a third example made of wood and possibly leather is a three-part device of a far more sophisticated construction. Previous researchers have classified all three as 'prostheses'.

A prosthetic device must satisfy certain criteria. The materials from which it is constructed must withstand biomechanical (bodily) forces. It must have a clear means of attachment to facilitate removal, washing and care with the interface with the body and must be in proportion to the wearer. Most importantly it must function effectively in the position intended. In the light of findings and comments published by previous researchers it was decided that further investigation of the prosthetic toes was overdue and a complete reappraisal of both examples was warranted.[6] At this point it seems appropriate to acquaint the reader with the history of these artefacts while also giving details of their construction.

The Greville Chester toe EA 29996

EA 29996 the Greville Chester great toe (see Figure 1.1) was purchased by the British Museum in 1881 from one of its principal scouts, the Reverend Greville Chester.[7] At this time the British Museum relied on unofficial and semi-official collectors to provide objects for its growing collections. He became one of their most skilled buyers, also supplementing the growing collections of the Victoria and Albert, Ashmolean and Fitzwilliam Museums.

EA 29996 arrived at the museum amongst a large miscellaneous collection of other antiquities amassed during Chester's latest travels in Egypt. The original entry under item 81.6.14, 77 now recorded as EA 29996 in the British

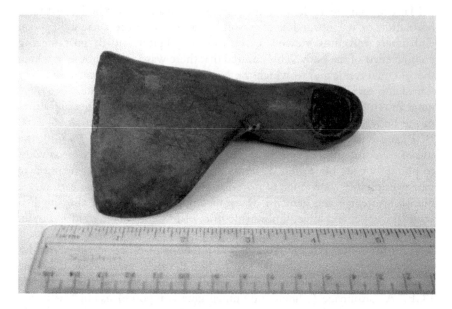

Figure 1.1 Dorsal view of EA 29996, the Greville Chester great toe made of
cartonnage, a composite material using linen and animal glue. Note areas
of wear on the proximal edge and in the first web space. Image courtesy
of J. L. Finch with permission from the British Museum, London.

Museum's Egyptian accessions register describes it as 'Leather artificial toe
from the right foot, nail wanting, from a mummy. 5in. From Thebes.'

Samuel Birch, Keeper of Oriental Antiquities at the British Museum, 1866–
1885, recorded and catalogued the expanding collection. His description of
this unique piece as 7029a (now EA 29996) for the manuscript slip catalogue
in their archives was:

> Object modelled in the shape of a great toe and portion of the right foot
> but no other toes, the nail which has been of some other material has
> been taken out. It is said to have come from a mummy probably from
> one the toe of which was wanting. At the left side of the toe are 8 small
> circular holes to sew it on or attach it to some part of a mummy. It is
> light brown colour. 4 1/2in[ches]l[ong]. Leather. Thebes.

Between 1989 and 1992, the British Museum's Department of Conservation
undertook an in-depth analysis of the artefact. Documents include a radiographic report with plates.[8] There is also a Conservation Research Section
Report on the filler and coating materials.[9] An X-ray defraction analysis of
the buff plaster, white inlay in the lace holes and the red coating along with
the infill in the toe nail cavity was also undertaken by Middleton and a final
report published.[10]

The body of the artefact is made of cartonnage, a composite material made of linen and animal glue. Textile analysis was undertaken by Granger–Taylor. Her findings assisted in dating the piece and were included in a paper written by Reeves who describes it as 'a rare and important object'.[11]

Granger–Taylor also notes that the textile examined in different areas appeared to be of a similar thread count. From this she concludes that they either came from similar pieces of cloth or were taken from one sheet torn into pieces.

Such was the craftsmanship of EA 29996 that it was selected to appear alongside many other wonderful pieces from the British Museum collection in the publication *Masterpieces of Ancient Egypt*.[12]

The cartonnage had been beautifully moulded to extend proximately, medially and laterally following the anatomy of the dorsum of the right foot. The layers of linen (3 mm) analysed by Granger–Taylor were clearly evident, the top coated in a light brown gesso (plaster, glue and red ochre), the underside was coated in a red resin type material, similar to but not identical to Dragon's Blood gum, a leaf stem exudate from *Dracaena draco* (Liliacae).[13]

The eight holes on the inner border showed distinct fragmentation indicative of some form of thread having been passed through them for securing the device onto the foot. The four holes on the outer border had been overpainted in antiquity. With experimentation, it was possible to reconstruct the lacing under the foot with a linen thread passing between these eight medial and four lateral holes providing a secure and comfortable double purchase.

Wear was recorded not only on the holes and in the web space but also at the toe tip and under the toe where abrasion had occurred with the ground or sandal. On the proximal edge where the top of the foot hits the top of the cartonnage as the foot flexes, 7.3 mm of the surface had fallen away exposing the linen below. There was also some cracking in the first web space between the big toe and second digit possibly indicative of a sandal thong passing up between the toes.

Excavation Number 453

In 1999 the German Institute of Archaeology, Cairo in conjunction with the Supreme Council of Antiquities in Egypt undertook extensive excavations in the necropolis of Thebes-West (Sheik Abdel-Gurna). Some seventy-three individuals were discovered in the large subterranean tomb complex in Theban Tomb 95 (TT95), the tomb of Meri, First Prophet of Amun. TT 95 was originally built in the 18th Dynasty (1550–1300 BCE) to house the deceased from the family of this high royal official. In subsequent periods, however, the tomb was usurped by others. At the end of a shaft originating from the transverse hall an additional burial chamber had been built. Yellow type coffin fragments and funerary pottery found here dated the chamber to the 21st– 22nd Dynasty (1065–740 BCE). Heavily disturbed by robbers in antiquity, few individuals could be reconstructed from the fragmentary remains.[14]

The body of one female of 50–60 years of age had been broken into several parts; skull, abdominothoracic torso, right thigh, shins, both arms. The left thigh and hands were missing but extensive linen bindings remained.[15] Excavation Number 453 was discovered attached to the mummy's right foot and was described as follows:

> The missing toe had been replaced by a wooden 'prosthesis' painted dark brown and made up of three separate components. The main component consisted of a longitudinal wooden corpus (12–3.5–3.5cm) and replaced the toe. This corpus was attached to two small wooden plates (together about 4–2.5–0.3cm). These plates were fixed to each other by seven leather strings. All wooden parts were delicately manufactured and the major corpus of the prosthesis perfectly shaped like a big toe even including the nail. A broad textile lace was fixed to the small plates and to the prosthetic corpus which was tied around the forefoot, fixing the toe in place. . . . Careful inspection revealed clear marks of use on the sole of the prosthetic toe.

Nerlich *et al.* describe this as possibly the oldest known 'intravital limb prosthesis' (see Figure 1.2).[16]

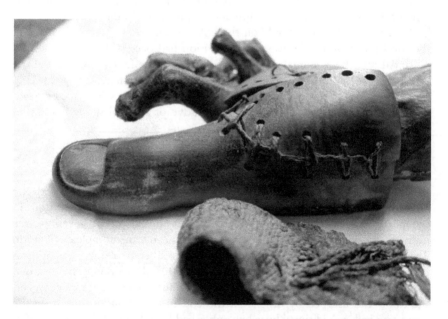

Figure 1.2 Side view of Excavation Number 453, made in three sections laced together using a series of marline hitches. The woven linen strap in the foreground secured it onto the right foot of the female mummy. Image courtesy of J. L. Finch with permission from the Egyptian Museum, Cairo.

Re-examination showed that the craftsman had used chisels to follow the anatomy of the foot when carving the sections A and B as one piece. Using a bow drill twenty-nine holes were made, then the sections were separated and a leather top piece cut. Although some of the lacing had disintegrated, these three sections were laced together using an overhand knot to secure a series of marline hitches. This configuration is commonly used to lash sails or sheaves of wheat together. The two sections had been sanded using abrasive blocks or stones. Under high magnification clear figuring in the form of tangential bands was revealed, suggestive of *Ulmaceae*, elm.

The plantar aspect under the toe had been shaved flat to provide stability with the ground. The proximal edge where the foot flexes during push off had been deliberately rounded for comfort. Between parts A and B there was some indication of a hinge. The leather top section was pierced with four holes which would have attached to the eight medial holes on the inner border of section A, a similar arrangement to that suggested for the attachment of EA 29996.

Methodology

A prosthetic toe must function efficiently and assist the wearer to walk effectively. If these were indeed true prosthetic devices it was essential to assess how they would have performed on the wearer. The rarity of these artefacts precluded their use in a laboratory trial; thus it was deemed necessary to co-opt volunteers and to construct working models which were design copies of the originals. These copies also had to be comfortable for the volunteers to wear in the controlled environment of a Human Performance (gait) laboratory. Plaster casts of their feet were required, onto which the replicas could be built. Working with the general public and in a clinical setting involved submitting documentation for NHS Research Ethics Approval and obtaining a site specific Honorary Research Passport. Consultants in these fields were contacted and gave generously of their expertise and time.

Only participants presenting with complete but stable disarticulation at the first metatarsal phalangeal (MPT) joint at the base of the right toe could be included in the research. Finding suitable volunteers with a stable pathology, lacking complicating contradictions in the affected or contralateral limb (deformity, ulcers or neuropathy) proved extremely difficult and it became apparent that fragile pathologies rendered some unsuitable for the study. Following collaboration with the subregional Manchester Disablement Services Centre, a press release was issued from the University of Manchester Media Office. This attracted a great deal of interest worldwide and yielded some eighteen respondents. Each was contacted, their histories taken and images of their affected right foot requested. Due to the logistics of travel, time constraints inherent in the project plus the cost of consumables, two volunteers (referred to as V1 and V2) were contacted. They were informed of the project through

Letters of Invitation. Research Participation Information Sheets were then made available prior to medical screening.

V1 was a 68-year-old male (height 1.65 m, mass 60.3 kg, shoe size 40); period since loss was 51 years.

V2 was a 53-year-old female (height 1.69 m, mass 80 kg, shoe size 41); period since loss was 31 years.

Foot status and stability of the stump were assessed plus medical history recorded by Consultants in Rehabilitation Medicine. Detailed neuro-circulatory foot assessments were conducted and cadence and step were observed. Only when the clinicians, participant and researcher were satisfied with the overall suitability of the patient were Research Participant Consent Forms offered. Throughout the whole of the consultation process and subsequent trial period it was stressed that the individuals were free to withdraw from the research at any time. V1 and V2 never met each other during the course of the research.

Producing the replicas

Negative impressions of both feet and the left big toe were taken from each volunteer using plaster of Paris bandage. 3D plaster positive models were made from these and were subsequently vacuum-moulded to produce polypropylene negative impressions. Stable polyurethane foam positive models were then cast. These were used for the formation of the cartonnage replica and formed the template for the carving of the articulated wooden replica. The materials were fully researched, to provide as close a match as possible.

Replica of the Greville Chester toe (P1)

For the construction of the cartonnage Ramie Trinity White linen (114 cm wide) was obtained from Whaleys (Bradford, UK) Ltd with an approximate warp: weft thread count of 30 per cm. It was washed to remove any surface treatment. Animal glue is thermally reversible which makes manipulation of the final product easier. Liberon Italian rabbit skin glue (Axminster Tools, UK) was mixed 1:1.8 parts by weight with water to glue respectively and heated to 60°C. The right big toe was reconstructed using modelling clay and positioned onto the model of the right foot. Its proportions were checked against the model taken of the left toe and was allowed to harden. The positive model of the right foot was coated in Vaseline™ and the linen overlaid to a depth of 3 mm and then left twenty-four hours to harden. This was removed and trimmed to conform to the original. Eight medial (inner side) and four lateral (outer side) holes were punched, diameter 2.5 mm. Ten coats of Winsor and Newton acrylic gesso primer were applied allowing one hour drying time between coats. The final surface was sanded with a series of graded glass papers. Three coats of acrylic gesso mixed with powdered red and yellow ochres gave the desired surface colour. A thin wash of Havannah Lake mimicked the inner red resin coating.

Replica of Excavation Number 453 (P2)

Ulmus laevis was used for parts A and B, the heartwood of this species of elm was deemed to be the nearest identifiable match to the original ancient timber. The skin for part C was natural russet cowhide obtained from A. L. Maugham, Liverpool, UK. The cord for lacing the parts together was 'S' twisted natural linen 5/8 supplied by Somac Threads Ltd, Chester, UK. This was split to give a cord of 2/8, giving it the slightly looser appearance of the original.

An expert in carving in the round was eventually co-opted onto the team. This individual was the 2007 British Bird Carving Champion and was able to provide invaluable insight into the type of wood used in the original and the way that the sections had been orientated in terms of the grain. He believed that parts A and B had been carved as one piece. Thus, an outline of both sections was drawn on the timber in the correct alignment with the grain and the residual timber trimmed. The trimmed shape was checked against the positive model, and then the false toe and external surfaces of the piece were carved out from the trimmed block. To ensure a snug fit with the positive model of the foot the internal surface was chiselled out. 'Smoking', a method used by gunsmiths, was then used to finish the inner surfaces. This involved coating the surface of the positive model foot with a brown dye. Where the dye touched, the wood was sanded down until the dye no longer made any contact with the inner surface.

Referring to images of the original artefact a series of twenty-nine holes was drilled using a 3 mm drill bit. A pyrographic wood burning tool was used to separate the two sections from each other ensuring that there was the correct alignment in the area of the hinge. This method of separation, although not deemed to be authentic to the original method, provided a clean-cut edge. The top edge was sanded smooth to ensure comfort when flexing the foot and the plantar aspect of the toe was shaved flat, thus conforming to the original. The sections were coated with linseed oil inside and out over a period of weeks. Section C was cut from russet cow hide and the required holes punched.

The lacing pattern holding the sections together was elucidated by an ex–Royal Naval engineer. The form of lacing used between the parts A and B was replicated by firstly securing the cord with a round turn plus overhand knot. Then a sequence of round turns with marline hitches was continued according to the pattern on the original (see Figure 1.3). It was gratifying to find that on completion the pattern produced on the inner surface of the replicas matched those on the original.

A pair of replica sandals was made for each volunteer modelled on E14504, Musée du Louvre, France. Montembault made detailed studies of the Louvre collection of ancient Egyptian footwear. E14504 is an example of her Class 1 Type A, a simple leather sandal.[17]

The straps are fixed to two earlike flaps which are on each side of the ankle and are integral to the sole. The sole is made of one thickness of leather. The

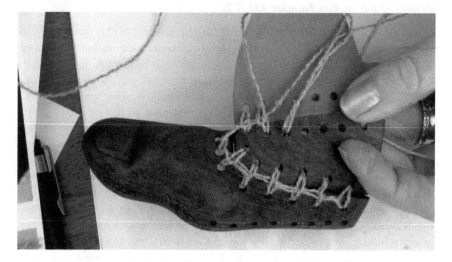

Figure 1.3 Replica of Excavation Number 453 (P2) showing the series of round
turns and marline hitches used to connect the sections together. Image
courtesy of J. L. Finch.

sandal is supported on the foot by two laces going through these flaps which
are then locked under the sole at the position of the first web space (between
the great and first toe). This simple type of footwear changed little throughout
Pharaonic history so was deemed an appropriate example on which to model
our replica sandals. Russet cow hide was used, the same as that used for section
C on Excavation Number 453.

Preliminary fitting of P1 and P2

It was deemed prudent to have preliminary fittings of both replicas plus sandals
before the final trials were undertaken. During this process adjustments were
made and any areas of discomfort were noted and addressed. The lacing
pattern under the foot was finalised and checked for comfort (see Figure 1.4).

Collecting the data

Gait is defined as any method of locomotion, characterised by periods of
loading and unloading of limbs. Gait includes running, hopping and skipping
but the most frequent method used is walking. The gait cycle consists of a
sequence of support and swing phases of the legs. In the support or stance
phase the foot is in contact with the ground, in the following swing phase it
is in the air. In walking, there is a period when both feet are in contact with
the ground. One complete gait cycle from heel strike to the next heel strike
with the same foot is called a stride. Two steps make a stride. Each stance and

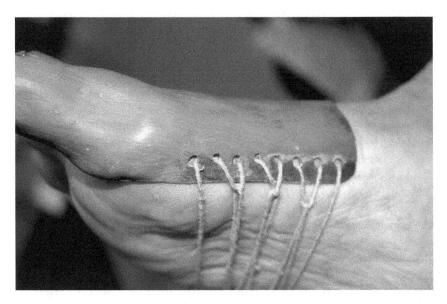

Figure 1.4 Showing the method of attachment of P1 to the foot. A series of loops
along the medial (inner) edge provides a double purchase across to the
four holes on the lateral (outer edge). This method was also used in
attaching P2 to the foot. Image courtesy of J. L. Finch.

each swing phase can be subdivided, but when fitted together they produce
a continuous sequence.

The first aim of the study was to establish if the designs of these two toe
'prostheses' were able to give a satisfactory level of function when walking
either when worn on their own or when worn with a typical Egyptian thong
sandal. The biomechanics of walking is a complex subject requiring a level of
expertise found only in specialist departments. I was most fortunate indeed to
enlist the invaluable help of Dr Glyn Heath, the then-Directorate of Prosthetics
and Orthotics at the University of Salford. The amount of data collected in
such trials can be overwhelming. I remain greatly indebted to Andrey Aksenov,
University of Salford who spent inordinate hours manipulating the data to
make it meaningful. Thanks to this very supportive team I was able to secure
the essential laboratory time in the Human Performance Research Gait
Laboratory at the University of Salford.

Motion or kinematic data

There are twenty-six bones in the foot, many overlapping and making mapping
of movements of all impossible. Kinematic data records the movement of the
foot throughout the gait cycle and in this case was limited to that in the sagittal
plane which divides foot into right and left portions. This provided information

regarding spatial and temporal changes. Optoelectronic motion capture records the movement of infrared reflective markers attached to specific body segments. The reflection from these positions on the foot when processed provides the 3D coordinates of each point.

Ten stationary integrated cameras along a 10 m walkway made up the Qualysis Proreflex Track Manager system (Gotenburg, Sweden). The shutters of these cameras open at exactly the same time enabling video fields from separate cameras to be synchronised. Each volunteer had four 10 mm reflective markers placed on each foot: R1/L1 on the distal phalanx, R2/L2 on the proximal phalanx, immediately distal to the MTP joint, R3/L3 on the sustentaculum tali and R4/L4 on the medial malleolus or ankle bone (see Figures 1.5 and 1.6).

As sagittal plane motion is the most useful indicator of big toe flexion, when the principles of trigonometry are applied motion of the foot can be calculated. The data was exported to Visual3D™ (C-Motion, Inc, Germantown, USA). Angular changes in the right foot wearing the replica toe were compared to those recorded from the left, this being used as a comparator or control. The angular changes can then be manipulated to form a time line, the sequence of one gait cycle performed by both the left foot (control) and right foot (replica). The amount of time taken for various phases of the gait cycle to be completed were calculated including the amount of flexion achieved when the replica toe pushed off compared to that achieved by the normal left or contralateral toe. The effect of wearing a sandal with the device was also determined from the data.

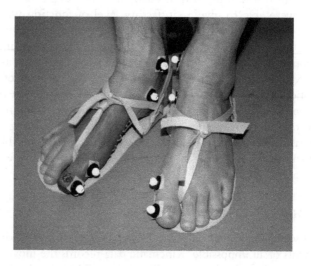

Figure 1.5 Replica P1 with replica Egyptian sandals worn by Volunteer V1. Note the placement of the four reflective markers. Image courtesy of J. L. Finch.

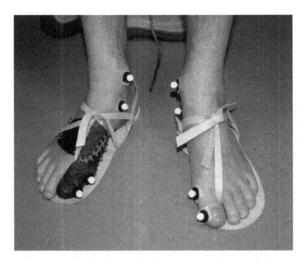

Figure 1.6 Replica P2 with replica Egyptian sandals worn by Volunteer V1. Image courtesy of J. L. Finch.

Pressure or kinetic data

The second aim of this study was to record kinetic data which involves changes in the pressure distribution under the foot, the strike pattern and the way the pressure moves across the foot as the heel strikes the floor and eventually pushes off. Most people strike the ground using the outside of the heel and then roll inwards pushing forward from under the big toe. An unduly high pressure in certain areas is interpreted as producing a level of discomfort. Over prolonged periods this may lead to tissue damage. Measuring such changes in pressure required the Medilogic(r) Pressure Measuring System (T and T Medilogic Medizintechnik GmbH, Schönefeld, Germany). This consists of a mat placed on the walkway containing force sensitive resistors. Wireless transmission permits instantaneous display of pressure values. The pressure profile can then be displayed either as contours (isobars) connecting areas of equal pressure, as 3D mountain plots or as colour-coded pixels. The strike pattern and duration, associated heel and push-off pressures are recorded. How long the foot has remained on the ground (contact time) can also be determined.

Questionnaire

A questionnaire was also provided for each volunteer. This was to assess if the working environment (the gait laboratory) with all the associated equipment had influenced their performance. In such trials information recorded by the cameras and pressure mat may not necessarily correlate with the comfort and performance perceived by the subject. The questionnaire asked the volunteers to rate on a scale of one to ten how they perceived each device to be performing.

Results

It is beyond the scope of this paper to discuss the results in full.[18] Analysis of the motion and kinetic data showed that each volunteer responded differently to the variables, and thus the results were highly subjective. This is a major drawback when undertaking such a study and even if a greater cohort had been co-opted the same variability in the results would probably have been noted. It was, however, very encouraging that both volunteers were able to walk wearing the replicas, albeit within the confines of a laboratory.

Both volunteers felt that neither the walkway, the presence of the ten integrated cameras, nor the presence of the technicians had compromised their performance during the trials. They also felt that the replicas were not too heavy to wear. It was noted by V1 that replica P1 (the cartonnage device) felt very inflexible and seemed to throw the foot to the right. With the sandal, it was a little more comfortable but the problem was perceived to persist. V1 therefore gave P1 a low score for comfort and ease of walking. V2 also found this replica inflexible and likewise gave it a disappointing score for comfort.

Comments regarding replica P2 (the three-part device) were in sharp contrast. Describing its performance, V1 commented that with time he could have got used to using the device, it was also thought very comfortable especially when wearing a sandal. V2 likewise thought replica P2 was exceedingly more compliant and thus more comfortable against the skin and remarked it felt softer to walk on. Both volunteers scored this device very highly indeed for comfort. These subjective comments are extremely valuable and to some degree in sharp contrast to the kinematic/motion data and kinetic/pressure collected in the laboratory.

The kinematic results showed that P1 and P2 performed exceptionally well for V1, especially when supported by a sandal. The stages in the gait cycle did not appear to be unduly compromised, although there was hesitation and thus some delay in pushing off from the ground with the replica toe strapped in place. An impressive amount of dorsiflexion was achieved as the foot swung forward: V1 wearing P1 plus the sandals achieved eighty-seven per cent flexion, while wearing P2 V1 achieved seventy-eight per cent flexion; left toe as the control was deemed to be one hundred per cent. Although a lesser degree of flexion was achieved by V2 it was still an impressive sixty-two per cent and sixty-three per cent, wearing P1 and P2 respectively. It was interesting also to note from the kinetic/pressure data that no excessive pressures were recorded under the right foot when wearing either of the devices with or without a sandal and there was no significant loading passed onto the normal left side.

Although walking under limited conditions cannot mimic completely conditions experienced in the 'normal outside world', it becomes apparent that both devices appeared to be performing well, especially with a sandal, and were not producing undue discomfort.

Conclusion

The purpose of the research was to evaluate the functionality of the design of two ancient Egyptian artificial restorations of the right big toe. The proposal was complex and it necessitated a large highly skilled team. Many problems were encountered and compromises made.

It was difficult to locate suitable volunteers in the Manchester area. The press release attracted numerous individuals worldwide but due to the limited time of the study, limited resources and funding, and the risk of data overload from co-opting a larger number of volunteers, only two were eventually selected. Ideally the research should have invited more respondents to become part of the trial. The pathology and foot anatomy of the owner of EA 29996 remains unknown; therefore the foot presentation of the female mummy found wearing Excavation Number 453 was used as a guide in the selection process. This individual presented with complete disarticulation of the right first MTP joint. It was suggested that she may also have suffered from diabetes. Visits to Diabetic Foot Clinics did reveal several suitable patients but because of their peripheral neuropathy there could have been an increased risk of ulceration when undertaking the trials. None were therefore considered for inclusion. The two volunteers selected were of different sexes, ages, heights, body masses and shoe sizes.

Due to the rarity of the original artefacts it was necessary to make and test replicas. These were design copies made specifically for the volunteers co-opted. The data generated from this study must only be viewed as an indication of how the particular design performed under the trial conditions. The actual fit and comfort of the original artefacts for their respective owners will always remain unknown.

Although the materials and techniques were thoroughly researched many compromises had to be made. Experimental replication cannot always be expected to follow exactly those processes undertaken by the ancient Egyptians. Present-day materials were selected to provide the nearest match to the original (linen, animal glue, gesso, wood, cordage) and techniques were adapted using modern tools (steel saws, chisels and pyrograph cutting tool).

EA 29996 was constructed out of cartonnage. The use of this material was widespread, producing mummy masks, mummy cases, anthropoid coffins and other funerary items. Mummy cases were usually moulded with an opening down the back. After placing the deceased into it, the case was laced down the back.[19] From the beautiful anatomical conformity shown by this artefact it seems plausible to suggest that the wet cartonnage had been laid directly over the foot of the intended wearer, possibly with some form of grease applied first to aid its removal.

Three independent wood experts suggested that Excavation Number 453 had been carved from a species of *Ulmus*, elm. This was based on the configuration of the transverse section of the vessels showing the presence of undulating tangential bands. This manifests as a ripple effect across the wood. No sections could be taken so this conclusion was based on visual inspection and comparison with specimens of *Ulmus* in the University of Oxford Herbarium. *Ulmus* is a genus of the Middle East, Anatolia and the Caucuses. This wood is not found in Egypt, examples are rare, occasionally being used for chariot hubs due to its strength under compression.[20] A selection of bronze or copper chisels had been used probably with a wooden mallet and the surface made smooth using sand and abrasive blocks. It was suggested that the sections had been drilled and then separated using a bow drill. This was a fundamental tool of the carpenter. The revolving drill cap enabled pressure to be exerted while the rapid passage of string wound round the shaft achieved a considerable number of revolutions per unit time. The reciprocating bow drill had string attached at both ends of the shaft, making it more efficient. The skills necessary to produce this beautifully crafted object may well have been handed down.

The volunteers were asked to perform under laboratory conditions only. No data from quiet standing was done. The study only focused on the performance of the replicas during walking. The volunteers were not given much time to acclimatise to wearing the replicas before the day of the trial although there was time given for a preliminary fitting. This may have been useful, although more difficult to monitor.

A radiograph of the foot may have been useful to determine whether the sesamoid bones under the first metatarsal head (base of big toe) were still in place. These two small bones can be lost during amputation. When present they help stabilise the medial longitudinal arch and assist flexion of the hallux. V1 had intact arches and excellent relative dorsiflexion on the right side. His foot pathology may also have been a factor. The original lacing pattern under the foot was suggested from the wear apparent on the holes on EA 29996. A similar method of lacing was used for both replicas. This interpretation may have been incorrect. In all seven variables were chosen and each data set consisted of the best ten trials under those conditions. Problems of repeatability arose in some variables.[21]

The sandal thong was moved from the first to the second web space on the right foot of V2 to help V2 keep the sandal in place. The thong was not moved over on the left foot. Locating the exact foot segment and positioning the reflective markers required the expertise of specialists in gait analysis. Such assistance was crucial to ensure that reliable kinematic data was obtained. The reflective markers fell off during some of the trials and had to be carefully repositioned and the trial repeated. This was time-consuming.

Statistical tests were undertaken to see if there was any significant difference in the data obtained from the right and left sides, this being determined by the varying conditions under which the volunteers were asked to walk. The standard deviation(s) for some data sets indicated there to be a high degree of variation. Doing more repeats, however, may have been tiring for the volunteers and their performance may have been adversely affected. The overall scores for P1 and P2 in the questionnaire seem to have been influenced by their own individual perception of which design would best satisfy that of a functional prosthetic device.

Although a great toe is not essential in walking, some clinical benefit would have been gained by wearing either device, whether in reducing plantar pressure distribution or in producing a more symmetrical walking pattern. Wearing such a prosthesis would also protect the amputation site from further damage.

The quality of execution of both the original artefacts is, however, indisputable. In both examples, great care has been taken to mimic the anatomy of the foot. The selection of materials is also intriguing, firstly the use of cartonnage and secondly the non-indigenous wood, *Ulmus*. It seems reasonable to assume that fashioning these replacement toes would have required the skills and expertise only afforded by elite members of Egyptian society. How well the originals fitted their owners will remain unknown but some consultation process may have taken place during the preliminary phases of construction and then during the final fitting, inferring some sort of prescriptive and iterative process.

We must now address the question, 'If they were worn in life, by whom were they worn, why and where?' The owner of the EA 29996 remains a mystery. However, the three-part device was found strapped onto the foot of Tabaketenmut, the elderly daughter of the priest Bakamon, dated between 950–710 BCE. Thebes at this time was ruled by pontiffs who bore the titles of High Priests of Amun. During these years, known as the 22nd and 23rd Dynasties, the chief dignitaries came from powerful families. If the identification of her father is correct, she too may have also been involved in temple duties and rituals. With an incomplete body, although arguably only slightly impaired, performing rituals in front of the gods may have been seen as unacceptable. Replacing her missing big toe may not have been solely for practical purposes but also for ideological reasons. In the ancient world completeness and perfection of the body is often deemed a prerequisite for undertaking temple rituals.[22]

In his paper 'Techniques of the body', Mauss puts forward some interesting ideas regarding 'habitus'. He proposes that habits that are developed throughout an individual's lifetime such as walking, swimming, climbing and the care of the body emerge and evolve in response to the society in which the individual lives, and are greatly influenced by their level of education, the proprieties demanded by that society as well as his or her status within that society. [23] Tabaketenmut appears to have been a priestess, and born into a priestly family.

She would certainly have been expected to abide by a particular code of ethics, these dictated according to her duties within the temple and according to her involvement in cultic ceremonies. The prosthetic toe appears to have been rounded off on its proximal edge and exhibits abrasion marks on the underside, thus suggesting it was designed to be worn and was worn. We do not know at what age the amputation occurred nor whether her gait was greatly affected. The wearing of sandals may have been obligatory and coupled with the prosthesis to reaffirm her bodily perfection, stability and a more fluid efficient gait would have been re-established. Such was the quality and importance of the object that the embalmers included it in her burial. Her body could then be presented to the gods complete and her resurrection as a transfigured spirit would be assured.

Despite the many pitfalls and unanswered questions, undertaking experimental archaeology remains a powerful tool and can be shown to extend our understanding. There can be a tendency to underperform and there may be arrogance to overinterpret. Just because a successful outcome is achieved does not necessarily mean that that was the way it was originally conceived and constructed.

Prior to this research the earliest known classical device was thought to be Roman, known as the Capua leg and securely dated to 300 BCE. Although the artefact, housed in the Royal College of Surgeons, London, UK was destroyed in a bombing raid in May 1941, a replica exists in the Science Museum, London, UK. A detailed examination of the original was undertaken in 1920 by Sudhoff, the eminent medical historian and a paper was published by von Brunn of Rostock in 1926.[24] Techniques in gait analysis advance rapidly. I am certain that if experimental archaeology were to be carried out to explore the functionality of the design of this lower limb prosthesis, it would further our understanding of this branch of science.

To date it seems reasonable to suggest that these two rare and beautiful objects from ancient Egypt are tangible examples of the earliest extant extremity prosthetic devices. The beautifully crafted three-part wooden device, at least 400 years earlier than the Capua leg, shows us that a prosthetic practitioner (albeit unwittingly) of this branch of science may well have been living in the Nile Valley between 950–710 BCE.

Notes

1 The reconstruction of a New Kingdom loom was achieved by co-opting the skills of Herbert G. Farbrother, OBE, formerly of the Cotton Research Corporation. Details of the processes involved and the consequent problems which were encountered can be found in Kemp and Vogelsang-Eastwood, 2001, pp. 405–426.

2 Taylor, 2001, pp. 14–32.

3 References made to restorative practices in the Pyramid Texts, Coffin Texts and Book of the Dead can be found in Finch, 2009, pp. 66–67.

4 Finch, 2009, pp. 50–63 for a discussion on the various types of bodily restorations with illustrations.

5 The CT density suggests it to be made from ceramic, Wagle, 1994.

6 Finch, 2011.

7 Dawson *et al.*, 1995, p. 96 for the biography of Reverend Greville Chester.

8 Lang, 1989. The false toe was possibly filled with mud and a fourth attachment hole on the lateral side is visible.

9 Shashoua, 1991. The red coating on the inner surface was similar to Dragon's Blood gum from leaf stem resins of *Dracaena* species.

10 Middleton, 1992. The buff plaster had the characteristic morphology and geological makeup of the Theban area. Regarding ancient quarries, see Harrell, 1992.

11 Reeves, 1999. The linen was fine plain tabby weave, all threads plied or doubled, a characteristic of yarns produced up to 600 BCE when this method was superseded by draft spinning.

12 Strudwick, 2006, p. 268.

13 Edwards *et al.*, 1997 explains the characterisation of Dragon's Blood gum.

14 Nerlich and Zink, 2003.

15 Nerlich *et al.*, 2000. This paper includes images of the mummy, right foot and prosthesis strapped to the foot.

16 Nerlich *et al.*, 2000. See endnote 15.

17 Montembault, 2000. Classification of Class 1 Type sandals p. 82. E14504 appears on p. 88.

18 Results and discussion from this study can be found in Finch *et al.*, 2012.

19 Taylor, 1988 describes how cartonnage mummy cases were constructed.

20 Gale *et al.*, 2000. The characteristics of *Ulmus* plus examples of the wood forming parts of ancient Egyptian chariots are described on p. 346. Details of woodworking techniques can be found pp. 356–358.

21 See Finch *et al.*, 2012, p. 187, Table 3.

22 Finch, 2012/2013, pp. 111–132 provides a comprehensive account of the concept of perfection in the ancient world.

23 Mauss, 1973. This transcript of his lecture given on 17 May 1934 to the Société de Psychologie puts forward the notion of 'habitus' and the influence of society and status on how an individual manipulates his or her bodily actions, pp. 73–75.

24 Bliquez, 1996 provides a comprehensive account of classical prosthetic devices including a full description with accompanying images of the Capua leg, pp. 2640–2676.

Bibliography

Bliquez, L. J. (1996) 'Prosthetics in Classical Antiquity: Greek, Etruscan and Roman Prosthetics', in *ANRW* II 37.3, pp. 2640–2676.

Dawson, W. R. *et al.* (1995) *Who Was Who in Egyptology*. London: Egypt Exploration Society.

Edwards, H. G. M., Farwell, D. W. and Quye, A. (1997) 'Dragon's Blood I-Characterization of an Ancient Resin using Fourier Transform Ramen Spectroscopy', *The Journal of Ramen Spectroscopy* 28.4, pp. 243–249.

Finch, J. L. (2009) *The Significance of Two Ancient Egyptian Hallux Restorations to the History of Prosthetic Medicine: Evaluation of the Original Artefacts and the Biomechanical Assessment of Replicas*. Manchester: University of Manchester, Ph.D. thesis.

Finch, J. L. (2011) 'The Ancient Origins of Prosthetic Medicine', *The Lancet* 377.9765, pp. 548–549.

Finch, J. L., Heath, G. H., David, A. R. and Kulkarni, J. (2012) 'Biomechanical Assessment of Two Artificial Big Toe Restorations from Ancient Egypt and their

Significance to the History of Prosthetics', *The Journal of Prosthetics and Orthotics* 24.4, pp. 181–191.

Finch, J. L. (2012/2013) 'The Durham Mummy: Deformity and the Concept of Perfection in the Ancient World', in David, R. (ed.) *Bulletin of the John Rylands University Library Manchester* 89 Supplement 2012/2013 *Ancient Medical and Healing Systems: Their Legacy to Western Medicine*, pp. 111–132.

Gale, R. *et al.* (2000) 'Wood', in Nicholson, P. N. and Shaw, I. (edd.) *Ancient Egyptian Materials and Technology*. Cambridge: Cambridge University Press, pp. 334–371.

Harrell, J. A. (1992) 'Ancient Egyptian Limestone Quarries: A Petrological Survey', *Archaeometry* 34, 2, pp. 195–211.

Kemp, B. J. and Vogelsang-Eastwood, G. (2001) *The Ancient Textile Industry at Amarna*. London: Egypt Exploration Society.

Lang, J. (1989) 'Radiographic Examination of an Artificial Toe (Late New Kingdom?)', in Middleton, P. A. (ed.) *Internal British Museum Department of Scientific Research Report number 6042*. London: British Museum.

Mauss, M. (1973) 'Techniques of the Body', *Economy and Society* 2.1, pp. 70–81. Transcript of a lecture given at a meeting of the Société de Psychologie, 17 May 1934.

Middleton, A. P. (1992) *Internal British Museum Department of Scientific Research Report Number 6042*. London: British Museum.

Montembault, V. (2000) *Catalogue des Chaussures de l'Antiquité Égyptienne*. Paris: Réunion des Musées Nationaux.

Nerlich, A. G., Zink, A., Szeimies, U. and Haghedorn, H. G. (2000) 'Ancient Egyptian Prosthesis of the Big Toe', *The Lancet* 356.9248, pp. 2176–2179.

Nerlich, A. G. and Zink, A. (2003) 'Anthropological and Paleopathological Analysis of Human Remains in the Theban Necropolis: A Comparative Study on Three Tombs of the Nobles', in Strudwick, N. and Taylor, J. H. (edd.) *The Theban Necropolis, Past Present and Future*. London: British Museum Press, pp. 218–228.

Reeves, C. N. (1999) 'New Light on Ancient Egyptian Prosthetic Medicine', in Davies, V. (ed.) *Studies in Honour of Egyptian Antiquities. A Tribute to T. G. H. James, Occasional Paper 123*. London: British Museum Press, pp. 337–356.

Shashoua, Y. (1991) 'The Identification of the Filler and Coating Materials on an Egyptian Prosthetic Toe Registration Number EA 29996', in *Conservation Research Section Report 1991/34*. London: British Museum.

Strudwick, N. (2006) *Masterpieces of the British Museum*. London: British Museum Press.

Taylor, J. H. (1988) 'The Development of Cartonnage Cases', in D'Auria, S., Lacovara, S. P. and Roehrig, C. (edd.) *Mummies and Magic: The Funerary Arts of Ancient Egypt*. Boston, MA: Museum of Fine Arts, pp. 166–168.

Taylor, J. H. (2001) *Death and the Afterlife in Ancient Egypt*. London: British Museum Press.

Wagle, W. A. (1994) 'Toe Prosthesis in an Egyptian Mummy', *The American Journal of Roentgenology* 162.4, pp. 999–1000.

2 A very distinctive smile: Etruscan dental appliances

Jean MacIntosh Turfa and
Marshall Joseph Becker

Introduction

During the second half of the first millennium BCE, a few Etruscan and Italic noblewomen wore false teeth made with golden bands; they were buried with these prostheses in place, tempting items for modern *tombaroli* to extract. Few such dental appliances have come to us with proper contextual information, but even those separated from their owners' bodies, including several that became Victorian collectors' items, can still furnish a wealth of information about those who wore them and the technology used to construct them. They also pose some tantalising paradoxes and challenges to what we know about ancient technology and Etruscan and Italic society. In the past these appliances were studied somewhat haphazardly, as curiosities or as illustrations of the supposed advances in dentistry of an ancient civilisation. In some cases, nineteenth-century museums and private collectors commissioned copies of these ancient specimens for study or display. Many of these copies came to be treated as genuine, leading to great confusion in scholars' attempts to tabulate and measure all the known examples. Further confusion has accrued because many authors over the last 200 years have simply repeated past scholarship and few had actually handled the original pieces. We attempt to correct this in our book, *The Etruscans and the History of Dentistry: The Golden Smile*, with Becker's autopsy of all extant prostheses and study of the information from a few specimens that now are lost or unavailable for examination. The sophistication of Etruscan goldsmiths and the startling social traditions behind these appliances mark the only time in the history of dentistry prior to the modern era that such prostheses were developed and used. Our study of 20 band-appliances has found that the phenomenon has virtually nothing to do with medical practice or professional dentistry. The known wire appliances (W1-W7) are an entirely different category of prosthesis.

Dental appliances formed from thin gold bands, with inserted replacement front teeth, began to be used in Italy during the seventh century BCE. They are documented by relatively few examples, all apparently buried with their owners. These represent a range of several hundred years, perhaps down to the second century BCE, followed by a brief period in the first centuries

Table 2.1 Dental appliances (Etruscan and Italic)

	Name, Location Measurements	Provenance, Date (BCE)	Sex	Jaw region	Type, Function
1	Barrett I Formerly collection of Dr. Wm. C. Barrett, Buffalo, NY location unknown L. 20 mm	Etruria 5th c.?	F?	Maxilla left central incisor plus two more teeth	Simple band, three spaces, stabilising
2	Barrett II as No. 1 L. 25 mm	Bisenzio, tomb on Capodimonte 500–480	F	Maxilla left second premolar to central incisor?	Simple band, five spaces, stabilising
3	Van Marter Obtained by Dr James Gilbert Van Marter in Italy location unknown L. 25 mm	'Lake of Valseno' (Bolsena?) 600??	F??	Maxilla?	Ring series, three spaces, central false tooth
4	Copenhagen, National Museum inv. 8319 L. 21.6 mm	Orvieto(?) 500–490	F	Maxilla left central incisor to right lateral incisor	Three welded loops, no rivet, one false tooth (right central incisor)
5	Poggio Gaiella Florence Museo Archeologico inv. 11782 L. 42 mm	Chiusine necropolis Poggio Gaiella tomb of 4th–3rd c.?	F 25–40 years	Maxilla left first premolar to right first premolar. Now in wrong skull and mandible	Single, complex band, eight spaces, stabilising. Now in two pieces
6	Populonia Florence, Museo Archeologico, inv. 84467 – lost in 1966 Florence Flood	Populonia, San Cerbone necropolis tomb of 4th c.	?	Maxilla? (all four incisors?)	Four-ring series, four spaces, one rivet, one false tooth
7	Ghent, University Museum, looted by German forces, WW II L. 27 mm	'near Orvieto' tomb? of 6th c. or later	?	Maxilla (all four incisors?)	Complex band, three loops, four spaces
8	Bruschi I Tarquinia, Museo Nazionale Archeologico, Ex Bruschi-Falgari L. 32 mm	(probably Tarquinia) 5th c.?	F	Maxilla all four incisors	Narrow band, four spaces, stabilising

Table 2.1 continued

	Name, Location Measurements	Provenance, Date (BCE)	Sex	Jaw region	Type, Function
9	Bruschi II Tarquinia, Museo Nazionale Archeologico, Ex Bruschi-Falgari Missing since 1916–1925 transfer. L. 29 mm	Territory of Tarquinia? date unknown	F???	Maxilla (all four incisors?)	Four rings, one rivet (one false tooth, right central incisor?)
10	Bruschi III Tarquinia, Museo Nazionale Archeologico, Ex Bruschi-Falgari L. 36.8 mm	Territory of Tarquinia? 2nd c.??	F	Maxilla? Teeth displayed are not original	Four braces, five spaces, no rivets, stabilising
11	Corneto I Tarquinia Museo Nazionale Archeologico Missing since 1916–1925 transfer. L. 28 mm	Tarquinia Probably excavated 1876–1877 530–510?	??	Maxilla? Left canine to right lateral incisor	Braced? band, five spaces, two rivets, one false tooth (right central incisor)
12	Corneto II Tarquinia Museo Nazionale Archeologico Missing since 1916–1925. L. 62.5 mm	Tarquinia Possibly excavated c. 1875 500?	F??	Maxilla? (left second premolar to right canine?)	Compound: seven rings, eight spaces, three rivets (animal tooth replaces central incisors; false left first premolar missing)
13	Liverpool I Liverpool World Museum inv. 10334, ex Joseph Mayer L. 30.9 mm	unknown date unknown collected before 1857	F?	Maxilla all four incisors	Band with four spaces, two rivets, two false teeth (central incisors)
14	Liverpool II Liverpool World Museum inv. 10335, ex Joseph Mayer L. 28.2 mm	unknown date unknown collected before 1857	F? 45+ years	Maxilla all four incisors	Band with four spaces, two rivets, two false teeth (central incisors, missing)
15	Valsiarosa Civita Castellana, Museo Archeologico dell'Agro Falisco Ex Villa Giulia 1515 L. 38 mm	Valsiarosa necropolis of *Falerii Veteres* Tomb 20 4th c.?	F?	Maxilla all four incisors Displayed on ancient skull that is not original owner's.	Four welded loops, four spaces, one rivet (false right central incisor missing)

Table 2.1 continued

	Name, Location Measurements	Provenance, Date (BCE)	Sex	Jaw region	Type, Function
16	Teano Berlin, Institut für Geschichte der Medizin, Humboldt University L. 47 mm Not Available	Teano (Campania), Fondo Gradavola necropolis, Tomb 18 4th–3rd c.	F	Maxilla left to right canines	Six rings, no rivets, stabilising
17	Praeneste (Palestrina) Villa Giulia inv. 13213 L. 31 mm	Praeneste, Sporadic find in necropolis date unknown	F 35–45 years*	Maxilla all four incisors	Band, four spaces, two rivets (false central incisors missing)
18	Satricum Villa Giulia inv. 12206 L. 29 mm	Satricum, Borgo Le Ferriere, Tumulus C 7th c./c. 630	F 50 years	Maxilla left lateral incisor to right canine	Band, five spaces; gold tooth (right central incisor)
19	Bracciano Vienna, Museum of Natural History inv. 24.296 (catalogued c. 1990) L. 24 mm, estimated Not available	Near Lake Bracciano, tomb 7th c.?	F?	Maxilla left central incisor to right lateral incisor	Band, three spaces, one rivet holds false tooth (cut-down right central incisor)
20	Tanagra Athens National Museum: Lambros Collection inv. 358 L. 43.3 mm	Tanagra, Boeotia 4th–3rd c.?	F? 45 ± 10 years*	Maxilla left to right canines	Compound band, two loops, no rivets, stabilising
21	Sardis Ankara, Turkey: Collection of Dr Ilter Uzel (L. 48 mm) Not available	Salihli 'ancient Sardis' found in a tomb 3rd c??	F 25–40 years	Mandible skull, some teeth found	Band, four loops, two rivets (in two false teeth, human or bovine central incisors)

For more complete data, see Becker and Turfa, 2017, or the bibliography cited in endnote 2.
Almost all of the known gold bands are now slightly distorted (or worse) from burial and modern handling.

Where noted, sex has been assigned based on (small) tooth size, determined by the spaces in appliances.

*age estimate based on dental wear of extant teeth.

L. = length of appliance as preserved.

M = male; F = female.

? = some uncertainty in identification of sex, age or date.

?? = serious uncertainty.

BCE and CE when Roman authors (especially satirists) speak of society women trying to hide the effects of age with white false teeth. From that era, only a single prosthesis has ever been found in Rome (No. W7 below) and that belonged to a cremated woman in her fifties.[1] Her prosthesis, however, was made in a different technique from the Etruscan appliances – using gold wire rather than flat bands. Although often cited in Roman literature, this technique previously had been known from only six other cases, all found in the eastern Mediterranean, Levant and Egypt (Nos. W1–W6). While the Etruscan appliances were the work of goldsmiths, not dentists, the Hellenistic and Roman wiring technique reveals true dentistry.

Many issues can be raised with regard to these appliances, but we have few ready explanations. A disconnect between actual finds of prostheses and the facile comments of Roman authors is surprising. The earlier gold band-appliances are linked to Etruscan technology; in fact, they betray quite sophisticated metallurgy (below), although they were never as efficient as modern bridges or braces. As a social phenomenon Etruscan appliances are even more puzzling: all examples with true contexts came from the burials of affluent women, and even the orphaned appliances, according to the measurements of their gold loops, are so small that they probably were fashioned for female teeth. The reasons why Etruscan women of the ruling classes should have needed to replace one or more of their upper front teeth are difficult to discover and have led us to consider parallel ethnographic evidence for dental evulsion: rites of passage and mourning rituals heretofore undocumented for ancient Etruria. Other questions arise concerning the availability of dental treatment in ancient Etruria, or in general in the Mediterranean world and Near East during (or before) the first millennium BCE. A survey of documented dental appliances will begin our discussion of these issues; basic data has been condensed into Table 2.1.[2]

The phenomenon of wire appliances

The most recent find of a gold dental appliance, No. W7, comes from excavations at a necropolis in Rome. This wire appliance is fashioned from gold, as are all but one of the Near Eastern appliances. One wire appliance, from Lower Egypt, is made from drawn silver, from a necropolis of Ptolemaic or Roman date. The Near Eastern examples all post-date the invention of Etruscan gold band-appliances, and range in date from the fourth century BCE to the early Imperial period. Five appear to have been installed in the mandible, in contrast to the Etruscan band-appliances. Five of these apparently used the owner's teeth as replacements.

Table 2.2 Wire appliances (Hellenistic and Roman)

Item, Dimensions	Provenance, Location	Date	Sex/Age	Replacement Material	Type/Design
W1. Sidon I L. 34 mm	Sidon, Tomb XI, Room 1, fosse b (1861 excavations) Louvre	1st 1/4 4th c. BCE	F	two human incisors, two holes drilled in each	mandibular?? wire binding six teeth
W2. Sidon II L. 35 mm (estimated)	Sidon, Tomb I, 'Ain Hilweh, East sarcophagus American Univ. Museum, Beirut	5th–4th c. BCE	M? middle aged	–no–	mandible, with decayed teeth
W3. Alexandria L. 25 mm	Ibrahimieh, Tomb Greco-Roman Museum, Alexandria	Roman 1st c. CE	?	–no–	mandible poor condition
W4. El-Qatta L. 43 mm(broken)	El-Qatta Tomb No. 90 reused mastaba, shaft 5 (Cairo Museum?)	Roman	?	R central incisor, drilled	maxilla, wire deformed
W5. Tura el-Asment silver wire L. 27 mm	Tomb T-121 in Ptolemaic necropolis Cairo/Museum?	Ptolemaic	M?? young adult?	R central incisor returned to mouth with root modified	maxilla severe malocclusion, necrotic abscess of R central incisor
W6. Eretria L. 49 mm (estimated)	tomb at Eretria Athens National Archaeological Museum	4th c. BCE	F???	–no–	mandibular complex pattern binding 6 teeth incomplete?
W7. Rome L. 39 mm	tomb in Collatina necropolis, partially cremated skeleton. Rome, Soprintendenza	Imperial Roman, 2nd c. CE	F 50?	original tooth: R central incisor, root missing (drilled, wired)	mandibular: adjacent teeth damaged by periodontal disease

All gold wire except W5, which is silver wire.

Discussion of known ancient dental appliances

Provenance

Although provenance information on several pieces is unconfirmed, the majority of band-type appliances came from southern Etruria and environs. Three early finds of Etruscan appliances collected in the 1880s (Nos. 1–3) came from the region of Lake Bolsena in the south Etruscan heartland, including the site of Bisenzio (Visentium, an early settlement in this rich region of trade and metal working). Another example, now in Copenhagen (No. 4) came from nearby Orvieto, the major Etruscan city of Volsinii. A lost specimen once in Ghent was also attributed to Orvieto (No. 7). Five examples, the largest group, came from unidentified tombs in the necropoleis of Tarquinia (Nos. 8–12). Two pieces in Liverpool (Nos. 14–15), found early in the nineteenth century, may have come from Vulci. Northern Etruria is represented by a bridge from the region of Chiusi (No. 5), and a lost specimen from the early city of Populonia (No. 6). The Italic zone of central Italy produced the earliest archaeologically datable appliance, which is also the only bridge with a gold false tooth, from a necropolis at Latin-speaking Satricum (No. 18). Other Italic necropoleis represented include Latin Praeneste/Palestrina (No. 17), the Faliscan city Falerii Veteres (Civita Castellana, No. 15), and Campanian Teano (No. 16). Provenance cannot be verified for a bridge said to have been excavated at Bracciano in southern Etruria (No. 19) and made known around 1990.

Two examples of these appliances are outliers: a stabilising appliance using gold bands to brace loose teeth was found in Tanagra (Boiotia), and is now in the Athens National Museum (No. 20): its technique of construction is Etruscan in origin. Some Greek medical writers had spoken of the use of metal to stabilise loosened teeth (see below) but the band-construction matches all the Etruscan/Italic examples. One possible specimen, said to be from a tomb at Sardis, was published in two brief articles in dental journals and said to be in a private collection. As it has not been made available for study, we cannot verify its authenticity or provenance.[3] Obviously the dates of Etruscan appliances preclude any connection to the Herodotean fiction of a Lydian migration![4]

Etruscan dental appliances: dating

Some complex band-appliances were used as braces for living teeth. These range in estimated date (mostly based on descriptions of artefacts found with them) from the early fifth century (Nos. 1, 2, 'Etruria' and Bisenzio) through the fourth and third century (Nos. 5, 8, 16, 20) to possibly the second century (No. 10, Tarquinia?). This implies that this use began distinctly later than the single bridges with one or two false teeth. The earliest known appliance (No. 18, from Satricum) is a band with one replacement front tooth in gold;

it comes from a Latin town with a strong flavor of Etruscan culture. Although the tomb was disturbed and could not be reconstructed, all ambient evidence points to burial during the seventh century. The appliance was constructed earlier still, perhaps in the first half of the seventh century.[5] It is the only example of a false tooth constructed in gold, and all other bridges seem to have employed human or animal teeth or ivory. If the scanty evidence is correct, the bridges, with replacement teeth, range in date (of the tomb in which their wearer was found) from this example (No. 18) of the seventh century to the fourth–third century (Nos. 6, 15). Three other band-appliances may perhaps be dated to the sixth and early fifth century BCE (Nos. 11, 12, 3). All are one-of-a-kind constructions for individual situations. These vary from three loops of which the middle example holds the one central incisor replacement tooth (Nos. 3, 19), to the band with five spaces in which is found the unique gold tooth (No. 18), to an example spanning eight spaces into which have been inserted three false teeth (No. 12). The wire appliances also were used for both replacement and stabilising, and range from the fourth century BCE (Sidon, Nos. W1–2) to the second century CE (Rome, No. W7).

Dental appliances: technique of construction

All twenty (or twenty-one) band-appliances associated with Etruscan technology were constructed using thin sheet gold cut and hammered into a narrow band that encircled the teeth, either in a continuous loop (thirteen examples) or a set of rings (eight examples). In those few cases where the false teeth are preserved, the 'replacement teeth' were trimmed and smoothed from human teeth, probably the wearer's own, or were carved from animal teeth (see No. 12). It is possible that some specimens from which the replacement tooth is missing (as No. 14) had false teeth carved from ivory or other organic materials. The sole exception is the oldest dated example, the bridge from Satricum (No. 18) which has a gold replacement tooth welded to its gold band. Most replacement teeth were attached by one small cylindrical rivet each, also of gold, set horizontally through the drilled tooth. Where we believe the person's own teeth were used, the roots had been trimmed. The whole structure was then fitted into the mouth (in what must have been a ticklish process) by anchoring a loop around a sound, rooted tooth on each side and tightening the band to keep everything in place. In cases where the band-appliance functioned as a brace for loosened teeth, and there was no replacement tooth, the technique was the same, to encircle or wrap the relevant teeth with a thin gold band.

Using flat bands for the construction must have been a well-reasoned choice: Etruscan jewellery, from the earliest days (*circa* 700 BCE) employed wire, even though making it was a laborious and time-consuming process. Wire had to be made by cutting sheet metal, then twisting, hammering and annealing in multiple iterations – draw plates for wire making were not yet known to be

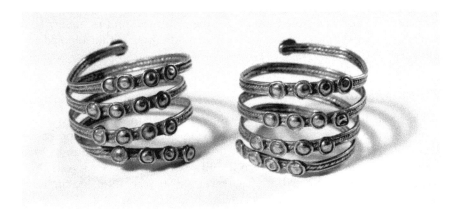

Figure 2.1 Etruscan gold hair spirals constructed with plain and twisted wire and stamped discs of gold sheet, late seventh–early sixth century BCE, University of Pennsylvania Museum, inv. MS 3346A and B. Image courtesy of the University of Pennsylvania Museum.

in use, nor was steel for tools (see Figure 3.1). Presumably the display of wire in filigree ornaments and chains contributed to the symbolic value of jewellery, since observers would appreciate the labour-intensive process. But wire does not stand out in a smiling mouth the way a band of gold could.

Advanced metallurgical techniques

The metallurgical skill of the Etruscan goldsmith is shown in these appliances to be considerable; in fact, both Liverpool appliances, analysed in May 2015, show an exceptionally high degree of purity in the gold. The Liverpool World Museum generously made them available for Matthew Ponting and Pablo Fernandez-Reyes (University of Liverpool) to test by scanning electron microscope with energy dispersive spectrometry (SEM-EDS): a full report of these test results is in Becker and Turfa (2017: Appendix VII). Both the gold bands and the rivets of these two examples were found to be at least ninety-eight per cent gold, which could only have been attained by assiduous refining processes to remove the naturally occurring silver and other metals from the original: a process called 'parting'. The process of achieving a higher purity than that found in most (seventh–sixth century BCE) Etruscan jewellery or artefacts of other Mediterranean cultures at such an early date may be remarkable. Of course, these two examples may be of later date, after the processes for parting gold had become more common. Even after that process had been perfected, jewellery of great purity is not common. These findings regarding the two Liverpool appliances call for the immediate analysis of all the other appliances, particularly those believed to be of the earliest dates. There is no indication that the non-toxic aspect of gold or silver was recognised at this date. The earliest datable appliance, the five-space/socket example from Satricum, is a real masterpiece simply for the construction of its hollow gold replacement tooth, made of two pieces beaten into shape within a mould and affixed to the band.

Dental appliances: anatomical details

All band-appliances may be shown by their tooth size to have been worn by women.[6] The condition of wear on the living 'anchor' teeth can sometimes yield information for the age-at-death of the wearer and these seem to have been mature women, aged between 25–40 years (No. 5), 35–45 years (No. 17), 45 ± 10 years (No. 20, from Greece), or 50 years (No. 18, the early example from Satricum). Only two wire appliances, Nos. W2, W5 (silver) from Sidon and Ptolemaic Egypt, have been tentatively associated with men, but all the wire appliances relate to dental issues rather than Etruscan ornamentation.

The 'false teeth', replacements for missing teeth, vary in number from one (as in No. 3, composed of three rings with the replacement in the central ring) to a nominal three (see No. 12). Invariably only the incisors (central and/or lateral) are replaced. In virtually all well-documented examples, they were worn in the upper jaw (maxilla). Unfortunately, in many cases, especially those found in the nineteenth century, museums or dealers chose to display them in lower jaws (mandibles) or even in different skulls entirely (for instance, Nos. 5, 10 and 15). In some examples, this resulted in damage to appliance or skull/remaining teeth, and caused great confusion among scholars who studied the phenomenon only through publications and photographs.

Seven bridges replaced a single tooth each, while five replaced two adjacent teeth; only one (No. 12) replaced three teeth, and used an ingenious method to do so (below). Some show more sophisticated or difficult techniques of creating or joining the loops needed to encircle the teeth. At least one tooth on each side of the replacement was rooted and living, and anchored the appliance in place; thus No. 3 (Bolsena?) had three spaces for a central replacement tooth framed by a single anchor tooth on each side. Some examples replaced two front teeth (central incisors or a central and a lateral incisor), centred between a single anchor tooth on each side (Nos. 13, 14, 17). The original Etruscan examples were intended to replace one or both upper central incisors – deliberately removed – with an ornamental false tooth. Later adaptations used this 'bridge' technology to provide loose-tooth stabilisation or replacements for lost teeth. Since upper central incisors would be among the last teeth to be lost in the natural decay process, it is not surprising that the adaptations of Etruscan techniques would be applied to teeth other than the upper central incisors.

The basic design of the early Etruscan examples is well illustrated by two appliances now in the Liverpool World Museum. Both were obtained in the early nineteenth century for Joseph Mayer, a Liverpool goldsmith whose varied collection formed the core of the first Liverpool Museum. The bulk of his Etruscan antiquities came by various routes from the Bonaparte excavations at Vulci, but the appliances cannot be surely assigned to this group. Liverpool I (No. 13, see Figures 2.2 and 2.3) is a gold band with two replacement central incisors, each held by a single rivet. The incisors appear to have been carved from two human incisors, perhaps those of the owner, with the roots filed away and carved to fit snugly against the gums. The original, rooted lateral

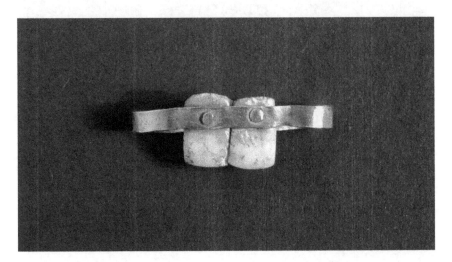

Figure 2.2 Liverpool I appliance, frontal view, inv. 10334. Image courtesy of the National Museums Liverpool.

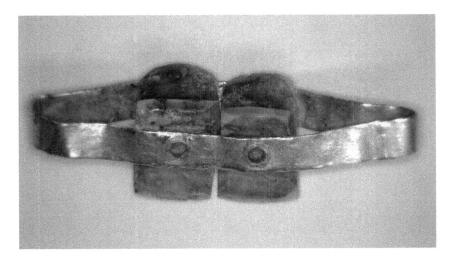

Figure 2.3 Liverpool I appliance, lingual (interior) view, inv. 10334. Image courtesy of M. Gleba with permission from the National Museums Liverpool.

incisors are missing, so we cannot confirm that the replacements represent the wearer's own teeth. Liverpool II (No. 14, see Figures 2.4 and 2.5) is constructed in the same fashion, with riveted replacements for the central incisors set into a gold band, and presently retaining, on either side, teeth with long roots.

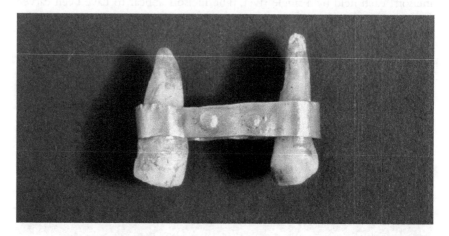

Figure 2.4 Liverpool II appliance, frontal view, inv. 10335. Image courtesy of the National Museums Liverpool.

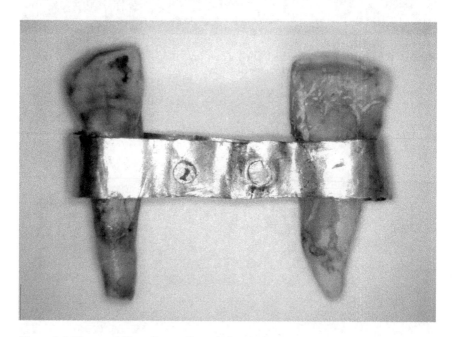

Figure 2.5 Liverpool II appliance, lingual (interior) view, inv. 10335. Image courtesy of M. Gleba with permission from the National Museums Liverpool.

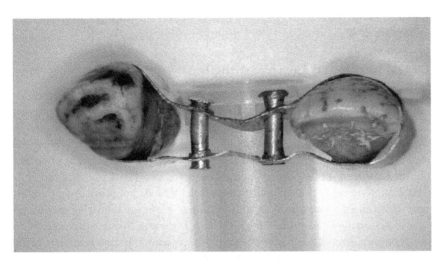

Figure 2.6 Liverpool II appliance, view of rivets (gold band now deformed), inv. 10335. Image courtesy of M. Gleba with permission from the National Museums Liverpool.

These may have been inserted by the nineteenth-century dealer, but we believe that they are probably the owner's teeth; of the replacement teeth only the fine gold rivets remain (see Figure 2.6). Possibly the false teeth were made of some material softer than tooth enamel.

Some cases of surviving appliances had more than one living human tooth encircled on each side. For instance, in the Satricum example (No. 18), the living teeth adjacent to the gold replacement must have been loose or fragile, so the band was designed to encircle the next teeth as well, and thus covered all four incisors and one canine, with the artificial gold tooth replacing an incisor. Some goldsmiths employed more ingenious solutions, as in the most complex of the Etruscan prostheses. One appliance from Tarquinia, possibly dating to the sixth century (No. 12), was a compound construction of seven rings encircling eight tooth spaces, three of which held replacements. One loop encompassed two spaces to surround the 'central incisors' but these replacement 'teeth' were actually a single piece, carved from an animal tooth to resemble two separate teeth and affixed with two rivets, looking just like appliances with two individual human teeth, each held by a rivet. Unfortunately, the appliance, probably excavated in the Corneto necropolis around 1875, is missing.

A similar situation applies to the band-appliances worn either to stabilise loose teeth or to serve as pure ornamentation (Nos. 1, 2, 5, 8, 10, 16[?], 20). These examples have no rivets, being a simple loop of gold or set of golden rings tightly surrounding part of a row of teeth. These teeth surrounded by these simple bands range in number from two (No. 20, Tanagra) or three (No. 1), to four, five or six teeth (No. 16, Teano). In some cases, where the appliance is no longer associated with the jaw and the teeth are missing, it is difficult to identify the exact locations of the braced front teeth.

Dental health and Etruscans' teeth

The diet of Etruria was quite healthy, and until the later centuries of the first millennium low in the refined foods such as bread that contribute to dental caries: most skeletons of the eighth–seventh centuries (and earlier) have teeth worn from chewing coarse foods and not infected with cavities.[7] In central Italian (and other) populations, the molars are the teeth most likely to be lost during midlife, followed by the other more medial teeth. Features such as dental calculus imply poor hygiene as a factor.[8] The dental profile of a middle-aged Chiusine noblewoman, Seianti Hanunia Tlesnasa, whose skeleton and sarcophagus have been studied in the British Museum, shows the results of an old injury causing a TMJ (temporomandibular joint) dysfunction that made hygiene difficult, resulting in loss of molars and a chronic abscess of a second premolar.[9] But neither Seianti nor other Etruscan or Italic skeletons that have been studied show the loss of front teeth, nor did an elderly woman buried in a rich tomb at Narce in the sixth century BCE, and the list could go on.[10] While increasing luxury in food choices affected the dental health of Etruscans and their Italic neighbors, front teeth were rarely lost during life. The need for replacements of front teeth is puzzling. The rare evidence of Roman extractions, namely eighty-five extracted molars (and one premolar) recovered from a dentist's shop in the Roman Forum shows a similar profile of tooth loss. It would appear that the lost front teeth of Etruscan women of the upper classes wearing ornamental appliances may reflect a deliberate phenomenon.[11]

A note on alleged ancient dentistry

Numerous 'histories of dentistry' refer to alleged ancient Egyptian burials found 'with gold teeth', appliances or fillings in place. Unfortunately, all of these are archaeological fantasies. There is absolutely no physical evidence for these finds representing any form of dentistry, and no examples of dental work performed, or even of deliberately extracted teeth, are known from among the ancient Egyptians.[12] It is surprising that, of the thousands of known Egyptian mummies, many of whom obviously suffered or even died as a result of dental abscesses, there is no evidence of intervention, even when a diseased tooth could have been extracted by hand. A few jaws show holes, similar (in some scholars' eyes) to the surgical procedure of drilling at the apex of a root to create drainage for an abscess, but these are in fact the natural process of an infection eroding out to the surface, and not surgical scars at all.[13] Masali suggested Sumerian use of gold wires *post mortem* as cosmetic attempts to keep loose teeth in place, but again, no examples of wire appliances have ever been found in Mesopotamian burials.[14]

Ancient sources on dental prostheses and related matters

No direct reference to the Etruscan gold-band prostheses is preserved in Greek or Roman literary or epigraphic sources; Etruscan literature has not survived. Perhaps the best reference is from the Roman *Law of the Twelve Tables*. Its text is known from fragments of a posting made in the early fifth century BCE, but believed, on account of its archaic language, to derive from a much older source.[15] The new Roman Republic had enacted sumptuary laws to limit the outflow of wealth from its economy, forbidding burial of riches in tombs (in contrast to Etruscan 'princely tombs' that held fortunes in gold ornaments, furniture and vehicles). *Table X* of this set of laws, as preserved in a quote by Cicero, in *On the Laws* 2.24.60, stated: '*neve aurum addito*' ('nor shall anyone add gold') from one law, and '*At cui auro dentes vincti escunt, ast im cum illo sepeliet uretve, se fraude esto*' ('But whoever has had teeth fastened together with gold, if someone shall bury or cremate him, this shall be with impunity'). For Cicero, this signalled the humane intentions of the law.

The earliest medical reference to dental appliances seems to come to us from the Hippocratic text *On Joints*:

> If the teeth at the point of injury are displaced or loosened, when the bone is adjusted fasten them to one another, not merely the two, but several, preferably with the gold wire, but failing that, with thread, until consolidation takes place.[16]

The term translated 'gold wire' (*chrysiō*) in the original Greek means 'with gold', and it is logical to assume the form would be wire. The term for 'with thread' (*linō*) can mean 'with linen thread'.

Several works of poetry and satire offer confirmation of the use of dental appliances, with a comment by Horace (65–8 BCE, *Satire* 1.8.48–50) that seems to imply false teeth worn by one Canidia as she indulges in some witchcraft on the Esquiline late at night: 'Canidia's teeth, the tall hairpiece of Sagana you will see them with much laughter and fun fall out, along with the herbs and charmed love-knots [they carry]'.[17]

Other references to false teeth come from satirists of the first century CE. The Greek Lucillius, patronised by Nero, wrote an epigram criticising use of cosmetics and false parts: 'You bought hair-braids, seaweed-rouge, honey, wax, and teeth. For the same expense you could have bought a face'.[18]

The Roman poet Martial (40–104 CE) mocked men and women who had bad or missing teeth, and had worse in store for courtesans who used dentures:

> You yourself are at home, Galla, but you are being made up in the middle of Subura [Rome's slum]. Your hair is manufactured in your absence. Nor do you lay aside your teeth at night any differently than you do your silk dresses, and you lie packed away in a hundred boxes. Nor does your

face sleep with you. You flirt with an eyebrow that is brought to you in the morning . . .[19]

Because of my verses, Fidentinus,
do you think you are a poet, and want to be believed?
In the same way Aegle imagines she has teeth,
having bought them in bone and Indian horn . . .[20]

Thais has black teeth, Laecania snow-white ones.
What is the reason? This one has bought teeth, the other her own.[21]

You use teeth and hair that are bought and you are not embarrassed.
What will you do about your eye, though, Laelia? They don't sell them.[22]

Martial's *Epigram* 10.56 derides a dentist, Cascellius, perhaps practising on the Aventine in Rome around 80 CE, who extracts or repairs aching teeth, but no author describes the fashioning of a bridge or appliance.

Roman-era medical texts suggest treatments for sore gums, toothache or trauma, and offer various pharmaceutical prescriptions to alleviate pain or swelling and prevent infection, but do not describe the use of dental bridges. Celsus notes, following the Hippocratic texts, the use of gold to temporarily hold teeth loosened by trauma, and discusses the problems of incomplete tooth extraction.[23] Galen and others, in surviving works, concentrate on medication or other treatment for wounds or infections of the mouth, not replacement of teeth.

Perhaps the last Roman reference to dental appliances, according to Waarsenburg, is from the second century CE author Lucian of Samosata. In the *Professor of Public Speaking* (*Rhētarōn Didaskalos / Rhetorum praeceptor* 24), a low-life says he pretended to love 'a seventy-year-old woman who had only four teeth remaining and all of them fastened with gold'.[24]

One last reference to false teeth comes to us from a different culture entirely. The Talmudic writings imply that the Hebrews of the Late Hellenistic period were making some type of dental appliances, using gold, silver and wood.[25] References to these *schen zahar* ('gold, false') teeth distinguish them from a removable type, *schen-tothebeth*, which according to Rabbi Zera (279–320 CE) were not to be 'carried' (worn) on the Sabbath.[26] The Palestine Talmud notes a young girl who was ashamed to ask a *nagor* ('turner' of wood) to make her another appliance of ivory.[27] The term *Rarash*, or worker in wood, stone or metal, also is found associated with the craft of producing dentures. An exhaustive study of Talmudic dental references would certainly clarify the situation for the Late Roman period, although to date no such appliances have been discovered.

Conclusion

It seems that ancient authors took it for granted that artificial bridges and braces were options for affluent persons, especially women. Although they did not describe wearing such objects, the satires worked because readers were already familiar with the practice. Although gold appliances could be buried legally on the owner, very few have ever been found, and most were made long before the Roman satirists' society evolved. But what early Etruscan or Italic rituals caused the earliest appliances with false teeth to be needed? It seems very unlikely that several affluent women, who would not be training at arms, riding horseback, or performing heavy household chores, should happen to lose their front teeth when the rest of the population never did . . . they must have lost them deliberately. We can only allude to ethnographic studies for possible parallels.

Ceremonial tooth removal (dental ablation or dental evulsion) is documented in the archaeological record as well as from modern ethnographic studies, although not specifically for Etruscan society.[28] Geographically the custom can be found from North Africa (prehistoric to modern) and India, the Arctic and beyond. In Hawaiian society for instance, tooth ablation was part of formal mourning rituals.[29] In parts of ancient China, one or more incisor was removed from boys at puberty and from girls at marriage.[30] In fact, there are examples of tooth removal in Italian Neolithic women, but there is a gap of millennia between that period and the age of Etruscan culture.[31]

There is one difference between the Etruscan phenomenon and all the ethnographic parallels: only the women of first-millennium central Italy availed themselves of gold-banded replacements for their lost teeth. Lacking Etruscan literature, and noting that this custom was limited to a small number of high-ranking women, we do not yet have enough data to develop a reasonable explanation. It seems likely that certain women had one or two front teeth removed, fashioned into dental bridges and installed in their mouths: they would have been better able to eat and speak, but what rite of passage had they undergone that others never did? Whatever it was, their families must have proudly commissioned the goldsmith to create for them a prestigious new smile.

Authors' note

We gratefully acknowledge the generous help of several scholars, especially: Larry Bliquez: Georgina Muskett and Chrissy Partheni of Liverpool World Museum; Matthew Ponting and Pablo Fernandez-Reyes of University of Liverpool; and Cynthia Reed and Margarita Gleba, whose technical examination and photography were indispensable.

Notes

1   Catalano *et al.*, 2007; Minozzi *et al.*, 2007; Becker, 1997. On Jewish dental prostheses, see Lehmhaus, this volume.

2   The foremost and most complete study hitherto on Etruscan and related dental appliances is Bliquez, 1996. For surveys including all appliances in the Tables, see the following, which include earlier references for the original publications of individual pieces: Becker, 1997, 1998, 2002, 2003; Bliquez, 1983, 1996; Emptoz, 1987; Hoffman-Axthelm, 1970, 1981, 1985; Naso, 2011; Teschler-Nicola *et al.*, 1998; Waarsenburg, 1991.

3   Terzioğlu and Uzel, 1986, 1987. Collectors in the dental profession have often been targets for the sale of copies or forgeries; items from unauthorised excavations carry other uncertainties. If an Etruscan-style gold-band prosthesis were to be found in a controlled excavation at Sardis, it could be evidence of an Etruscan woman abroad, or the movement of an Etruscan goldsmith at a time (third century BCE) when fortunes were falling in his or her central Italian homeland. Only the skull of this skeleton, if the find is genuine, may survive, but identification of ethnicity through DNA or other biochemical analyses has been prevented.

4   For sensible recent research in that field, see Ghirotto *et al.*, 2013.

5   Waarsenburg, 1991.

6   See Ditch and Rose, 1972; Kieser, 1990; Rösing *et al.*, 1995; Teschler-Nicola, 1992; Teschler-Nicola and Prossinger, 1998; Becker, 2002.

7   See Becker *et al.*, 2009, Table 6; Turfa, 2012, pp. 136–163 on diet; Turfa and Becker, 2013 on general health.

8   See a man from Archaic Chiusi, Becker *et al.*, 2009, pp. 78–79 no. 18.

9   Lilley, 2002; Stoddart, 2002; Swaddling and Prag, 2002.

10 Becker *et al.*, 2009, pp. 59–61 no. 8.

11 Becker, 2014.

12 See Leek, 1972; Foreshaw, 2010.

13 Miller, 2008; Foreshaw 2010, p. 73.

14 Masali, 1985.

15 See Warmington, 1938, pp. xxvi–xxxi, pp. 502–503.

16 Hippocrates, *On Joints* 33.7–11 (trans. E. T. Withington): καὶ ἢν μὲν διεστραμμένοι ἔωσιν οἱ ὀδόντες οἱ κατὰ τὸ τρῶμα καὶ κεκινημένοι, ὁπόταν τὸ ὀστέον κατορθωθῇ, ζεῦξαι τοὺς ὀδόντας χρὴ πρὸς ἀλλήλους, μὴ μοῦνον τοὺς δύο, ἀλλὰ καὶ πλέονας, μάλιστα μὲν δὴ χρυσίῳ, ἔστ᾽ ἂν κρατυνθῇ τὸ ὀστέον, εἰ δὲ μή, λίνῳ.

17 Horace, *Satires* 1.8.48–50: *Canidiae dentes, altum Saganae caliendrum/Excidere atque herbas atque incantata lacertis/Vincula cum magno risuque iocoque videres.* Latin translations by Turfa unless otherwise noted. On prosthetic hair, see Draycott, this volume.

18 Lucilius, *Epigrams* 11.310 (trans. W. R. Paton): Ἠγόρασας πλοκάμους, φῦκος, μέλι, κηρόν, ὀδόντας· τῆς αὐτῆς δαπάνης ὄψιν ἂν ἠγόρασας.

19 Martial, *Epigrams* 9.37.1–6: *Cum sis ipsa domi mediaque ornere Subura, fiant absentes et tibi, Galla, comae, nec dentes aliter quam Serica nocte reponas, et iaceas centum condita pyxidibus, nec tecum facies tua dormiat, innuis illo quod tibi prolatum est mane supercilio, et te nulla movet cani reverentia cunni quem potes inter avos iam numerare tuos. promittis sescenta tamen; sed mentula surda est, et sit lusca licet, te tamen illa videt.* On prosthetic hair, see Draycott, this volume.

20 Martial, *Epigrams* 1.72.1–4: *Nostris versibus esse te poetam, Fidentine, putas cupisque credi?sic dentata sibi videtur Aegle. emptis ossibus Indicoque cornu . . .*

21 Martial, *Epigrams* 5.43: *Thais habet nigros, niveos Laecania dentes. Quae ratio est? emptos haec habet, illa suos.*

22 Martial, *Epigrams* 12.23: *Dentibus atque comis – nec te pudet – uteris emptis. Quid facies oculo, Laelia? Non emitur.*

23 Celsus, *On Medicine* 7.12.
24 Lucian, *A Professor of Public Speaking* 24 (trans. A. M. Harmon): γυναικὸς ἑβδομηκοντούτιδος τέτταρας ἔτι λοιποὺς ὀδόντας ἐχούσης, χρυσίῳ καὶ τούτους ἐνδεδεμένους.
25 *Shabbot* 64b, 65a; also *Palestinian Shabbot* VI: 5; *Shabbot* 65a; *Palestinian Shabbot* VI: 8c. On Jewish dental prostheses, see Lehmhaus, this volume.
26 Talmud, *Nedarim* 66a, 66b.
27 *Shabbat* VI: 8c.
28 See Pietrusewsky and Douglas, 1993; Milner and Larson, 1991; Singer, 1952; Briggs and Margolis, 1951.
29 Pietrusewsky and Douglas, 1993.
30 Kanaseki, 1962.
31 Robb, 1997; other cultures: Pietrusewsky and Douglas, 1993; Milner and Larson, 1991; Singer, 1953; Briggs and Margolis, 1951; Kanaseki, 1962.

Bibliography

Baggieri, G. (1999) 'Appointment with an Etruscan Dentist', translated and edited by J. K. Whitehead, *Etruscan Studies* 6, pp. 33–42.

Baggieri, G. (2001) 'Le Protesi Dentarie Etrusche in Lega Aurea. Archeometallurgicia della Biocompatibilità', *Studi Etruschi* (1998), pp. 321–329.

Baggieri, G. (2005) *Odontoiatria dell'antichità in reperti osteo-dentari e archeologici*. Rome: MelAMi.

Becker, M. J. (1994) 'Early Dental Appliances in the Eastern Mediterranean', *Berytus* 42, pp. 71–102.

Becker, M. J. (1998) 'Etruscan Gold Dental Appliances: Evidence for Cultural Processes', in Guerci, A. (ed.) *Health and Diseases: Historical Routes, Volume 2 of the Proceedings of the 1st International Conference on Anthropology and History of Health and Disease*. Genoa: Erga edizioni, pp. 8–19.

Becker, M. J. (2002) 'Etruscan Female Tooth Evulsion: Gold Dental Appliances as Ornaments', in Carr, G. and Baker, P. (edd.) *Practices, Practitioners and Patients: New Approaches to Medical Archaeology and Anthropology*. Oxford: Oxbow Books, pp. 236–257.

Becker, M. J. (2003) 'Etruscan Gold Dental Appliances: Evidence for Early "Parting" of Gold in Italy through the Study of Ancient Pontics', in Tsoucaris, G. and Lipkowski, J. (edd.) *Molecular and Structural Archaeology: Cosmetic and Therapeutic Chemicals*. Dordrecht: Kluwer Academic (NATO Science Series, 117), pp. 11–27.

Becker, M. J. (2014) 'Dentistry in Ancient Rome: Direct Evidence Based on the Teeth from Excavations at the Temple of Castor and Pollux in the Roman Forum', *International Journal of Anthropology* 29.4, pp. 209–220.

Becker, M. J., Turfa, J. M. and Algee-Hewitt, B. (2009) *Human Remains from Etruscan and Italic Tomb Groups in the University of Pennsylvania Museum* (Biblioteca di Studi Etruschi 48). Pisa: Fabrizio Serra.

Becker, M. J. and Turfa, J. M. (2017) *The Etruscans and the History of Dentistry: The Golden Smile*. London: Routledge.

Bliquez, L. J. (1983) 'Classical Prosthetics', *Archaeology* 36, pp. 25–29.

Bliquez, L. J. (1996) 'Prosthetics in Classical Antiquity: Greek, Etruscan, and Roman Prosthetics', in *ANRW* II 37.3, pp. 2640–2676.

Briggs, L. C. and Margolis, M.-L. (1951) 'Remarques sur la coutume d'avulsion dentaire chez les peuples préhistoriques de l'Africa du Nord et du Sahara'. In

Association Française pour l'Avancement des Sciences: Congrés de Tunis (9–16 Mai), pp. 115–22.

Catalano, P., Minozzi, S., Musco, S., Fornaciari, G. (con la collaborazione di Caldarini, C., Colonnelli, G., Fornaciari, G., Grandi, M., Minozzi, S., Pantano, W., Torri, C. and Zabotti, F.) (2007) 'Le prime evidenze di odontotecnica nella Roma Imperiale: una protesi dentaria in oro rinvenuta in una tomba monumentale', [Poster]. *XVII Congresso dell'Associazione Antropologica Italiana, 26–29 Settembre 2007*, Cagliari.

Ditch, L. E. and Rose, J. C. (1972) 'A Multivariate Dental Sexing Technique', *American Journal of Physical Anthropology* 37.1, pp. 61–64.

Emptoz, F. (1987) 'La Prothèse Dentaire dans la Civilisation Étrusque', in *Archéologie et Médecine: VII Recontre Internationale d'Archéologie et d'Histoire (Antibes 1986)*. Juan-les-Pins: Editions A. P. D. C. A., pp. 545–560.

Foreshaw, R. J. (2010) 'Were the Dentists in Ancient Egypt Operative Dental Surgeons or were they Pharmacists?', in Cockitt, J. and David, R. (edd.) *Pharmacy and Medicine in Ancient Egypt. Proceedings of the Conferences held in Cairo (2007) and Manchester (2008)*. BAR IS 2141. Oxford: Archaeopress, pp. 72–77.

Ghirotto, S., Tassi, F., Fumagalli, E., Colonna, V., Sandionigi, A., Lari, M., Vai, S., Petiti, E., Corti, G., Rizzi, E., De Bellis, G., Caramelli, D. and Barbujani, G. (2013) 'Origins and Evolution of the Etruscans' mtDNA', *PLoS ONE* 8.2, e55519. Doi: 10.1371/journal.pone.0055519.

Gnade, M. (ed.) (1991) *Stips Votiva: Papers Presented to C. M. Stibbe*. Amsterdam: Allard Pierson Museum, University of Amsterdam.

Hoffmann-Axthelm, W. (1970) 'The History of Tooth Replacement', *Dental Science and Research* 8.9, pp. 81–87.

Hoffmann-Axthelm, W. (1981) *A History of Dentistry* (from first edition) translated by H. M. Koehler. Chicago: Quintessence Publishing Company.

Hoffmann-Axthelm, W. (1985) *Die Geschichte der Zahnheilkunde* (second edition). Berlin: Quintessenz Verlags-GmbH.

Kanaseki, T. (1962) 'The Custom of Teeth Extraction [Ablation] in Ancient China', in *VIe Congrés International des Sciences Anthropologiques et Ethnologiques (Paris 1960). Volume I: Rapport général et Anthropologie*. Paris: Musée de L'Homme (Palais de Chaillot), pp. 201–205.

Kieser, J. A. (1990) *Human Adult Odontometrics: The Study of Variation in Adult Tooth Size*. Cambridge: Cambridge University Press.

Leek, F. F. (1972) 'Did a Dental Profession Exist in Ancient Egypt during the 3rd Millennium B.C.?' *Medical History* 16.4, pp. 404–406.

Lilley, J. D. (2002) 'Seianti Hanunia Tlesnasa: Some Observations on the Dental Features', in Swaddling, J., and Prag, J. (edd.) *Seianti Hanunia Tlesnasa. The Story of an Etruscan Noblewoman*. London: British Museum Occasional Paper Number 100, pp. 23–26.

Masali, L. (1985) 'La cura dei denti presso i popoli mesopotamici', in Vogel, G. and Gambacorta, G. (edd.) *Storia della odontoiatria*. Milan: Ars Medica Antiqua Editrice, pp. 47–50.

Menconi, A., and Fornaciari, G. (1985) 'L'odontoiatria etrusca', in Vogel, G. and Gambacorta, G. (edd.) *Storia della odontoiatria*. Milan: Ars Medica Antiqua Editrice, pp. 89–97.

Miller, J. (2008) 'Dental Health and Disease in Ancient Egypt', in David, R. (ed.) *Egyptian Mummies and Modern Science*. Cambridge: Cambridge University Press, pp. 52–70.

Milner, G. R. and Larsen, C. S. (1991) 'Teeth as Artifacts of Human Behavior; Intentional Mutilation and Accidental Modification', in Kelley, M. A. and Larsen, C. S. (edd.) *Advances in Dental Anthropology*. New York, NY: Wiley-Liss, pp. 357–378.

Minozzi, S., Fornaciari, G., Musco, S. and Catalano, P. (2007) 'A Gold Dental Prosthesis of Roman Imperial Age', *The American Journal of Medicine* 120.5, e1–e2.

Naso, A. (2011) 'Protesi dentarie auree in Etruria e nel Lazio', in Rafanelli, S. and Spaziani, P. (edd.) *Etruschi: Il privilegio della bellezza*. Sansepolcro: Aboca, pp. 146–154.

Pietrusewsky, M. and Douglas, M. T. (1992) 'Tooth Ablation in Old Hawai'i', *The Journal of the Polynesian Society* 102.3, pp. 255–272.

Robb, J. (1997) 'Intentional Tooth Removal in Neolithic Italian Women', *Antiquity* 71, pp. 659–669.

Rösing, F. W., Paul, G. and Schnutenhaus, S. (1995) 'Sexing Skeletons by Tooth Size', in Radlanski, R. J. and Renz, H. (edd.) *Proceedings of the 10th International Symposium on Dental Morphology*. Berlin: C. and M. Brünner GbR, pp. 373–376.

Singer, R. (1952) 'Artificial Deformation of Teeth', *South African Journal of Science* 50, pp. 116–122.

Stoddart, R. W. (2002) 'Remains from the Sarcophagus of Seianti Hanunia Tlesnasa: Pathological Evidence and its Implications', in Swaddling, J. and Prag, J. (edd.) *Seianti Hanunia Tlesnasa. The Story of an Etruscan Noblewoman*. London: British Museum Occasional Paper Number 100, pp. 29–38.

Swaddling, J. and Prag, J. (edd.) (2002) *Seianti Hanunia Tlesnasa. The Story of an Etruscan Noblewoman*. London: British Museum Occasional Paper Number 100.

Terzioğlu, A. and Uzel, I. (1986) 'Etruskische Goldbandprothese in Westanatolien entdeckt', *Apotheker Journal* 8.12 (15 December 1986), pp. 34, 36.

Terzioğlu, A. and Uzel, I. (1987) 'Die Goldbandprothese in etruskischer Technik. Ein neuer Fund aus Westanatolien', *Phillip Journal für restaurative Zahnmedizin* 4, pp. 109–112.

Teschler-Nicola, M. (1992) 'Sexualdimorphismus der Zahnkronendurchmesser. Ein Beitrag zur Geschlechtsdiagnose subadulter Individuen anhand des frübronzezeitlichen Gräberfeldes von Franzhausen I, Niederösterreich', *Anthropologischer Anzeiger* 50, pp. 51–65.

Teschler-Nicola, M., Kneissel, M., Brandstätter, F., and Prossinger, H. (1998) 'A Recently Discovered Etruscan Dental Bridgework', in Alt, K. W., Rösing, F. W. and Teschler-Nicola, M. (edd.) *Dental Anthropology: Fundamentals, Limits, and Prospects*. Vienna: Springer, pp. 57–68.

Teschler-Nicola, M., and Prossinger, H. (1998) 'Sex Determination Using Tooth Dimensions', in Alt, K. W., Rösing, F. W. and Teschler-Nicola, M. (edd.) *Dental Anthropology: Fundamentals, Limits, and Prospects*. Vienna and New York, NY: Springer Verlag, pp. 501–518.

Torino, M., Menconi, A. and Fornaciari, G. (1996) 'Le Protesi dentarie etrusche: errori di interpretazione', in Laquidara, L. (ed.) *Quaderni internazionale di Storia della Medicina e della Sanità. Numero speciale: Atti del 1 Congresso Nazionale della Società Italiana di Storia dell'Odontostomatologia*, Anno V, n. 1, pp. 119–125.

Torino, M., Menconi, A. and Fornaciari, G. (1997) 'Le protesi dentarie auree nei gruppi umani a cultura Etrusca: nuove acquisizioni'. In *Atti del XIX Convegno di Studi Etruschi ed Italici (Volterra, 15–19 ottobre 1995): Aspetti della cultura di Volterra etrusca fra l'età del ferro e l'età ellenistica e Contributi della ricerca antropologica alla conoscenza del popolo etrusco*. Florence: Olschki, pp. 535–544.

Turfa, J. M. (2012) *Divining the Etruscan World: The Brontoscopic Calendar and Religious Practice*. Cambridge: Cambridge University Press.

Turfa, J. M. (ed.) (2013) *The Etruscan World*. London and New York, NY: Routledge.

Turfa, J. M. and Becker, M. J. (2013) 'Health and Medicine in Etruria', in Turfa, J. M. (ed.) *The Etruscan World*. London and New York, NY: Routledge, pp. 855–881.

Vogel, G. and Gambacorta, G. (edd.) (1985) *Storia della odontoiatria*. Milan: Ars Medica Antiqua Editrice.

Waarsenburg, D. J. (1991) '*Auro dentes iuncti*: An Inquiry into the Study of the Etruscan Dental Prosthesis', in Gnade, M. (ed.) *Stips Votiva: Papers Presented to C. M. Stibbe*. Amsterdam: Allard Pierson Museum, University of Amsterdam, pp. 241–247.

Warmington, E. H. (ed.) (1938, reprinted 1967) *Remains of Old Latin. Volume III: Lucilius. The Twelve Tables*. Cambridge, MA: Harvard University Press.

Weinberger, B. H. (1948) *An Introduction to the History of Dentistry,* Volume 1 (Saint Louis: C. V. Mosby, 1948) [Special edition by Gryphon Editions in Birmingham, Alabama, 1981].

3 Prosthetic hair in ancient Rome

Jane Draycott

Introduction

This chapter will examine the use of prosthetic hair in the form of wigs and hair pieces in the Roman Republic and Empire. It will survey the importance of hair as a social and symbolic presentation of self in Roman society, investigate the reasons for and ramifications of hair loss for Roman men and women, and determine the extent to which prosthetic hair was utilised as a means of addressing these, before assessing the importance of prosthetic hair as an alternative social and symbolic presentation of self in Roman society.

Wigs and hair pieces are deliberately excluded from Lawrence Bliquez's survey of the literary and archaeological evidence for prostheses in ancient Greece and Rome on the grounds that they served a cosmetic rather than a practical purpose.[1] Admittedly, they might not be the first items that come to mind when considering prostheses but in actual fact, as this chapter will show, in ancient Rome prosthetic hair was the only type of ancient prosthesis that even came close to serving a similar purpose to the contemporary prosthesis, in not only acting as a substitute for the lost body part in a cosmetic sense but also in a practical one.[2] An ancient Roman wig or hair piece was usually (although, as we shall see, not always) made from human hair and this meant that it could be not only worn as such but also styled as such.

Hair has been described as offering 'a unique opportunity to examine the interface between the body and material culture'.[3] Theoretically, an individual's hairstyle told someone looking at them everything they needed to know through semiotics or 'hair codes'.[4] There is a substantial amount of literary and archaeological evidence for both the appearance and significance of hair and hairstyles in the Roman Republic and Empire. While an ancient Roman was born with a particular hair type, he or she chose, or had chosen for them, a particular hairstyle which could vary according to their gender, stage of life (both age and position), social class, status, political affiliation, religious belief and profession: hair played a crucial role in the social and symbolic presentation of self and it made a significant contribution to the language of the body.[5] Consequently, premature hair loss, whether experienced by a man or a woman, whether the result of natural or unnatural processes, was potentially not just an impairment but also a disability as it affected their ability to present them-selves in the appropriate manner.[6] Under these circumstances, using prosthetic hair, whether in the form of a wig or a hair piece, could ameliorate the severity of the condition and its negative impact upon the sufferer's life.

Premature hair loss in ancient Rome

Today the most common type of hair loss is male pattern baldness, which starts in the late twenties or early thirties, with most men having experienced some degree of hair loss by their late thirties and around half of all men having experienced male pattern baldness by the age of fifty.[7] In the Roman Republic and Empire, it was recognised that nothing could prevent men from losing hair as they aged and baldness was frequently utilised in literature and art as a signifier of the elderly man.[8] However, victims of premature hair loss – and presumably victims of male pattern baldness were included in this – were publicly mocked.[9] Not even dictators or emperors were immune from this treatment.[10] Today female pattern baldness is far less common than male pattern baldness and normally starts after the menopause, although up to half of all women who give birth experience post-partum hair loss, that is more hair loss than usual.[11] In the Roman Republic and Empire, victims of female pattern baldness or other types of hair loss were certainly mocked, but they were also subjected to moralising regarding the particular aspects of their lifestyle or their own actions that were perceived to have contributed to or even caused their hair loss. Seneca (4–65 CE), in his discussion of basic principles, heavily influenced by his Stoic philosophical leanings, observes that new diseases have developed over time as a direct result of changes in lifestyle, and he explicitly links the supposedly new disease of female hair loss to women behaving less like women and more like men:

> The illustrious founder of the guild and profession of medicine [Hippocrates] remarked that women never lost their hair or suffered from pain in the feet; and yet **nowadays they run short of hair and are afflicted with gout**. This does not mean that woman's physique has changed, but that it has been conquered; in rivalling male indulgences, they have also rivalled the ills to which men are heirs. They keep just as late hours, and drink just as much liquor; they challenge men in wrestling and carousing; they are no less given to vomiting from distended stomachs and to thus discharging all their wine again; nor are they behind the men in gnawing ice, as a relief to their fevered digestions. And they even match the men in their passions, although they were created to feel love passively (may the gods and goddesses confound them!). They devise the most impossible varieties of unchastity, and in the company of men they play the part of men. What wonder, then, that we can trip up the statement of the greatest and most skilled physician, when **so many women are gouty and bald!** Because of their vices, women have ceased to deserve

the privileges of their sex; they have put off their womanly nature and are therefore condemned to suffer the diseases of men.[12]

Ovid (43 BCE–17/18 CE) devotes an entire poem to the subject of Corinna's hair loss, a direct result of her attempts to follow fashion and increase her physical attractiveness by dying it a supposedly more desirable colour. Their differing responses to her hair loss are notable.[13] She is bereft, he takes a certain amount of delight in pointing out that her hair loss is entirely her own fault and uses the episode as an opportunity to warn against female adornment and vanity:

> I said: 'Stop dyeing your hair!' **Now you've no hair left to colour.** Since it was so luxuriant, why not have let it be? It stretched right down, and touched your sides . . . Alas, what suffering [your hairs] had to bear! How they offered themselves patiently to the steel and fire, as their waves were twisted and tied in ringlets! I cried: 'That's wicked, wicked to scorch your hair! It's fine as it is: go carefully with the steel! Take the pressure away! No one ought to burn it: your hair itself teaches others how to pin theirs' . . . Why search your neat hair for what's vilely lost? Silly girl why hold the mirror sadly in your hand? It's no use contriving to stare at yourself: you need to forget about yourself, to please. No mistress of magic herbs has wounded you, no Thessalian witch soaked you in treacherous water: no illness's power has touched you – perish the thought! – No evil tongue has thinned your dense hair. Your hand did it and you're paying for your crime . . . Alas! She scarcely contains her tears and with her hand hides her delicate cheeks painted with blushes. She holds her former hair in her lap, and stares at it, ah me, a tribute not fitting for that place! Calm yourself, doing your face! The harm's reparable. Shortly your natural hair will be seen again.[14]

Considering the cultural and social importance of hair to the ancient Romans, it is hardly surprising that hair loss does not seem to have been simply accepted. One way in which the emperor Domitian (51–96 CE) coped with his premature hair loss was to author the treatise *On the Preservation of the Hair*, while in response to Dio Chrysostom's (*circa* 40–120 CE) treatise *In Praise of Hair*, the balding Synesius (*circa* 337–414 CE) authored the treatise *In Praise of Baldness*.[15] There were a variety of ways of dealing with hair loss. Surviving recipes for preparations designed to thicken thinning hair or encourage hair growth so as to restore hair lost entirely indicate that one might have recourse to medicine or cosmetics, although interestingly many of these require that first any existing hair be shaved off.[16] Considering that some types of hair loss were understood as part of the natural aging process and thus, perhaps, inevitable no matter how many medicinal or cosmetic preparations were utilised, it is not surprising that there is also evidence for attempts to secure assistance from a deity, with divine intervention perhaps considered the only

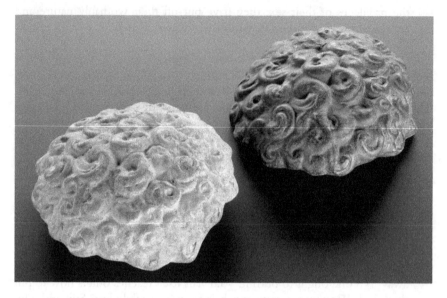

Figure 3.1 Terracotta scalp votives, Science Museum inv. A114891 and A634932. Image courtesy of the Wellcome Library, London.

means of arresting the process or restoring hair that had already been lost. At least one individual, Heraieos of Mytilene, sought the assistance of the god Asklepios to cure his baldness; his miraculous healing following the application of a drug to his head is recorded among the *iamata* from the sanctuary of Asklepios at Epidauros.[17] Perhaps these terracotta scalps (see Figure 3.1 for two Roman terracotta scalp votives) are evidence of votive offerings made by individuals afflicted with male pattern baldness, while this marble head (see Figure 3.2 for a Roman marble head) is evidence of a votive offering made by an individual afflicted with alopecia areata.

Ultimately, however, when potions and prayers had failed, the only remaining alternative was utilising some sort of disguise. Although Martial (*circa* 38–41 CE – 102–104 CE) describes Phoebus' initial attempts to paint hair onto his bald head, he later observes that Phoebus has resorted to a kid-skin wig instead.[18] Thus the most viable options were covering up the head or utilising a wig or hair piece.[19]

Wigs and hair pieces in ancient Rome

Prosthetic hair is the most frequently mentioned type of prosthesis in ancient Greek and Latin literature. While the ancient Greeks do not seem to have utilised prosthetic hair outside of the theatre, there were several different types of prosthetic hair available to ancient Romans.[20] A full wig was known as a *capillamentum* or a *caliendrum* while a hair piece used to supplement one's own

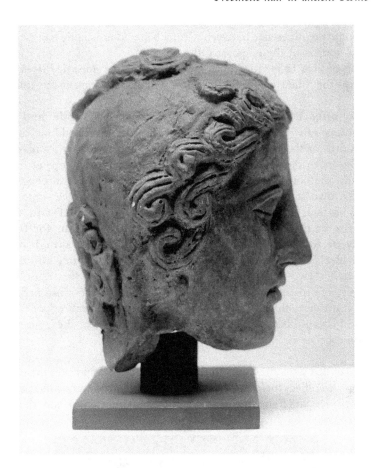

Figure 3.2 Marble head, Antiquarium Comunale. Image courtesy of the Wellcome
　　　　Library, London.

hair was known as a *galerus* or a *galerum*. A full wig was significantly more
time-consuming for a wig-maker to create than a hair piece such as an
extension or a braid, so it would have been commensurately significantly more
expensive to purchase.[21] This probably restricted use of full wigs – or at least
high quality full wigs – to the wealthier members of ancient Roman society.
Ancient literature records both men and women wearing them. While nothing
is known about the manufacture of wigs and hair pieces, according to Ovid
and Martial they could be purchased near the Porticus Philippi, in front of the
temple of Hercules and the Muses.[22] According to Suetonius (*circa* 60–122
CE), the emperor Otho had thinning hair and wore a wig of such high quality
that nobody could distinguish it from his natural hair, and presumably such a
wig was specially made by an artisan at the height of their powers.[23] It is worth
noting, however, that portraits of Otho, whether on coins or carved in the

round, do depict a very peculiar hairstyle that might well be intended to demonstrate the difference between natural hair and prosthetic hair (see Figure 3.3 for a portrait of the emperor Otho, 69 CE).

Tertullian (*circa* 155–240 CE), in his polemic *On the Apparel of Women*, gives us perhaps the fullest description of prosthetic hair in ancient literature:

> **You affix I know not what enormities of subtle and textile perukes**; now, after the manner of a helmet of undressed hide, as it were a sheath for the head and a covering for the crown; now, a mass drawn backward toward the neck. The wonder is that there is no open contending against the Lord's prescripts! It has been pronounced that no one can add to his own stature. *You*, however, *do* add to your *weight* some kind of rolls, or shield-bosses, to be piled upon your necks! **If you feel no shame at the enormity, feel some at the pollution; for fear you may be fitting on a holy and Christian head the slough of some one else's head, unclean perchance, guilty perchance and destined to hell**. Nay, rather banish quite away from your 'free' head all this slavery of ornamentation. In vain do you labour to seem adorned: in vain do you call in the aid of all the most skilful manufacturers of false hair. God bids you 'be veiled'. I believe he does so for fear the heads of some should be seen![24]

He believes that women who convert to Christianity should alter their physical appearance to reflect their newfound religiosity since modesty will ensure their salvation.[25] He differentiates between things worn (*cultus*) and things that

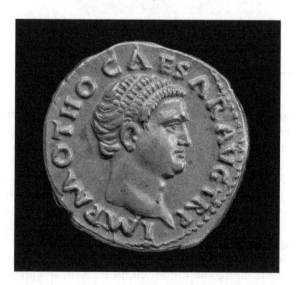

Figure 3.3 Coin of the emperor Otho, British Museum inv. R.6333. Image courtesy of © The Trustees of the British Museum.

beautify (*ornatus*), and includes false hair in the latter category.[26] Tertullian's contemporary Clement of Alexandria (*circa* 150–215 CE) also criticised women for wearing wigs and hair pieces.[27] Tertullian's and Clement's rather specific objections, influenced by their adherence to Christianity, aside, the wearing of wigs and hair pieces is frequently strongly criticised in male-authored ancient literature due to the artifice involved, criticisms that are likewise found in male-authored discourses about cosmetics.[28] Ancient medical practitioners divided cosmetics into those that preserved beauty (*kosmetikon*) and that unnaturally embellished it (*kommotikon*).[29] The former was acceptable; the latter was not.[30] While Ovid is merely snide about his mistress' wig-wearing, Martial is overtly critical about the women of his acquaintance that do likewise. He opines that Laelia should be ashamed of resorting to wearing a wig, and presumably Galla, who not only wears false hair but also false eyebrows, should feel twice as much shame as Laelia.[31]

People (usually, but not always, women) were thought to utilise wigs and hair pieces to deceive and pretend to be something they were not. This might be young and beautiful, but also, and potentially more significantly, healthy.[32] Hair was considered an important component of female sexual attractiveness, and women were considered to be much less sexually attractive as a result of hair loss.[33] Roman writers such as Horace (65–8 BCE), Ovid, Martial and Lucillius (*floruit* 60s CE) give examples of women who wear wigs to either appear much younger than they are or to hide signs of debilitating illness.[34] Lucian (*circa* 125–180 CE) goes one further and presents the courtesan Philematium, who is not only aging and going grey, but has also been so ill that her hair has fallen out; her profession necessitates that men find her attractive, hair is necessary for sexual attractiveness, hence the wig.[35] This deception and pretence extended to the use of wigs and hair pieces as a means of disguising one's identity to facilitate misbehaviour. Thus, Juvenal (*floruit* late first–early second century CE) claims that the empress Messalina wore a blonde wig to spend the night in a brothel competing with the prostitutes that worked there and Cassius Dio (*circa* 155–235 CE) tells a similar story of the emperor Elagabalus, while Suetonius claims that the emperors Gaius and Nero wore wigs to roam the streets and cause trouble at night.[36] Yet such criticisms are entirely stereotypical and formulaic, so not entirely trustworthy.[37]

What is clear, however, is that wigs and hair pieces were risky. The prospect of someone's wig coming loose and either slipping or falling off entirely is frequently presented as a source of amusement.[38] Avienus (*circa* fourth century CE) tells a story of a horseman whose wig fell off during his routine and when he was faced with public ridicule turned the situation to his advantage through a display of wit: 'As the horseman saw that he was the laughing-stock of so many thousands, he shrewdly brought cunning to his aid and turned away the jest from himself. "Why be surprised," he remarked, "that my assumed locks have gone, when my natural hair deserted me first?"'[39] The spectacle of someone wearing a bad or unsuitable wig is also played for laughs.[40] Ovid tells of an occasion where he interrupted a woman dressing and she was in such a

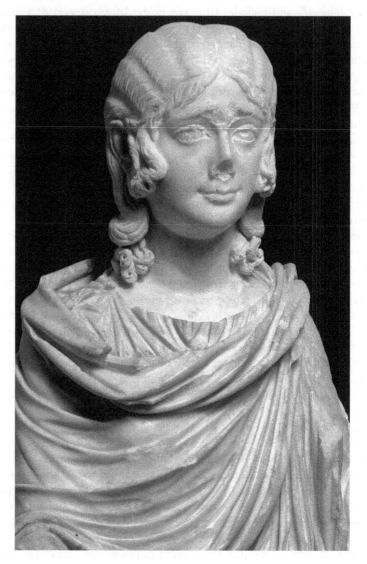

Figure 3.4 Marble bust of a young girl, British Museum inv. 1879, 0712.13. Image
   courtesy of © The Trustees of the British Museum.

hurry that she put her wig on back to front.[41] While amused, he was also
repulsed: 'Ugly is a bull without horns; ugly is a field without grass, a plant
without leaves, or a head without hair'.[42]

   Until recently, scholars assumed that wigs and hair pieces were necessary to
create the elaborate hairstyles of the late first and second centuries CE attested
by surviving portraiture, and that the wearing of wigs and hair pieces was
somewhat normalised in Roman society.[43] However, recent experimental

archaeological research into ancient Roman hairdressing has suggested that wigs and hair pieces were not, in fact, necessary, and that hairstyles could be constructed out of the individual's own hair and sewn into place.[44] If this was in fact the case, perhaps wigs and hair pieces were not so widely used. This raises the question of whether, regarding hair, Romans, both male and female, were caught between a rock and a hard place: did they either need their own hair, or a wig that was of such high quality that no one knew they were wearing it? This perhaps explains the rare examples of statues in which wigs are visible, the difference between someone choosing to wear a wig yet not needing to, and someone having to wear one while pretending not to. A case in point is a curious marble portrait bust of a young girl wearing a wig despite seemingly abundant natural hair, perhaps in imitation of the empress Julia Domna, an extreme example of the practice of fashionable hairstyles on young girls as a means of demonstrating their sexual desirability and commensurate readiness for marriage (see Figure 3.4, a marble portrait bust of a young girl, *circa* 210–230 CE).[45] Thus the wearing of wigs and hair pieces was yet another means for the Roman elite to demonstrate their conspicuous consumption and *luxuria*.[46]

Relatively few Roman wigs and hair pieces have survived in the archaeological record due to the very specific conditions necessary for the preservation of the organic materials that they were normally made from (hair, leather, plant fibres, etc.). However, examples of hair pieces made from human hair have been recovered from several locations around the Roman Empire. Three comprising dark brown and blonde sections of hair attached to pieces of leather and dating from the second century CE were recovered from burials excavated at Les Martres-de-Veyre in France.[47] One comprising a piece of plaited hair was found inside a cremation urn at Rainham Creek in Britain.[48] Another comprising a section of blonde hair in conjunction with two cantharus-headed jet pins which remain in situ threaded through the hair dating from the late third century to the early fifth century CE was found inside a lead sarcophagus at York in Britain (see Figure 3.5, the hair piece with the pins still in situ).[49]

Two more comprising of hair attached to pieces of linen were found in tandem with the mummified bodies of their owners in the necropolis of Dush in the Kharga Oasis in Egypt.[50] One of the mummies was a woman approximately twenty years old, the other was a child approximately seven years old, both had very short and sparse growth of natural hair, and it has been suggested that this was a side-effect of typhoid, so the hair pieces served as a means of disguising this.[51] Another was found at Gurob in the Fayum and comprises a piece of plaited hair that would have been fixed to the wearer's head with 62 bronze pins in the 'orbis' hairstyle that dates from either the late first or the first half of the second century CE (see Figure 3.6, the hair piece).[52] The length and styles of these hair pieces indicate that they were worn to supplement existing hair, although it is impossible to say for certain. The frequency with which the hair pieces are discovered braided and/or in

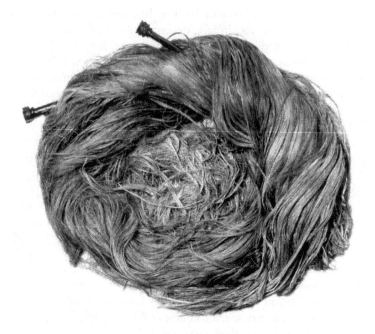

Figure 3.5 Hair piece with jet pins in situ, Yorkshire Museum inv. YORYM: 1998.695. Image courtesy of York Museums Trust: https://yorkmuseumstrust.org.uk: CC–BY–SA 4.0.

conjunction with hair pins indicates that they were styled and arranged just as an individual's own hair would be.

However, one example of a hair piece made from auburn hair has been recovered from a tomb on the Via Latina in Rome, and thanks to the preservation of the tomb's contents and the inscriptions on its marble sarcophagi, it is possible to state with certainty that this hair piece was worn by a wealthy woman named Aebutia Quarta, the daughter of Gaius Antestius Balbinus, in the late first and early second century CE.[53] Perhaps here we have an example of a woman who sought to follow fashion and amplify her natural beauty, or perhaps a woman whose own hair was for some reason lacking so she sought to disguise her deficiency by utilising the financial resources at her disposal, but either way her wealth enabled her to purchase and wear a hair piece of the highest possible quality in conjunction with her natural hair, and hold it in place with a golden hairnet.[54]

As ancient writers such as Tertullian recounted, wigs and hair pieces could be made of substances other than human hair, although we have to wonder how convincing such items were, assuming they were intended as imitations of wigs and hair pieces made from human hair rather than as a distinct category of objects in their own right. A wig made from linen and tinted a shade of chestnut was reportedly recovered from the tomb of a Christian woman on

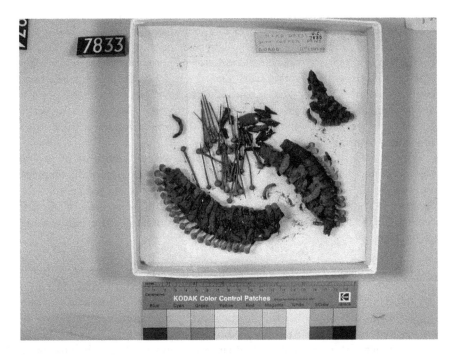

Figure 3.6 Hair piece with bronze pins in situ, Petrie Museum inv. UC7833. Image courtesy of the Petrie Museum of Egyptian Archaeology, UCL.

the Via Ostiensis in the early eighteenth century; unfortunately, its current whereabouts, if it even still exists, is unknown.[55] A wig in the form of corkscrew curls on a plaited base with a plait hanging down at the back, made from grass fibres coated in beeswax, was recovered from a house at Harit in Egypt.[56] Another contemporaneous wig from Egypt resembles the one from Harit but is made from date palm fibres.[57] A hair piece from Egypt made from string and linen was found attached to the mummy of a child.[58] Several other possible hair pieces made from plant fibres have been recovered from military sites in Britain, one from the Roman fort at Vindolanda in England, dating to the period 97–103 CE, and the other from the Roman fort at Newstead in Scotland, dating to around 86 CE.[59] However, there is some debate over whether they should be considered hair pieces at all, as opposed to hats or caps, or even baskets.[60]

Prosthetic hair in ancient Rome

Although we have no information about the manufacture of wigs and hair pieces in ancient Rome, as we have seen the ancient literary and archaeological evidence suggests that, for the most part, they were made from human hair. Where did this hair come from? One type of hair described as 'Indian hair' (*capelli Indici*) is known to have been imported from India because there is documentary evidence in the form of a record of customs dues being paid on it at Rome, and it was perhaps sought after because it was basic black in colour.[61] Yet there is a considerable amount of literary evidence for another type of hair, known as 'captive hair' (*captivis comis*) because it was taken from German prisoners.[62] This type of hair seems to have been particularly popular during the reigns of Augustus and Domitian, perhaps because there was a considerable amount of military activity on the Rhine frontier at these times and thus a plentiful supply of German prisoners.[63]

Why was German hair so popular? Martial wrote a series of poems to commemorate the opening of the Colosseum during the reign of the emperor Titus in 80 CE. One of these poems provides a fascinating insight into the diversity of the population of the city of Rome in the latter part of the first century CE, which evidently comprised peoples from both within and without the empire.

> What race is so remote, so barbarous, Caesar, that no spectator from it is in your city? That farmer of Rhodope has come from Orphic Haemus, the Samaritan fed on draughts of horses' blood has come, and he who drinks discovered Nile's first stream, and he on whom beats the wave of farthest Tethys. The Arab has sped hither, the Sabaeans too, and Cilicians have here been sprayed with their own showers. **Sicambrians have come with hair curled in a knot** and Ethiopians with hair curled otherwise. Diverse sounds the speech of the peoples, and yet it is one, when you are called true father of the fatherland.[64]

Ancient Roman conceptions of the world placed Rome at its centre, and Martial plays upon this idea here, enlisting the Sicambrians in the far north (a particular tribe among the many that inhabited Germania, located east of the Rhine and towards the coast) and the Ethiopians in the far south (a generic term used to refer to the inhabitants of sub-Saharan Africa) to emphasise his point that Rome draws in people from the farthest reaches of the known world.[65] The opposition of north and south had been a feature in ancient ethnographical writing since the composition of the Hippocratic treatise *Airs, Waters, Places* in the late fifth century BCE and the initial suggestion of environmental determinism, with the peoples that inhabited these extreme areas being subjects of special interest to ancient authors.[66] What is notable here, however, is that Martial does not just mention the Sicambrians and the Ethiopians by name as he does with the range of other exotic peoples he includes. Rather, he highlights a particularly distinctive feature of both peoples: their hair and hairstyles. It is clear from other ancient literary sources that discuss the Sicambrians and the Ethiopians that Martial was not alone in this, and it is clear from archaeological evidence that he was not exaggerating in his highlighting of Sicambrian hair.[67] The Sicambrians were known for their long blonde or red hair (*flavus; rutilus*) tied up in the style known as the

Suebian Knot (*nodus Suebicus*), the Ethiopians for their woolly black hair (Greek οὖλος; Latin *torta*).[68] Their hair, not just its colour and texture but also its chosen style, was one of the main differences between them and the Romans, and ultimately the transition from native hairstyle to Roman hairstyle was used as an indicator of the acquisition of *cultus*.[69]

There was likely a practical benefit to the use of German hair for wigs and hair pieces as, unlike the Romans, both German men and women wore their hair long. Perhaps more importantly, however, is the fact that Germans were famous for their blonde (*flavus*) or red (*rutilus*) hair, colours that were not only unusual in Italy, but also replete with positive connotations such as divinity.[70] The fact that these hair colours were particularly associated with Germanic tribes is made clear from first Caligula's and later Domitian's attempts to falsify the origins of the 'prisoners' paraded in their sham triumphs by colouring the participants' hair these shades.[71] Petronius (*circa* 27–66 CE) portrays Encolpius as being especially pleased once his shaven head is covered with a wig: 'in fact, I was even more handsome than before, because my new hair was bright blond'.[72] It was also in all likelihood widely seen as symbolic, as ownership of German hair represented ownership of German people, and exotic and luxury goods were seen to represent the fruits of Roman imperialism.[73]

However, there are some other things for us to consider here. First is the Roman understanding of the Germans and their physicality. The German tribes were famous for their vitality, strength, endurance, savagery, eagerness for war and courage.[74] In fact, the Germans occupied a special place amongst Rome's foreigners and were considered to be reminiscent of early Romans.[75]

Second is the Roman understanding of the special emphasis placed upon hair in Germanic culture, particularly in relation to the so-called 'Suebian knot' hairstyle.[76] This is explicated most fully by Tacitus in his *Germania*:

> **It is a characteristic of the [Suebi] to dress their hair on the side and bind it up tight in a knot**. This distinguishes the Suebi from the other Germani, and their free-born from their slaves. Among other tribes, whether through kinship with the Suebi or, as often happens, through imitation, this also occurs, but infrequently and only in youth, whereas among the Suebi it continues until the hair turns grey; they draw back their bristling hair and often tie it on the very top of their heads. The leading men have an even more ornate style. Such is their concern for their appearance, but blameless, since it is not to seduce or attract seduction: they arrange their hair into such a height to cause fear when they are about to go into battle, adorned for the eyes of their enemies.[77]

That the importance and significance of the Suebian knot was clear to the Romans is obvious from its frequent appearance in ancient literature and art. That the Suebian knot was a genuine hairstyle and these were not merely poetic or artistic licence is attested by two surviving bog bodies, the first known as 'Osterby Man' (see Figure 3.7), found in 1948 in the Köhlmoor

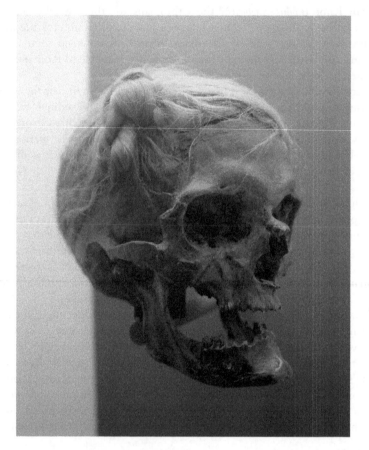

Figure 3.7 The skull of 'Osterby Man', Landesmuseum, Gottorf Castle, Schleswig, Schleswig-Holstein. Image courtesy of Andreas Franzkowiak, Halstenbek, Germany, Licence: CC-BY-SA-3.0, https://commons.wikimedia.org/wiki/File:Osterby_Man.jpg.

near Osterby in Germany and subsequently dated through radiocarbon dating to having died between 75 and 130 CE, and the second known as 'Dätgen Man', found in 1959 near Dätgen in Germany. Two other bog bodies with the hairstyle were reportedly found in the Netherlands and Lower Saxony during the nineteenth century.[78]

The Roman admiration for all things German and an awareness of the importance and the significance of the Suebian knot are combined in an anecdote concerning the emperor Caracalla provided by Herodian (*circa* 170–240 CE):

> He grew especially fond of the Germans in those regions; after gaining their friendship, he entered into alliances with them, and selected for

his personal bodyguard the strongest and most handsome young men. He frequently put off the Roman cloak and donned German dress, appearing in the short, silver-embroidered cloaks which they customarily wear, **augmented by a yellow wig with the locks arranged in the German style**.[79]

The Germans did not take exception to Caracalla's mimicry. Rather, Herodian describes them as being delighted and absolutely adoring him.[80] The Roman response to the emperor appearing in public dressed as a barbarian would in all likelihood not have been so positive.

Third is the transformation of German hair, on both men and women, as a result of Romanisation and the acquisition of *cultus/culta*.[81] This is demonstrated most clearly by funerary monuments recovered from the Rhine and Danube frontiers, upon which there is a tendency for men to represent themselves in Roman dress and women to represent themselves in ethnic dress, although some women do represent themselves in Roman dress and sport Roman hairstyles.[82] The barbarian hair that was once depicted on state monuments and coinage as long, loose and wild is now, in the case of men, cut short and, in the case of women, styled neatly.[83]

Just how appropriate (or inappropriate) would a Roman citizen dressing in the manner of a defeated and subsequently servile barbarian have been considered to be?[84] Related to that, what did it mean for a Roman man or woman to wear the hair of a defeated enemy renowned for his or her physicality to cover their own physical deficiency? On the one hand, this is one of the points, and one of the advantages, of Roman imperialism – to the victor, the spoils. On the other, utilising these spoils in such a supposedly trivial way is potentially a misuse of it, and that is something that a variety of ancient Roman authors rail against, and worry will result in Roman decline.[85]

Additionally, since most of our ancient literary sources are concerned with women using Germanic hair in their wigs and hair pieces, we should consider what the consequences for women might have been in relation to their use of 'captive hair'. It is important to remember that, according to Tacitus, in German culture, a woman's hair was shorn if she was an adulteress.[86] How familiar would the Romans have been with this custom? What might it have meant for a Roman woman to wear the hair of a German woman who, among her own people, would have been viewed as an adulteress? While such a practice might be considered appropriate for a courtesan or prostitute, it would certainly be inappropriate for a respectable woman. Thus, blonde or red hair might not only have been considered German or captive hair, but also, by some, immoral hair. That the hair used to make wigs and hair pieces might be tainted somehow is made clear by one of Tertullian's objections to Christian women wearing wigs and hair pieces; in his excoriation of feminine adornment he flags up the possibility that the hair used to make wigs and hair pieces might have come from the hair of a sinner and so contaminate the wearer.[87]

Conclusion

It is worth reiterating that, despite some literary and archaeological evidence for wigs and hair pieces made from other substances, most do, in fact, seem to have been made from human hair. Prosthetic hair is virtually unique amongst prostheses in that it can be made from a part of the human body, whether that body belongs to the intended user of the prosthesis or someone else entirely. In ancient Rome, the only other type of prosthesis where this was a possibility, the dental appliance, does not seem to have commonly capitalised upon this possibility in the way that wigs and hair pieces did.

Hair was a fundamental physical feature for both men and women in the Roman Republic and Empire, a means of expressing crucial information about gender, stage of life, social class, status, political affiliation, religious belief and even profession. Those who experienced natural hair loss were mocked while those who shaved their own heads or had their heads shaved by others were set apart from society. Since hair was so significant and the possession of it so important, it is not surprising that those who were lacking sought to hide their deficiencies. Prosthetic hair in the form of wigs and hair pieces was one way in which they could do this. The wearing of prosthetic hair, particularly prostheses made from the hair of defeated barbarians, provided a means of creating an alternative social and symbolic presentation of self that emphasised certain desirable qualities such as strength and vitality. It was not, however, without risk, as the wearing of wigs and hair pieces had negative connotations and often the hair utilised to make them did too.

Notes

1 Bliquez, 1996, p. 2641. For discussion of ancient cosmetic dental prostheses, see Turfa and Becker, this volume, and Lehmhaus, this volume. The tendency of scholars to dismiss forms of bodily adornment such as false hair and cosmetics as 'mundane, frivolous, and relevant only to women' is remarked upon by Fletcher, 2005, p. 3.
2 For discussion of the different types of contemporary prosthesis, and their forms and functions, see the Introduction.
3 Ashby, 2016.
4 Levine, 1995, p. 85.
5 According to Graeco-Roman writers, Roman men went long-haired and bearded until Publius Titinius Mena introduced barbers to the city of Rome from Sicily in 300 BCE, with their long hair and beards seen as signs of maturity and wisdom, see Varro, *On Agriculture* 2.11.10; this is reiterated by Pliny the Elder, *Natural History* 7.59; see also Cicero, *For Caelius* 33 for reference to Appius Claudius Caecus' shaggy (*horrida*) beard. On Greek and Roman barbers, see Nicholson, 1891; Kaufman, 1932; and Toner, 2015, pp. 93–95. By the time of the Late Republic adult male hair was expected to be short and neatly barbered but not overly styled; on male *cultus* in this period, see Ovid, *Art of Love* 1.514–522, 1.723–729, and *Remedies for Love* 679. Surviving portraiture from the first century BCE supports the texts, with mature men depicted clean-shaven and with closely cropped hair; Walker, 1991, p. 269 suggests that these types of portraits were intended to serve a didactic function, and p. 271 that this lasted from the first

century BCE to the second century CE; see Flower, 1996, pp. 10–11 on *imagines*. According to Zanker, 1995, p. 218 beards were avoided in official portraiture in this period. Younger men, however, seem to have favoured neatly trimmed 'dainty' beards (*barbula*), which were considered urbane and dissolute by their elders yet attractive by women, and longer hair; Cicero, *Letters to Atticus* 1.14.5, 1.16.11 and *For Caelius* 33; Olson, 2014. That this manner of approaching the practice of personal grooming was a distinctly Roman phenomenon is emphasised by Dio Chrysostom, *The Borysthenitic Discourse* 17; on beards being 'un-Roman', see Zanker, 1995, p. 218. According to Graeco-Roman writers, female hairstyles were rather more varied, with long hair accessorised in different ways depending upon the individual's stage of life; see Sebesta, 1994 on the costume of the Roman woman. Unmarried girls apparently wore their hair held back off their faces with woollen fillets and *vittae*, symbols of maidenly modesty; see Nonius, *Advantageous Learning* 236 M; Festus, *Latin Vocabulary* 353 L; Ovid, *Art of Love* 1.31–32; on the hair of virgins, see Levine, 1995, pp. 95–96; on *vittae*, see Olson, 2008; Fantham, 2008. On her wedding day, a woman would apparently arrange her hair in the *seni crines* hairstyle underneath a flame-coloured hairnet and veil; Propertius, *Elegies* 4.11.33–34; Festus 364 L, Paul's epitome of Festus, *Latin Vocabulary* 55 L, 454.23 L; on the hair of brides, see Levine, 1995, pp. 96–102; on the costume of brides, see La Follette, 1994; on the problematic nature of the evidence for the Roman wedding, see Hersch, 2010, particularly p. 73 on the bride's hairstyle and hair accessories. Apparently from that day forward, a married woman would pin up her hair using a woollen headband and hairnet and then cover it with a veil; Varro, *On the Latin Language* 5.130; Plautus, *The Braggart Soldier* 790–793' on the hair of wives, see Levine, 1995, pp. 102–105. Like brides, Vestal Virgins seem to have worn the *seni crines* hairstyle, but they covered it with a white veil rather than a flame-coloured one. The *flaminica Dialis* wore the *tutulus* hairstyle covered with a veil, with the addition of a twig from a fruitful tree; Ovid, *Fasti* 3.393–398, 6.226–234; see Olson, 2012 for an up-to-date overview, but note the point made about the discrepancies between literary references and artistic representations. Whether male or female, it seems that deliberately deviating from these standard hairstyles made a statement; a man or woman who left their hair long, loose and unstyled might be in mourning or involved in a similarly negative situation such as a court case; see Seneca, *Controversiae* 4.1, 7.3.7, 9.51 for appropriate mourning dress; see Martial, *Epigrams* 2.26.3 for a man growing his hair and beard for a court case. Those who deviated from what was expected for no good reason were criticised, with 'effeminate' men, those with long hair drenched in oils and perfumes, coming in for particular approbation; see Ovid, *Art of Love* 1.500 onwards for what men should not do regarding their appearance; see Williams, 1999, pp. 127–129; Corbeill, 1996, pp. 151–168; Gleason, 1995; Edwards, 1994 on the role that appearance played in politics in this period; Christenson, 2004; on this with regard to beards; Olson, 2014.

6 Individuals might voluntarily or involuntarily cut their hair or shave their heads and the response to such actions varied considerably depending upon the reason for them doing so. Miranda Aldhouse-Green has described enforced head shaving as a violation of body-space, a form of violent assault and an act loaded with meaning, in terms of power relations, on the one hand, and transformation, on the other, see Aldhouse-Green, 2004a, p. 301; see also Artemidorus, *The Inter-pretation of Dreams* 1.30: 'If a man dreams that his beard has fallen off, or that it has been shaved off or forcibly ripped off by anyone, it signifies, in addition to loss of his blood relations, harm together with shame'. Those who shaved their heads or cut their hair involuntarily included invalids, slaves and women accused of adultery; according to Celsus, invalids suffering from a variety of conditions ranging from insanity to epilepsy to ophthalmia should have their heads shaved as

part of their medical treatment; Celsus, *On Medicine* 1.4.1, 3.18.8, 3.20.4, 3.23.7, 4.2.6, 4.2.9, 4.11.8, 6.2.2, 6.6.8 E, 6.6.15, 6.7.1 D, 6.7.4, 6.7.8 B, 7.7.15 D; individuals who were enslaved lost personal autonomy and became property and so their heads might be shaved or their hair cut upon capture to indicate their servile position, and subsequently maintained for the sake of ease; Petronius, *Satyricon* 110; Achilles Tatius, *Leucippe and Clitophon* 5.17, 8.5; Apuleius, *Metamorphoses* 9.12; Cyprian, *Letters* 77.3; Thompson 2003, p. 241; see Aldhouse-Green, 2004a and b on captors' interaction with slaves and their hair as a sign of dominance; women accused of adultery might have their heads shaved or their hair cut as a punishment, but also as a visible sign of their disgrace; Tacitus, *Germania* 19; see also Paul, 1 *Corinthians* 11.4–8 for comparison, and the possibility that this was done in Jewish communities.

7 http://www.nhs.uk/conditions/hair-loss/Pages/Introduction.aspx (accessed January 2018).

8 See Cockayne, 2003, pp. 11–12 and pp. 14–16 and Parkin, 2003, pp. 82–83 on the role of baldness in the physical appearance of old age.

9 For understanding of hair loss, see Celsus, *On Medicine* 6.1.1. For mockery, see Martial, *Epigrams* 5.49. Conversely, see Martial, *Epigrams* 12.82 for an account of the sycophant Menogenes complimenting a virtually bald man on his luxurious head of hair and resultant resemblance to Achilles. For discussion of premature hair loss experienced by men and women in ancient Rome, see Draycott, 2018.

10 Suetonius, *Julius Caesar* 45.1–2, 51.1; Suetonius, *Galba* 21.1; Plutarch, *Galba* 13.4; Suetonius, *Domitian* 18.1, 18.2 in which Domitian's baldness is referred to as a 'disfigurement', discussed in Morgan, 1997.

11 http://www.nhs.uk/conditions/hair-loss/Pages/Introduction.aspx (accessed January 2018).

12 Seneca, *Moral Epistles* 95.20–21 (trans. R. M. Gummere): *Maximus ille medicorum et huius scientiae conditor feminis nec capillos defluere dixit nec pedes laborare; atqui et capillis destituuntur et pedibus aegrae sunt. Non mutata feminarum natura, sed victa est; nam cum virorum licentiam aequaverint, corporum quoque virilium incommoda aequarunt. Non minus pervigilant, non minus potant, et oleo et mero viros provocant; aeque invitis ingesta visceribus per os reddunt et vinum omne vomitu remetiuntur; aeque nivem rodunt, solacium stomachi aestuantis. Libidine vero ne maribus quidem cedunt, pati natae, di illas deaeque male perdant! Adeo perversum commentae genus inpudicitiae viros ineunt. Quid ergo mirandum est maximum medicorum ac naturae peritissimum in mendacio prendi, cum tot feminae podagricae calvaeque sint? Beneficium sexus sui vitiis perdiderunt et, quia feminam exuerant, damnatae sunt morbis virilibus.* See Edwards, 1994, pp. 87–89 for discussion of Seneca's use of nature and culture in this instance.

13 Zetzel, 1996, pp. 74–77 has interpreted this as a reference to Propertius' work on a similar theme in which he likewise warns his unnamed mistress against female adornment and vanity regarding her hair, clothing and use of cosmetics. See Olson, 2012, pp. 80–95 for full discussion of male criticisms of female adornment.

14 Ovid, *Amores* 1.14 (trans. A. S. Kline): *Dicebam 'medicare tuos desiste capillos!' Tingere quam possis, iam tibi nulla coma est. At si passa fores, quid erat spatiosius illis? Contigerant imum, qua patet usque, latus . . . Cum graciles essent tamen et lanuginis instar, heu, male vexatae quanta tulere comae! Quam se praebuerunt ferro patienter et igni, ut fieret torto nexilis orbe sinus! Clamabam: 'scelus est istos, scelus urere crines! Sponte decent; capiti, ferrea, parce tuo! Vim procul hinc remove! non est, qui debeat uri; erudit admotas ipse capillus acus' . . . Quid male dispositos quereris periisse capillos? Quid speculum maesta ponis, inepta, manu? Non bene consuetis a te spectaris ocellis; ut placeas, debes inmemor esse tui . . . Non te cantatae laeserunt paelicis herbae, non anus Haemonia perfida lavit aqua; nec tibi vis morbi nocuit — procul omen abesto! — Nec minuit densas invida lingua comas. Facta manu culpaque tua dispendia sentis; ipsa dabas capiti mixta venena tuo . . .*

Me miserum! lacrimas male continet oraque dextra protegit ingenuas picta rubore genas. Sustinet antiquos gremio spectatque capillos, ei mihi, non illo munera digna loco! Collige cum vultu mentem! reparabile damnum est. Postmodo nativa conspiciere coma. For discussion, see Zetzel, 1996; Papaioannou, 2006.

15 Suetonius, *Domitian* 18.2; Draycott, 2018.

16 On hair loss: Celsus, *On Medicine* 6.4; Pliny the Elder, *Natural History* 28.163–166; Galen 12.403–405 K; Aëtius, *Sixteen Books on Medicine* 6.65; Paul of Aegina, *Medical Compendium in Seven Books* 3.1.1–2; on encouraging hair growth: Galen 13.432–434 K.

17 *IG IV²*, 1, 19.

18 For Phoebus' attempt to paint hair on his bald head, see Martial, *Epigrams* 6.57; for his eventually resorting to a kid-skin wig, see Martial, *Epigrams* 12.45.

19 See for example Julius Caesar's attempt to hide his thinning hair with a laurel wreath, see Suetonius, *Julius Caesar* 45.2.

20 See Lee, 2015, p. 70 for wigs not being common in Greece prior to the Hellenistic period; Xenophon, *Cyropaedia* 1.3.2 describes wigs as a Median fashion, while they are utilised in scenes of male to female transvestitism, such as Aristophanes, *Women at the Thesmophoria* 258.

21 Fletcher and Salamone, 2016; experimental archaeological reconstruction of an ancient Egyptian wig by a professional wig-maker resulted in the estimation that such a wig would have taken around 200 hours or one month to create – if an ancient Egyptian wig-maker could only produce a maximum of twelve wigs per year, he or she would have needed to charge enough for each wig to make this limitation on their professional activities worth their while.

22 Toner, 2015, p. 95 states that barbers made wigs, but does not provide any evidence to support this claim. For wigs and hair pieces in the Porticus Philippi, see Ovid, *Art of Love* 3.167–168; Martial, *Epigrams* 5.49.12–13. Dalby, 2000, p. 241. For discussion of the experimental archaeological reconstruction of an ancient Egyptian wig (*circa* 1400 BCE) and what that can tell about the ancient process of wig-making, see Fletcher and Salamone, 2016; see also Cox, 1977.

23 Suetonius, *Otho* 12.

24 Tertullian, *On the Apparel of Women* 2.7.1–2 (trans. S. Thelwell): *Affigitis praeterea nescio quas enormitates sutilium atque textilium capillamentorum, nunc in galeri modum quasi uaginam capitis et operculum uerticis, nunc in ceruicum retro suggestum. Mirum quod non contra domini praecepta contenditur! Ad mensuram neminem sibi adicere posse pronuntiatum est. Vos sane adicitis ad pondus, collyridas quasdam uel scutorum umbilicos ceruicibus adstruendo. Si non pudet enormitatis, pudeat inquinamenti, ne exuuias alieni capitis forsitan immundi, forsan nocentis et gehennae destinati sancto et christiano capiti supparetis. Immo, omnem hanc ornatus seruitutem a libero capite propellite. Frustra laboratis ornatae uideri, frustra peritissimos quosque structores capillaturae adhibetis: Deus uos uelari iubet, credo ne quarumdam capita uideantur.*

25 Raditsa, 1985, p. 306.

26 For discussion, see Lawler, 1929, p. 22.

27 Clement of Alexandria, *The Instructor* 2.104.1, 2.107.3, 2.108.5, 2.115.1-2, 3.5.1, 3.5.4, 3.8.1-3, 3.26.3, 3.57.2. See also another contemporary, albeit a pagan one, who expressed similar views, Philostratus (*circa* 170–250 CE), whose *Epistle* 22 is discussed in the Introduction.

28 See Olson, 2009; for expanded discussion on Roman cosmetics, see Olson, 2012, pp. 58–80.

29 Galen, 12.434 K.

30 For discussion, see Olson, 2009, p. 294.

31 Martial, *Epigrams* 12.23, 9.38.

32 See for example Lucian, *Dialogues of the Courtesans* 39.11, in which a courtesan wears a wig over grey hair, presumably to allow her to continue working; and

compare with 39.12, in which a courtesan whose hair was cut off while she is ill now wears a wig, likewise presumably to allow her to keep working.

33 See Musonius Rufus, *Discourse 21 On Cutting the Hair* for discussion of the ways that women arrange their hair to appear more beautiful; Ovid, *Arts of Love* 3.135–158 goes into considerable detail about which hairstyle a woman should choose depending upon the nature of her physical attributes. See Ovid, *Arts of Love* 3.242–250; Apuleius, *Metamorphosis* 2.8 for the loss of hair making women less attractive. On hair and female attractiveness, see Sensi, 1980–81.

34 Horace, *Satires* 1.8.47–50; Ovid, *Amores* 1.14; Martial, *Epigrams* 9.38, 12.23; Lucillius, *Greek Anthology* 11.68, 11.310; Lucian, *Dialogue of the Courtesans* 11.4.

35 Lucian, *Dialogues of the Courtesans* 11.4.

36 Juvenal, *Satires* 6; Cassius Dio, *Roman History* 80.2; Suetonius, *Caligula* 11.1; Suetonius, *Nero* 26.1. For discussion of Messalina's purported transgression, see Joshel, 1995, pp. 77–78.

37 Bradley, 2009, pp. 172–174.

38 See for example the witch Sagana in Horace, *Satires* 1.8.47–50.

39 Avienus, *Fables* 11.7–12.

40 See Petronius, *Satyricon* 110, where Petronius depicts two of his *Satyricon* characters covering up their shaven heads with women's wigs.

41 Ovid, *The Art of Love* 3.244–247.

42 Ovid, *The Art of Love* 3.249–250.

43 Bartman, 2001.

44 Stephens, 2008.

45 Olson, 2008, pp. 146–147.

46 On conspicuous consumption and *luxuria* in ancient Rome generally, see Dalby, 2000; see pp. 206–207 and p. 241 on wigs and hair pieces specifically. For a discussion of prosthesis use as conspicuous consumption in the nineteenth century, see Warne, 2009; for a discussion of wig-wearing as conspicuous consumption in eighteenth-century France, see Kwass, 2006.

47 Audollent, 1921, p. 163; see also Audollent, 1923, pp. 311–312, pl. 8, nn. 3–6.

48 Wood, 1883, pp. 108; Black, 1986, p. 225.

49 Yorkshire Museum inv. YORYM:1998.695. On hair pins specifically, see Fletcher, 2016.

50 Fletcher, 1995, pp. 37–38. There was a tradition of wig-wearing in Egypt dating back to 3400 BCE, Fletcher, 2005, p. 3.

51 Woman: Mummy n. 58.2.2.4, see Dunand *et al.*, 1992, p. 142, pl. 33.3–4; Fletcher, 1995, Volume 1 pp. 37–38, p. 415; child: Mummy n. 20.2.1.4, see Dunand and Lichtenberg, 1994, pp. 92–93 (with photographs); Dunand *et al.*, 1992, pp. 51–52, pl. 24.1–4; Fletcher, 1995, Volume 1 p. 37, p. 415.

52 Petrie Museum inv. UC7833; Petrie, 1927, p. 5, pl. 4; Corson, 1965, p. 74; Fletcher, 1995, Volume 1 p. 416, Volume 2 p. 947, pl. 819, pl. 820. On the hair pins specifically, see Fletcher, 2016.

53 For full details of the tomb, see Rossignani *et al.*, 2005. For the hair piece, see Legrottaglie, 2005; for the reticulum, see Benecchi, 2005.

54 An Italian documentary about the excavation, *Carvilius, un enigna dall'antica Roma*, is available on YouTube: https://youtu.be/cwJ5nVvRNag (accessed January 2018). It contains a lengthy section on the wig and hairnet and uses an actress to demonstrate what Aebutia Quarta would have looked like with her hair arranged this way.

55 Boldetti, 1720, 297; see Bartman, 2001, p. 14, n. 69.

56 Cairo Archaeological Museum inv. JE.33434; Lucas, 1930, p. 194; Lucas and Taylor, 1962, p. 30; Fletcher, 1995, Volume 1 p. 415, Volume 2 p. 945, pl. 815, pl. 816.

57 Cairo Archaeological Museum inv. Temp.Reg.18:1:26:26; Lucas, 1930, p. 194; Lucas and Taylor, 1962, p. 30; Fletcher, 1995, Volume 1 p. 415, Volume 2 p. 946, pl. 817.
58 British Museum inv. EA.54051 (the hair piece is not currently visible in the photograph of the mummy case on the British Museum's website); Dawson and Gray, 1978, p. 40, n. 78, pl. 21b; Fletcher, 1995, Volume 1 p. 415, Volume 2 p. 946, pl. 818.
59 Vindolanda: Wild, 1993. Newstead: National Museum of Scotland inv. X.FRA 1183; Curle, 1911, p. 108, p. 358, pl. 15.
60 The Vindolanda Museum has labelled the Vindolanda example as a wig. The Newstead example was originally interpreted as a basket, see Curle, 1911, p. 108, pl. 15. However, today the National Museum of Scotland has it labelled as a hat.
61 *Digest* 39.4.16.7. According to Arrian, *Indica* 6.9, Indian hair was dark like Ethiopian hair but not woolly.
62 There is also evidence for hair dye consisting of 'German herbs'; see Ovid, *Art of Love* 3. 159–168. For discussion of Roman hair dye, see Bradley, 2009, pp. 170–174.
63 Military activity such as Drusus' campaign against the Cherusci, Suebi, and Sicambri in 11 BCE, recounted in Florus, *Epitome* 2.30.25. See also Ovid, *Amores* 1.14.45–46, *Art of Love* 3.163–168, 3.242–250; Martial, *Epigrams* 14.26 refers to 'Teutonic locks' (*teutonicos capillos*), Bartman, 1999, p. 39; Leary, 1996, p. 79. See also Martial, *Epigrams* 5.37.8, 5.68, 14.26; Juvenal, *Satires* 13.164–165; Claudian, *On the Fourth Consulship of the Emperor Honorius* 4.446–447, Eutropius, *Brief History of Rome* 1.383.
64 Martial, *On the Spectacles* 3 (trans. D. R. Shackleton Bailey): *Quae tam seposita est, quae gens tam barbara, Caesar, ex qua spectator non sit in urbe tua? Venit ab Orpheo cultor Rhodopeius Haemo, venit et epoto Sarmata pastus equo, et qui prima bibit deprensi flumina Nili, et quem supremae Tethyos unda ferit; festinavit Arabs, festinavere Sabaei, et Cilices nimbis hie maduere suis. Crinibus in nodum tortis venere Sugambri, atque aliter tortis crinibus Aethiopes. Vox diversa sonat populorum, turn tamen una est, cum verus patriae diceris esse pater.*
65 Edwards and Woolf, 2003, p. 1. On Germans in antiquity, see King, 1990; Wolfram, 1997; Carroll, 2001. On Ethiopians in antiquity, see Snowden, 1970, 1991.
66 Isaac, 2004, p. 83. Germans and Ethiopians were frequently set up as opposites in ancient literature: Vitruvius, *On Architecture* 6.1.3–4; Pliny the Elder, *Natural History* 2.80.189; Julius Firmicus Maternus, *Mathesis* 1.2.1, 1.5.1–2. For discussion of this dichotomy, see Snowden, 1970, pp. 173–176.
67 On the hair of Germanic tribes, see Krierer, 2004, pp. 100–111; Isaac, 2004, p. 65 and p. 432. On the hair of Ethiopians, see Snowden 1970, pp. 6–7; Isaac, 2004, p. 71 and p. 80.
68 For the Suebian Knot, see Tacitus, *Germania* 38; Krierer, 2004, pp. 100–111.
69 On *cultus*, see Shumka, 2008, pp. 176–177. According to Levine, 1995, p. 88, 'even in its most natural state, hair seems especially to demand the attentions of culture'.
70 Seneca, *On Anger* 3.26.3; *Moral Epistles* 124.22. See Barton, 1994, pp. 119–122 for the significance of colouring in ancient physiognomy.
71 For Caligula, see Suetonius, *Caligula* 47 and Persius, *Satires* 6.46–47; Tacitus, *Agricola* 39 and Cassius Dio, *Roman History* 67.7.4. For discussion, see Beard pp. 185–186.
72 Petronius, *Satyricon* 110 (trans. J. P. Sullivan): *immo commendatior vultus enituit, quia flavum conymbian erat.* Of course, this is a personal preference and entirely subjective – see Ovid, *Amores* 2.4.37–44 for the poet's discussion of the type of women he finds attractive.

73 On Ovid and images of empire, see Habinek, 2002, pp. 46–49. On luxury and Roman imperialism generally, see Dalby, 2000.
74 Caesar, *Gallic War* 4.1.8–9 sees Caesar describe the Suebi as the most warlike nation among the German tribes and emphasises their strength and stature. See also Seneca, *On Anger* 1.11, 2.1.5; Seneca, *Natural Questions* 6.7; Josephus, *Jewish War* 2.16.4, *Antiquities* 19.1.15.
75 Rives, 1999, p. 62; Isaac, 2004, p. 438; Gruen, 2011, p. 178.
76 On the 'Suebian knot', see Seneca the Younger, *On Anger* 3.26.3; Juvenal, *Satires* 13.164–165. On the 'Sigambrian knot' see Martial, *On the Spectacles* 3.9. On 'knots of the Rhine', see Martial, *Epigrams* 5.37.8. See also Aldhouse-Green, 2004a, pp. 301–305.
77 Tacitus, *Germania* 38.2–4 (trans. J. B. Rives): *discreti, quamquam in commune Suebi vocentur. insigne gentis obliquare crinem nodoque substringere: sic Suebi a ceteris Germanis, sic Sueborum ingenui a servis separantur. in aliis gentibus seu cognatione aliqua Sueborum seu, quod saepius accidit, imitatione, rarum et intra iuventae spatium: apud Suebos usque ad canitiem horrentes capilli retorquentur, ac saepe in ipso vertice religantur. principes et ornatiorem habent: ea cura formae, sed innoxia; neque enim ut ament amenturve, in altitudinem quandam et terrorem adituri bella compti, ut hostium oculis, ornantur.* See Rives, 1999, pp. 282–285 for discussion of this passage and who the Suebi people that Tacitus is referring to actually were.
78 Rives, 1999, p. 285.
79 Herodian, *Roman Histories* 4.7.3 (trans. E. C. Echols): ᾠκειώσατο δὲ καὶ πάντας τοὺς ἐπέκεινα Γερμανούς, ἔς τε φιλίαν ὑπηγάγετο, ὡς καὶ συμμάχους παρ' αὐτῶν λαβεῖν καὶ τοῦ σώματος ἑαυτοῦ φρουροὺς ποιήσασθαι, γενναίους τε καὶ ὡραίους ἐπιλεξάμενος. πολλάκις δὲ καὶ τὴν Ῥωμαϊκὴν ἀποθέμενος χλαμύδα ἠμφιέννυτο τὰ Γερμανῶν περιβλήματα, ἔν τε χλαμύσιν αἷς εἰώθασιν, ἀργύρῳ πεποικιλμένους, ἑωρᾶτο. κόμας τε τῇ κεφαλῇ ἐπετίθετο ξανθὰς καὶ ἐς κουρὰν τὴν Γερμανῶν ἠσκημένας.
80 Herodian, *Roman Histories* 4.7.3: τούτοις δὴ χαίροντες οἱ βάρβαροι ὑπερηγάπων αὐτόν.
81 On *cultus* and *culta*, see Shumka, 2008.
82 Rothe, 2012, p. 241.
83 See for example *CIL* 13 7067, the funerary monument of the married couple Blussus and Menimane.
84 See George, 2002 for discussion of slave disguise in ancient Rome, the entire premise of which relies upon the belief that slave and free members of society look and dress differently.
85 Recall the famous quote from Horace, *Epistles* 2.1.156–157 (trans. H. R. Fairclough): 'Greece, the captive, made her savage victor captive, and brought the arts into rustic Latium': *Graecia capta ferum victorem cepit et artes intulit agresti Latio.*
86 Tacitus, *Germania* 19.1. For discussion of this passage, some comparative evidence, and examples of female bog bodies with shorn hair, see Rives, 1999, pp. 203–204.
87 Raditsa, 1985, p. 312.

Bibliography

Aldhouse-Green, M. (2004a) 'Crowning Glories: Languages of Hair in Later Prehistoric Europe', *PPS* 70, pp. 299–326.
Aldhouse-Green, M. (2004b) 'Chaining and Shaming: Images of Defeat, from Llyn Cerrig Bach to Sarmitzegetusa', *OJA* 23.3, pp. 319–340.
Arena, V. (2012) *Libertas and the Practice of Politics in the Late Roman Republic.* Cambridge: Cambridge University Press.
Ashby, S. P. (2016) 'Archaeologies of Hair: An Introduction', *IA* 42: http://dx.doi.org/10.11141/ia.42.6.1 (accessed January 2018).

Audollent, A. (1921) 'Les tombes des Martres-de-Veryre', *Man* 21, pp. 161–164.

Audollent, A. (1923) 'Les tombes gallo-romaines à inhumation des Martres-de-Veyre (Puy-de-Dôme)', *Mémoires présentés par divers savants à l'Académie des inscriptions et belles-lettres* (Paris) 13, pp. 275–328.

Bartman, E. (1999) *Portraits of Livia: Imaging the Imperial Woman in Augustan Rome.* Cambridge: Cambridge University Press.

Bartman, E. (2001) 'Hair and the Artifice of Roman Female Adornment', *AJA* 105.1, pp. 1–25.

Barton, T. S. (1994) *Power and Knowledge: Astrology, Physiognomics, and Medicine under the Roman Empire.* Ann Arbor, MI: University of Michigan Press.

Benecchi, F. (2005) '*Il reticulum*', in Rossignani, M. P., Sannazaro, M. and Legrottaglie, G. (2005) *La Signora del sarcofago: una sepoltura di rango nella necropoli dell'Università cattolica: ricerche archeologiche nei cortili dell'Università Cattolica.* Milan: Vita e pensiero, pp. 103–116.

Black, E. W. (1986) 'Romano-British Burial Customs and Religious Beliefs in South East England', *AJ* 143, pp. 201–239.

Bliquez, L. J. (1996) 'Prosthetics in Classical Antiquity: Greek, Etruscan and Roman Prosthetics', in *ANRW* II 37.3, pp. 2640–2676.

Boldetti, M.-A. (1720) *Osservazioni sopra I cimiteri de'santi matiri ed antichi Christiani di Roma: 297.* Rome: Maria Salvioni Stampatore Vaticano.

Bradley, M. (2009) *Colour and Meaning in Ancient Rome.* Cambridge: Cambridge University Press.

Carroll, M. (2001) *Romans, Celts and Germans: The German Provinces of Rome.* Stroud: Tempus.

Christenson, D. (2004) 'Unbearding Morality: Appearance and Persuasion in "Pro Caelio"', *CJ* 100.1, pp. 61–72.

Cokayne, K. (2003) *Experiencing Old Age in Ancient Rome.* London: Routledge.

Corbeill, A. (1996) *Controlling Laugher. Political Humor in the Late Republic.* Princeton, NJ: Princeton University Press.

Corson, R. (1965) *Fashions in Hair: The First Five Thousand Years.* London: Peter Owen.

Cox, J. S. (1977) 'The Construction of an Ancient Egyptian Wig (c.1400 BC) in the British Museum', *JEA* 63, pp. 67–70.

Curle, J. (1911) *A Roman Frontier Post and its People: The Fort of New-stead in the Parish of Melrose.* Glasgow: James Maclehose and Sons.

Dalby, A. (2000) *Empire of Pleasures. Luxury and Indulgence in the Roman World.* London: Routledge.

Dawson, W. R. and Gray, P. H. K. (1968) *Catalogue of Egyptian Antiquities in the British Museum: 1. Mummies and Human Remains.* London: British Museum.

Draycott, J. L. (2018) 'Hair Loss as Facial Disfigurement in Ancient Rome?', in Skinner, P. and Cock, E. (edd.) *Approaching Facial Difference: Past and Present.* London: Bloomsbury, pp. 65–83.

Dundand, F., Heim, J.-L., Henein, N. and Lichtenberg, R. (1992) *La Nécropole de Douch (Oasis de Kharga).* Cairo: Institut français d'archéologie orientale du Caire.

Dundand, F. and Lichtenberg, R. (1994) *Mummies: A Voyage through Eternity.* New York, NY: Harry N. Abrams.

Edwards, C. (1994) *The Politics of Immorality in Ancient Rome.* Cambridge: Cambridge University Press.

Edwards, C. and Woolf, G. (2003) *Rome the Cosmopolis.* Cambridge: Cambridge University Press.

Fabre, G. (1981) *Libertus. Recherches sur les rapports patron-affranchi à la fin de la République Romaine*. Paris: École Française de Rome.

Fantham, E. (2008) 'Covering the Head at Rome: Ritual and Gender', in Edmondson, J. and Keith, A. (edd.) *Roman Dress and the Fabrics of Roman Culture*. Toronto: University of Toronto Press, pp. 158–171.

Fletcher, J. (1995) *Ancient Egyptian Hair: A Study in Style, Form and Function: Two Volumes*. Manchester: University of Manchester, PhD thesis.

Fletcher, J. (2005) 'The Decorated Body in Ancient Egypt: Hairstyles, Cosmetics and Tattoos', in Cleland, L., Harlow, M. and Llewellyn-Jones, L. (edd.) *The Clothed Body in the Ancient World*. Oxford: Oxbow, pp. 3–13.

Fletcher, J. (2016) 'The Egyptian Hair Pin: Practical, Sacred, Fatal', *IA* 42: http://dx.doi.org/10.11141/ia.42.6.5 (accessed January 2018).

Fletcher, J. and Salamone, F. (2016) 'An Ancient Egyptian Wig: Construction and Reconstruction', *IA* 42: http://dx.doi.org/10.11141/ia.42.6.3 (accessed January 2018).

Flower, H. I. (1996) *Ancestor Masks and Aristocratic Power in Roman Culture*. Oxford: Clarendon Press.

Gleason, M. (1995) *Making Men. Sophists and Self-Presentation in Ancient Rome*. Princeton, NJ: Princeton University Press.

George, M. (2002) 'Slave Disguise in Ancient Rome', *Slavery & Abolition* 23.2, pp. 41–54.

Gruen, E. (2011) *Rethinking the Other in Antiquity*. Princeton, NJ: Princeton University Press.

Habinck, T. (2002) 'Ovid and Empire', in Hardie, P. (ed.) *The Cambridge Companion to Ovid*. Cambridge: Cambridge University Press, pp. 46–61.

Hallpike, C. R. (1969) 'Social Hair', *Man* 4, pp. 256–264.

Isaac, B. (2004) *Racism in Antiquity*. Princeton, NJ: Princeton University Press.

Joshel, S. (1995) 'Female Desire and the Discourse of Empire: Tacitus's Messalina', *Signs* 21.1, pp. 50–82.

Kaufman, D. B. (1932) 'Roman Barbers', *CW* 2, pp. 145–148.

King, A. (1990) *Roman Gaul and Germany*. London: British Museum Press.

Krierer, K. R. (2004) *Antike Germanenbilder*. Wien: Verlag der Österreichischen Akademie der Wissenschaften.

Kwass, M. (2006) 'Big Hair: A Wig History of Consumption in Eighteenth-Century France', *AHR* 111.3, pp. 631–659.

La Follette, L. (1994) 'The Costume of the Roman Bride', in Sebesta, J. L. and Bonfante, L. (edd.) *The World of Roman Costume*. Madison, WI: University of Wisconsin Press, pp. 54–64.

Lawler, L. (1929) 'Two Portraits from Tertullian', *CJ* 25.1, pp. 19–23.

Leary, T. J. (1996) *Martial Book XIV the Apophoreta*. London: Duckworth.

Lee, M. (2015) *Body, Dress and Identity in Ancient Greece*. Cambridge: Cambridge University Press.

Legrottaglie, G. (2005) 'Considerazioni sulla pettinatura', in Rossignani, M. P., Sannazaro, M. and Legrottaglie, G. (edd.) *La Signora del sarcofago: una sepoltura di rango nella necropoli dell'Università cattolica: ricerche archeologiche nei cortili dell'Università Cattolica*. Milan: Vita e pensiero, pp. 97–102.

Levine, M. M. (1995) 'The Gendered Grammar of Ancient Mediterranean Hair', in Eilberg-Schwartz, H. and Doniger, W. (edd.) *Off With Her Head! The Denial of Women's Identity in Myth, Religion, and Culture*. Berkeley, CA: University of California Press, pp. 76–130.

Lucas, A. (1930) 'Egyptian Wigs', *Annales du Service des antiquités de l'Égypte* 30, pp. 190–196.

Lucas, A. and Harris, J. R. (1962) *Ancient Egyptian Materials and Industries*. London: Edward Arnold.

Morgan, L. (1997) 'Hair and Heroism According to Domitian', *CQ* 47.1, pp. 209–214.

Nicholson, F. W. (1891) 'Greek and Roman Barbers', *HSCP* 2, pp. 41–56.

Olson, K. (2008) 'The Appearance of the Young Roman Girl', in Edmondson, J. and Keith, A. (edd.) *Roman Dress and the Fabrics of Roman Culture*. Toronto: University of Toronto Press, pp. 139–157.

Olson, K. (2009) 'Cosmetics in Roman Antiquity: Substance, Remedy, Poison', *CW* 102.3, pp. 209–310.

Olson, K. (2012) *Dress and the Roman Woman*. London: Routledge.

Olson, K. (2014) 'Masculinity, Appearance and Sexuality: Dandies in Roman Antiquity', *Journal of the History of Sexuality* 23.2, pp. 182–205.

Papaioannou, S. (2006) 'The Poetology of Hairstyling and the Excitement of Hair Loss in Ovid, "Amores" 1, 14', *Quaderni Urbinati di Cultura Classica, New Series* 83.2, pp. 45–69.

Parkin, T, (2003) *Old Age in the Roman World: A Cultural and Social History*. Baltimore, MD and London: Johns Hopkins University Press.

Petrie, W. F. (1927) *Objects of Daily Use*. London: British School of Archaeology in Egypt.

Raditsa, L. (1985) 'The Appearance of Women and Contact: Tertullian's De Habitu Feminarum', *Athenaeum* 63, pp. 297–326.

Richlin, A. (1995) 'Making Up a Woman: the Face of Roman Gender', in Eilberg-Schwartz, H. and Doniger, W. (edd.) *Off With Her Head! The Denial of Women's Identity in Myth, Religion, and Culture*. Berkeley, CA: University of California Press, pp. 185–214.

Rives, J. B. (1999) *Tacitus* Germania. Oxford: Clarendon Press.

Rossignani, M. P., Sannazaro, M. and Legrottaglie, G. (2005) *La Signora del sarcofago: una sepoltura di rango nella necropoli dell'Università cattolica: ricerche archeologiche nei cortili dell'Università Cattolica*. Milan: Vita e pensiero.

Rothe, U. (2012) 'The "Third Way": Treveran Women's Dress and the "Gallic Ensemble"', *AJA* 116.2, pp. 235–252.

Sebesta, J. L. (1994) 'Symbolism in the Costume of the Roman Woman', in Sebesta, J. L. and Bonfante, L. (edd.) *The World of Roman Costume*. Madison, WI: University of Wisconsin Press, pp. 46–53.

Sensi, L. (1980–1981) 'Ornatus e status sociale delle donne romane', *Annali della Faculta di Lettere e Filosofia Perugia-Sezione Studi Classici* NS 4, pp. 55–102.

Shumka, J. (2008) 'Designing Women: The Representation of Women's Toiletries on Funerary Monuments in Roman Italy', in Edmondson, J. and Keith, A. (edd.) *Roman Dress and the Fabrics of Roman Culture*. Toronto: University of Toronto Press, pp. 172–191.

Snowden, F. M. (1970) *Blacks in Antiquity: Ethiopians in Greco-Roman Experience*. London: Belknapp.

Snowden, F. M. (1991) *Before Colour Prejudice: The Ancient View of Blacks*. Cambridge, MA: Harvard University Press.

Stephens, J. (2008) 'Ancient Roman Hairdressing: On (Hair)pins and Needles', *JRA* 21, pp. 110–132.

Thompson, F. H. (2003) *The Archaeology of Greek and Roman Slavery*. London: Duckworth.

Toner, J. (2015) 'Barbers, Barbershops and Searching for Roman Popular Culture', *PBSR* 83, pp. 91–109.

Walker, S. (1991) 'Bearded Men', *Journal of the History of Collections* 3.2, pp. 265–277.

Warne, V. (2009) '"To Invest a Cripple with Peculiar Interest": Artificial Legs and Upper-Class Amputees at Mid-Century', *Victorian Review* 35.2, pp. 83–100.

Wild, J. P. (1993) 'A Hairmoss Cap from Vindolanda', in Jaacks, G. and Tidow, K. (edd.) *Archäologische Textilfunde – Archaeological Textiles: Textilsymposium Neumünster 4.-7.5.1993 (NESAT V), Neumuenster 1994*. Neumünster: Textilmuseum Neumünster, pp. 61–68.

Wilken, G. A. (1886) 'Über das Haaropfer und einige andere Trauergebräucher bei den Völkern Indonesiens', *Revue Coloniale Internationale* 2, pp. 225–269.

Williams, C. A. (1999) *Roman Homosexuality: Ideologies of Masculinity in Classical Antiquity*. Oxford: Oxford University Press.

Wolfram, H. (1997) *The Roman Empire and its Germanic Peoples*. Berkeley, CA: University of California Press.

Wood, H. (1883) 'Roman Urns Found Near Rainham Creek, on the Medway', *Archaeologica Cantiana* 15, pp. 108–110.

Zanker, P. (1995) *The Mask of Socrates: The Image of the Intellectual in Antiquity*. Berkeley, CA: University of California Press.

Zetzel, J. (1996) 'Poetic Baldness and its Cure', *Materiali e discussioni per l'analisi dei testi classici* 36, pp. 76–100.

4 'An amputee may go out with his wooden aid on Shabbat': dynamics of prosthetic discourse in Talmudic traditions[1]

Lennart Lehmhaus

Introduction

While different kinds of ancient prosthetic devices are known to us through archaeological findings as artefacts, in illustrations, or in ancient texts, Talmudic traditions about prostheses are the only available source for ancient Jewish culture.[2] In the following chapter, some of the most central passages discussing such prosthetic devices, their materiality, their various functions and, most importantly, their role within the socio-religious world of the rabbinic discourse will be examined in detail. I argue that, on the one hand, prostheses within these texts are a prime example of a liminal category that the rabbis deployed as a 'scholastic' tool – prostheses are 'good to think' with.[3] On the other hand, the sample texts will show that the rabbis must have also felt a need to include this topic in their discussions, as a possibly rather common phenomenon in their lived experience. Thus, at times, their discourse about prostheses became also a 'prosthetic discourse' tending to the inclusion of persons with certain impairments and mitigating some of the physical and social hardships experienced.

What remains? Methodological and theoretical questions

The scholarly study into ancient material remains of common usage, and especially of such items as prostheses, is fraught with difficulties posed by the sparse archaeological evidence. Moreover, in any attempt to triangulate those findings with literary or artistic depictions of artefacts we must be aware of several pitfalls to this endeavour.[4] Since this chapter is going to discuss the topic of ancient prostheses from the perspective of the Talmudic traditions, one has to point out that the difficulties known to us from other cultures tend to multiply in the case of Jewish ancient history. Frequently, it seems impossible to judge whether an archaeological artefact was in fact 'Jewish', even if it has been found in a suitable context or at a Jewish site (such as a ritual bath or a synagogue).[5] Due to this lack of unambiguous material remains of 'Jewish prostheses', we have to base our discussion solely on the textual representation of such prosthetic aids in Talmudic texts. However, in addition to these general problems, one has to be aware of the many particularities of rabbinic texts and their specific ways of transmitting and representing knowledge about medicine and disabilities. If not, one will likely end up with a positivistic, totally fragmented reconstruction of the discourse on prostheses in Talmudic traditions freed of all contextual links that are crucial for the very understanding of Talmudic ideas and concepts.

First, the textual basis available for our research is rather small compared with Graeco-Roman and later Byzantine traditions. Talmudic literature as the mainstream of rabbinic traditions consists mainly of the early traditions Mishnah (M) and Tosefta (T) from the third century CE which were transferred, elaborated and commented upon in the two Talmudic traditions, the Palestinian or *Yerushalmi* (pT/y) and the Babylonian or *Bavli* (bT/b) stemming from the fifth to the seventh centuries CE. Those traditions were transmitted over decades or even centuries in a context of oral recitation and learning before, in Late Antiquity, being written down, compiled and edited into their later 'final' form which is more or less known to us today. These four works deal mainly with socio-religious laws, customs and norms and were regarded later on as the authoritative core traditions of rabbinic Judaism. Randomly, one finds in these works medical or other technical knowledge in different contexts.[6]

Second, in contrast to most Graeco-Roman works, but similar to ancient Egyptian or Mesopotamian ones, rabbinic literature in general has an anonymous and collective authorship. Although we find a polyphonic discourse and the inclusion of many different opinions, all rabbinic texts are biased and they provide only the information and worldviews that their authors or compilers included.[7] Finally, in striking contrast to ancient Egyptian, Mesopotamian and Graeco-Roman culture, we find no Jewish texts exclusively concerned with medicine and the body until the early medieval period.[8] However, both *Talmudim* (the plural of *Talmud*) and other rabbinic works contain many single and sometimes also complex and detailed medical teachings (about physiology, anatomy, therapies, remedies, diet and regimen) which were scattered throughout or clustered within those broader Halakhic discussions on (religious) norms.[9]

Elsewhere, based on Hector Avalos' model of ancient healthcare systems, I have outlined three rabbinic notions of impairment and disability: explanations and aetiologies of certain impairments, physical aspects of disability including technical aids (i.e., prosthetics) and cures, and the range of attitudes towards the disabled in Jewish society.[10] These three categories may help us to grasp the rabbis' understandings of physical impairments, which undergird their discussions of disability in various legal, ethical or theological frameworks. Due to the overarching focus of this volume, I will emphasise the second point presenting some instructive discussions on prostheses from Talmudic texts. The discussion will explain the broader context of the religious (*halakhic*) discourse that has shaped and triggered those elaborations on the topic at hand. In the following, I will discuss two types of prostheses that can be found in rabbinic texts. The Talmudic engagement with one type, dental prostheses, should be explored under the aspect of its aesthetic or cosmetic usage, while the discourse about the other type – wooden aids for legs, feet and hands – seems to stress rather the technical or mechanical aspects as well as the religious context in which such prostheses were used.

Body parts and textual bodies

For a discussion of ancient mechanical or technical aids for the disabled, it seems interesting that in Western culture(s) depictions of the human body in analogy to machines, buildings, landscapes and other non-human entities have become commonplace. Also, discourses on impairments and disability have adopted a 'mechanical' understanding of the human body whose malfunctions can be 'fixed' by scientific-technical solutions of all sorts (prostheses, medical aids, technical devices, prenatal diagnosis, genetic screening and engineering, etc.).[11] Understanding of the human body, including ability and disability, is an overtly culturally constructed category that shaped and was shaped by social realities in different cultural contexts and historical periods.[12]

Already in antiquity, human bodies were imagined and perceived in various political, socio-cultural and religious traditions in a very similar way to these modern approaches – either mirroring material entities and domains (i.e., instruments, houses, cities or landscapes)[13] or comparing them to certain socio-political structures (bureaucracy, political bodies),[14] attributing particular tasks or certain functions to specific bodily structures.

However, in many instances the true physicality that lies behind these metaphors is blurred by this very discourse.[15] Some authoritative rabbinic texts, however, do not try to veil this notion of impairment via metaphoric expressions. On the contrary, those passages make the physical aspect quite visible and put it into the focus of the Talmudic discourse on religious obligations.

Prosthetic discourse and Talmudic prostheses

Most prostheses described in those texts seem to have had technical or cosmetic functions as they were either used in case of different mobility impairments or as artificial teeth or eyes. In Talmudic texts, the loss of limbs is described most frequently as caused by accidents and only in rare cases by a deliberate surgical amputation. Detailed descriptions and explanations of several terms for certain physical conditions, of which some would have to necessitate the use of prostheses, can be found in a list of priestly blemishes in the seventh chapter of Mishnah *Bekhorot* ('*Firstlings*'), and in the respective Talmudic elaborations hereof. The discussions are based mainly on the ideal of priestly bodily perfection *vis à vis* the divine, based on the definition in Leviticus 21:16–23. The Mishnah discusses them within the context of an extended list of possible blemishes often referring rather to aesthetic than to functional aspects of a certain impairment.[16]

Prostheses for feet, legs and hands

One example for such a straightforward discourse on impairment, which is later on elaborated into a discussion about the permissibility of walking aids, can be found in the laws concerning the annual pilgrimage in Mishnah Hagiga 1:1:

> All are bound to appear [at the Temple],[17] except for a deaf man (*heresh*), a mentally impaired person (*shote*) and a minor, a person of unknown sex (*tumtum*), a double-sexed person (*androgynos*), women, unfreed slaves, the lame, the blind, the sick, the aged, and one who is unable to go up on foot (*u-mi she-eino yakhol la'a lot be-raglaw*).[18]

Although on the three annual pilgrimage festivals (Pessach/Passover, Shavu'ot, and Sukkot) every Jew is expected to appear at the holy precinct of the Temple in Jerusalem, the main focus of this passage is on a long list of exceptions or exemptions from this general commandment ('all are bound').[19] The last and rather large group of exempted persons is primarily defined by their physical impairments (lameness, blindness, sickness, old age, walking difficulties, etc.) that serve to exempt people from the fulfilment of a religious duty, which is closely linked to the very physicality and physical presence of the worshipper.[20]

As one might notice, although this passage stresses physical impairments such as difficulty walking, many other groups mentioned here do not fit squarely into this category. Thus, the elaboration on this brief passage in the Palestinian Talmud seeks, among several detailed definitions of each group (i.e., who is considered a minor, etc.), to inquire deeper into the logic of exemption from the pilgrimage underlying the ruling in the earlier tradition. Through a comparison with similar or contrary rulings regarding the different groups in biblical and rabbinic traditions, the text tries to support the strict exemption or to include some of the mentioned people in a different way (such as the minor who is obliged).[21] However, in the case of the mobility impaired, the sick and the old, the passage makes use of some biblical verses in order to argue for an exemption: a lame man is exempt because of his inability to walk, a sick man because he cannot rejoice, and an old man because he cannot walk, either. The line of argumentation seems to reflect a tendency to alleviate the duty for some of the impaired, while for many of the non-impaired groups (women, slaves) the strict exclusion is re-enforced via their gender or social status.

While the Mishnah excluded several groups of people based on their bodily and mental impairments as well as their inabilities to fulfil the commandment of a 'walking pilgrimage' proper, the later Palestinian Talmud tried to alleviate the 'burden' of socio-religious exclusion that comes with certain impairments. This ruling is then expanded in the Babylonian Talmud, where the discussion, however, seems to be even more aware of the contradiction between the actual statement that 'all are bound' and the following list of exemptions in the Mishnah. The text provides proof texts from Scripture for excluding certain people, and it emphasises explicitly the importance of the walking impairments in this context as including also those who use wooden prostheses as walking aids:

> R. Tanhum said: One that is **lame in one foot** (sing.: *regel/* חיגר ברגלו אחת) is exempt from appearing [at the Temple], as it is said: *Regalim* [on foot].[22] But this [word] *regalim/raglayim* is [also] **required to exclude people with wooden legs (ba'ale qavin/** לבעלי קבין)! That follows from [the word] *pe'amim* [steps/times] (Exodus 23:17). For it is taught: *pe'amim*, 'pe'amim' means only feet, and thus it is said: *The foot shall tread it down, even the feet of the poor, and the steps of* [Hebr. *Pa'ame ha-oni*] *the needy* (Isaiah 26:6). And it further says: *How beautiful are your feet/steps in sandals* [Hebr. *pe'amayikh*], *O prince's daughter* (Canticles 7:2). What is the meaning of that which is written, [in Cant. 7:2]: "*How beautiful are your feet/steps in sandals, O prince's daughter*"? [The first part means:] How comely are the feet of Israel (*ragleihen shel Yisrael/* רגליהן של ישראל) at the time when **they go up for the [walking] pilgrimage** (*ba-sha'ah she-olin la-regel/* בשעה שעולין לרגל)![23]

In the Palestinian Talmud, the exemption for the lame and the old is interpreted as alleviation or relief for certain groups who are exempt from the obligation. The Babylonian tradition, by contrast, even includes people who are able to walk but do so with the help of prosthetic walking aids, which are not further specified. The explicit exclusion of those using prostheses might be explained by biblical and rabbinic ideas about physical beauty and integrity surrounding the appearance before God in festivals and in the ritualistic realm. So, one can assume that 'the identification of disability in rabbinic thought straddles the line between identities that impair a person's social status and those that impair a person's physical or sensory capacity'.[24]

The ruling in the earlier Mishnah mentions only in general terms the lame (חיגר ברגלו) and 'one who is unable to go up/ascend on foot/on his feet'. Still, the Babylonian Talmud interprets the Hebrew term for festival (*regalim*/ רגלים) as indicating already the prerequisite for participating in it, namely 'on two feet' (the homograph could also be interpreted as a Hebrew dual form for 'feet' or 'legs': *raglayyim*/רגלים). Moreover, this interpretation is linked to a person lacking two natural legs or feet and is, thus, dependent on wooden walking aids (*le-ba'ale qavin*/לבעלי קבין). While this passage on the pilgrimage festivals mentions the prostheses only in passing, other texts provide some details about the actual shape and usage of these devices. In the sixth chapter of tractate Shabbat we find, as mentioned in the following regarding the artificial teeth, an extensive discussion on ornaments and devices that people, especially women, may go out with on Shabbat. Among those items, we find the following:

> An amputee (הקטע) may go out [on Sabbath] with his [wooden] leg/ [hollowed out] prosthesis (*qab*/קב) [since this is considered his shoe]. This is Rabbi Meir's statement, while Rabbi Yosse forbids it.[25] And if it has a receptacle for pads (*beit qibbul ketutin-ketitin*/כתותין -כתותין בית קיבול) it is ritually impure (טמא). One's supports (*semukhot*/סמוכות) are ritually impure as *midras*-impurity (טמאין מדרס; for example, by treading, sitting or leaning), but one may go out with them on the Sabbath, and enter the Temple precinct while wearing them [these are not considered as shoes][26]. One's stool/chair and supports (*kisse u-semukhot*/כסא וסמוכות) are ritually impure as *midras*, and one may not go out with them on the Sabbath, and one may not enter the Temple precinct with them. *Anqatmin* are ritually pure (טהורין), but one may not go out with it [on Sabbath].[27]

This discussion of prosthetic devices for walking impairments appears in the same chapter of Mishnah Shabbat as the teachings about artificial teeth, which will be examined in the following section. In both cases, the rabbinic discussion seems to be triggered by the very action of 'wearing' a prosthesis, which may involve or prompt some other actions (like carrying a prosthesis around or re-adjusting it after it has fallen off). Interestingly, the discussion about the different prostheses shifts quickly to issues of ritual purity.

Since biblical times, Jewish religious lore has applied a clear distinction between states of 'ritual purity' (Hebrew: *tohara*/תהרה) and 'ritual impurity'

(Hebrew: *tum'a*/טומאה) to persons or objects in various contexts. The latter state excludes persons from certain religious duties (prayer/participation in certain rituals) or prohibits objects from the use in religious and other contexts. Moreover, the state of ritual impurity brings about certain restrictions for the social and family life (for example, prohibition of sexual relations during the menstruation period called *niddah*).[28] The return to a state of purity can be achieved by waiting a specific time period and by immersion in a ritual bath (*mikweh*). Impurities might be caused by direct contact with or proximity (under one roof) to a corpse; by contact with unclean (dead) animals; by certain bodily fluids (seminal emission/menstrual blood/fluxes); by child-birth; or by contact with an object or liquid that functions as a source or a carrier of such a state of (ritual) impurity. In contrast to biblical purity law, which is based on a concept of direct conveyance, rabbinic traditions developed the concept of an indirect and attenuated chain or circle of impurity that affects its various links or realms in different ways, and creates hierarchies of impurity. One of these indirect modes of contracting or conveying impurity, mentioned in our source, is called *midras* (literally 'treading'), which works basically through leaning, lying or sitting of a source of impurity on objects or surfaces (e.g., on benches, saddles, carpets, in a boat).[29]

This is the basis for the discussion of five different types or parts of prosthetic devices.[30] First, we find a hollowed-out prosthesis (*qab*), probably made of wood, for the amputee which may have at times some space for pads or rags. This might refer to some kind of peg leg or stilt that was fitted to the shape of the remaining leg or foot. It seems advisable to equip such a hard prosthesis with some kind of rag or pad in order to enhance its wearing comfort.[31] A clear distinction is made between these devices and the so-called 'supports' (*semukhot*). This designation may subsume different types of possibly detachable (leather) supports to cover the stump(s) for one who is missing one or both legs.[32] The text remains vague about the stool or chair and its supports (*kisse u-semukhot*/כסא וסמוכות), which seem to have been used in order to relieve pressure from the legs.[33] The last prosthesis is alluded to in even more nebulous terms using a rare word (*'nqtmyn*/אנקטמין), which is only explained in later Talmudic elaborations.[34]

The Tosefta Shabbat 5:1–2 on this passage adds only some minor details. Regarding the prosthesis with pad-receptacles the text simply allows one to go out, while any prosthesis without a hollowed-out receptacle is forbidden:

> R. Eliezer used to say: As for the prosthesis of an amputee (קב של קיטע) [the rule goes as follows]: If [the prosthetic device] has hollowed out receptacles (*beit qibul ketitin*/בית קבול [כתיתין]), one may go out [with it]. But if not, one is not allowed to go out with it. The stumps [of an

amputated limb] are [considered as] ritually impure (הגדמין טמאין), one may not go out with them.[35]

The Tosefta discusses the aspect of purity or impurity again with regard to the actual stumps of an amputation. The text considers them as ritually impure and one should not go out with them, although in this case there is no aspect of 'carrying' or 'wearing' involved. We cannot but speculate if the prohibition of going out without any prosthetic aids or cover for the stumps was motivated by medical reasoning (for example, the danger of inflammation and injury) or if this was due to a feeling of general discomfort such a pitiable sight would have triggered. It seems that the last comment in the Tosefta rather reiterates the ruling in the Mishnah regarding the prostheses called *'nqtmyn*, as a manuscript witness indicates.[36]

The Talmud Yerushalmi, in Shabbat 8:8, 8c, by contrast, addresses certain obscurities and possible contradictions in the Mishnaic ruling:

> Shmu'el said: One may go out with [a *qab*-prosthesis] since [it serves as a] shoe, and one enters with [it] into the Temple court. R. Yanai points to a difficulty or inconsistency: One goes out with [a *qab*-prosthesis] since [it serves as a] shoe – thus, it is considered a shoe. [However,] when one may enter to the Temple court it is not [considered as] a shoe? Rabbi Ba'a (MS variant: Mana) stated: Instead of pointing to a difficulty in Shmuel's teaching you could [already] point to a difficulty in the Mishnah itself – "His supports (*semukhot*/סמוכות) are ritually impure with *midras*-impurity (indirectly, through pressure), but one may go out with them on the Sabbath, and enter the Temple court while wearing them." R. Mana said: Quote [better] the end [of the Mishnah] where one cannot find any disagreement – "His stool/chair and supports (*kisse u-semukhot*/כסא וסמוכות) are ritually impure as *midras*, and one may not go out with them on the Sabbath, and one may not enter the Temple court with them. *Anqatmin* are rituly pure, and one may not go out with it." What are these *anqatmin* [considered to be] ritually pure? R. Abahu said: *honos qitemin* – [this means] 'donkey handle' (lit. 'ass for the hands' in Aramaic).[37]

The Palestinian tradition starts with an explanation by Shmuel who refers to the third prosthetic device, the supports (*semukhot*), with which one may go out on Shabbat and even enter the Temple court, although they convey the *midras*-impurity. Throughout this discussion, the sages point to the caveats and inconsistency of this ruling and they prefer to deal with the other prosthetic aids for which the Mishnah already stated unambiguous regulations. Moreover, the Talmudic passage provides a multilingual explanation for the devices called *anqatmin*. Abahu first refers to *honos qitemin* using the Greek word '*onos*' for 'ass' or 'donkey' and the Hebrew word for 'lopped limbs' (*qittemin*/קיטמין) – thus forming the meaning 'ass/donkey for a lopped limb'. An Aramaic translation (חמרא ידיי) with a similar meaning follows: 'ass for the hands'/'donkey handle'. We may assume that both designations refer to some type of prosthetic device used by amputees for locomotion. It is open to speculation if this refers to some sort of crutches or rather a kind of glove to support someone without legs. It might also describe a little stool or (wooden) base on which one could 'ride' (as if on a donkey) while moving along on one's hands.[38]

The discussion of the first part of the Mishnah in the Babylonian Talmud commences with a rather complicated and in parts hardly understandable debate about the right attribution of opinions to earlier sages (i.e., was it really R. Meir who permitted and R. Yose who restricted?), which is not of great interest to our discussion. However, regarding the uncleanness of the receptacles of the prosthesis, the Talmudic discussion seeks to determine in greater detail which type of ritual impurity applies, since this detail is not mentioned in the earlier traditions:

> [Mishnah] "And if it has receptacles for pads/hollow spaces for rags (*beit qibul ketitim*/בית קיבול כתיתים), it is subject to ritual impurity".

> [Talmud-Gemara] Abaye said: "It has the ritual impurity of a corpse, but not *midras* impurity". Raba said: "It is ritually impure even as *midras* (lit. 'treaded on'; indirect ritual impurity as if through pressure)". Said Raba: "Whence do I know it? For we have learnt: A child's carriage (*agala shel qatan*/עגלה של קטן) is ritually impure as *midras*". But Abaye said: "There he [the child] leans upon it, but here he [the person with amputated leg(s)] does not lean upon it". Abaye said: "How do I know it? Because it was taught: A walking cane of old men is completely [ritually] pure". And [what may] Raba [have answered]? — "There it is made to facilitate his steps; whereas here it is made to lean on, and he does so".[39]

The Babylonian rabbis debate if the mentioned impurity of a (wooden) prosthesis with pads-receptacles is to be likened to direct 'corpse impurity' or indirect '*midras*-impurity', since both categories effect the contractor of impurity differently regarding grade, time of the actual status and modes of purification. Whereas Abaye bases his conclusion on comparing the prosthetic device to a ritually pure cane providing indirect support to an old person, his interlocutor Raba emphasises the leaning on the prosthesis as being equal to a carriage transporting an infant which is deemed ritually impure. Although the disagreement between the sages seems to be based solely on the actual usage of both technical walking aids – indirect assistance versus full 'leaning' or transportation

– another line of thinking might be implicated here. The distinction may reflect, in fact, the crucial importance of intention and subjectivity invested to an object that determines its susceptibility for becoming impure, as recently discussed in studies by Yair Fürstenberg and Mira Balberg. Balberg has pointed out that the rabbinic impurity/purity discourse perceives the human body as a 'modular mechanism'. As such, certain realms (internal parts, hidden bodily areas), components (hands) or 'appendages' (hair, nails, teeth) can be either physically or conceptually separated or detached from the core-body, which is defined by those '*parts through which the person's bodily self is defined*' or 'that what one is fastidious about'.[40] Accordingly, the cane seems to be regarded by the rabbis as an external tool, which is separable from a person's body. The prosthetic *qav*, however, appears as a part of a person's core-body. Substituting the foot or leg, the prosthesis thus, *becomes* the limb actually missing, since the person invests it with a high degree of subjectivity.

In another tractate of the Babylonian Talmud, one finds some additional aspects of wearing prostheses on certain religious festivals, while also returning to the ambiguities of the rules in the base Mishnah:

> Rami b. Hama raised an objection [against various previous examples of rabbis making for themselves different types of shoe-like footwear, quoting]: 'An amputee may go forth with his artificial foot', according to R. Meir, while R. Jose forbids it (Mishna Shabbat 6:8). Both agree, however, that he must not go forth with it on the Day of Atonement (*Yom ha-Kippurim*). Said Abaye: In this case, the reference is where it [the prosthesis] has pads/receptacles (*ketitin*/ כתיתין), and [the prohibition to go out with them on the Day of Atonement is] due to the comfort (*ta'anug*/ תענוג). Said Raba to him: But if it be no object of wear, would the pads cause it to be one? And, moreover, is any comfort except for that coming from shoes forbidden on the Day of Atonement? Did not Rabbah b. Bar Hunah used to tie a cloth around his legs and go forth? Furthermore, since the conclusion [of that teaching] reads: 'If it [the prosthesis] has receptacles made of pads (כתיתין), it is capable of acquiring ritual uncleanness', it follows that the first portion deals with a prosthesis without such pads (כתיתין)? — Rather, said Raba: In truth, all agree [that an artificial leg] is considered a shoe, but in the case of the Sabbath they differ on the following point: One rabbi holds: we decree [a prohibition lest] it may fall off and cause him to carry it four cubits in a public domain; whereas the other sage holds: we do not decree [any prohibition].[41]

This passage introduces the aspect of comfort or pleasure provided by pads as parts of the wooden device to the Talmudic discussion on prostheses. In order to understand this, one has to consider the context in which these musings are embedded. Specific restrictions apply on the High Holiday of *Yom Kippur* (Day of Atonement), which includes long fasting and a 'poor' attire similar to that during the period of mourning. The preceding discussion scrutinises several kinds of footwear (e.g., sandals made of various materials) with regard to the prohibition of wearing full (leather) shoes on the Day of Atonement. The reference to the non-permissibility of wooden prostheses considered as shoes is made in order to exclude also the aforementioned types of sandals worn by certain rabbinic sages. Abaye, however, specifies that it is not the wood but the soft pads that render the prostheses prohibited. But his interlocutor Rabba takes pains to demonstrate that not comfort or pleasure is forbidden (as exemplified by the soft bandages of Rabba b. Bar Huna) but the wearing of shoes, as which wooden prostheses are perceived in other halakhic teachings.

Also in the context of marriage laws and family relationships, one finds another discussion of two prostheses we already know from the earlier text as well as the mentioning of a new prosthetic device. The discussion pivots on the question which items are acceptable for a valid performance of the *halitzah*-ritual, in which a childless widow refuses to marry her brother-in law in order to have children with him ('levirate marriage'):

> [Mishnah] "But if with a sock it is invalid etc." This then teaches that a sock is not regarded as a shoe; and so it has been also taught: [. . .]

> It has been taught in agreement with Raba: [If a sister-in-law] performed *halitzah* (the ceremonial release from levirate marriage) with a torn shoe which covered the greater part of the [levir's] foot, with a broken sandal which contained the greater part of his foot, with a sandal of cork or of bast, with an artificial foot of the disabled/walking impaired (*be-qab ha-qite'a/*בקב הקיטע), with a felt sock, with a support of the legs/feet (*be-semikhat ha-raglayim/*בסמיכת הרגליים), or with a leather sock, and also where she performed *halitzah* with an adult whether he was standing, sitting or reclining, and also if her *halitzah* was performed with a blind man, her *halitzah* is valid. [. . .] with a broken sandal which does not hold the greater part of his foot, with a support of the hands (*be-semikhat ha-yadayim/*בסמיכת הידיים), or with a cloth sock, and if her *halitzah* was performed with a minor, her *halitzah* is invalid.[42]

Since the *halitzah*-ritual includes the taking off of the woman's shoe (*halitzah* meaning 'to strip, to take off') as a symbolic act, the rabbis discussed which footwear and what materials are deemed permissible for this action.[43] While those devices made for the stump of a leg or a foot (i.e., the hollowed out *qab* and the 'support') are considered to be approved for being in the right place (like the shoe), any 'supports' used for the upper limbs (one's hands) are certainly not allowed.[44] This would point at a line of thinking that elaborates upon notions of the body as a 'modular mechanism' with detachable extensions. On the one hand, it conceptualises the prostheses for legs or feet (and hands/arms) as a kind of 'natural' extension and part of one's body. On the other hand, however, the discussion is fully aware of the artificial aspect of the prosthetic limb, which is 'worn' like a shoe and as such is detachable from the body.

Artificial teeth and eyes

The first sample text is embedded within a larger chapter of the tractate of the Shabbat laws that is concerned with things permitted to be carried in public on Shabbat (Mishnah Shabbat 6:1: 'With what may a woman go out and with what may she not go out?'). The act of carrying would be perceived in several instances as work and, thus, the action would be forbidden. However, rabbinic law knows many contexts in which carrying of certain items in the public domain is allowed, as the following passage shows:

> A woman may go out with braids [made] of hair (*hutei se'ar*/בחוטי שער) whether of her own [hair], or of another woman, or of an animal. [She may go out] with a frontlet [on her forehead] (*totephet*/ובטוטפת), or with bangles (*sanbutin*/ובסנבוטין) if they are sewn [to the cap]; with a cap [under the head-dress] (בכבול) or with a wig (נכריתובפאה) into the courtyard; with wool in her ears (במוך שבאזנה), or with wool in her shoe (ובמוך שבסנדלה), or with wool [rag] she has prepared for [examining] her menstruation (ובמוך שהתקינה לנדתה); or with a pepper (בפלפל), or with a grain [of] salt (ובגרגיר מלח), or with whatever else she [is accustomed to] put in her mouth (ובכל דבר שתתן לתוך פיה), provided she does not first put it [into her mouth] on Shabbat. And if it falls [out of her mouth] she may not replace/return it. [With regard to a] **artificial tooth (*shen totevet*/שן תותבת)** or a **golden tooth (*shen shel zahav*/ושן של זהב)**, Rabbi allows [one to go out/one to replace it?], but the Sages prohibit [it] (רבי מתיר, וחכמים אוסרים).[45]

The fifth Mishnah commences with a statement about braids that are allowed to be 'worn' by women as long as they do not need to be re-adjusted during Shabbat. It follows a sequence about other items worn on the head or the body for ornamental (cap, wig, frontlet, bangles) or pragmatic (wool in the ear or shoe, testing rags for menstrual blood) reasons. After this list, the text mentions two prosthetic devices for one's mouth: an artificial tooth and a tooth made of gold. Although one should refrain from applying modern medical terminology to ancient texts, some material findings allow for describing these devices with terminology understandable to the modern reader. Depending on the actual shape, which is not mentioned, both types of artificial teeth might be compared to several prosthodontic, restorative devices. First, one may understand it as a replacement for missing teeth or parts of them: a crown, a bridge or even an inlay (filling). Second, one could also think of a tooth cap or cover, which is primarily made for temporary use and is only loosely joined or attached to the teeth and gums. As recent studies have shown, most of the artefacts found consist of gold rings, bands and wires used to either anchor loose teeth or to provide a scaffold for dental prostheses. These inserts were sometimes of human origin; most likely the lost teeth of the subject or they may have been taken from the jaw of a deceased person. In some rare instances, animal teeth were also used, while often material such as bones, ivory, stones, metal, or even wood served to re-compensate for a tooth. Artificial teeth made entirely of gold seem to be a rare exception, while the use of gold for caps or crowns with a predominantly cosmetic purpose was more common.[46]

The associative link to the artificial teeth in the Mishnah is built by the reference to 'whatever else [a woman is accustomed] to put in her mouth' mentioning a peppercorn or a grain of salt as examples. In contrast to all preceding items on that list, however, the Mishnah presents two conflicting opinions regarding the artificial teeth. While one sage, Rabbi, takes a lenient stance on the matter, the majority of the rabbis prohibit the use of those prostheses. Since the Mishnah itself offers no explanation whatsoever for either decision, we may speculate about the possible line(s) of argumentation. Rabbi's point seems to be that no one would be interested in removing such a tooth in public because this may be considered an impolite behaviour or not aesthetic at all. Such a behaviour might have been considered indecent. In any case, the risk seems quite high that this small, but presumably costly item could get lost. Recalling the rule regarding other objects in the mouth, the sages on the other hand clearly seem to argue that especially because of the practical, daily usage of these devices for the consumption of food and as a cosmetic prosthesis those teeth might have fallen out of the mouth quite often. The re-adjustment of them would be regarded as forbidden action on Shabbat.[47]

The discussion in the Palestinian Talmud, in tractate Shabbat 6:5, elaborates exactly upon those aspects:

> Rabbi Mana said: "I have heard an explanation [regarding the tooth] from R. Shmuel in the name of R. Ze'ira, but I do not know what I have heard". How can one explain [the issue]? R. Yosse said: "It can be

explained by **a tooth made of gold** (*shen shel zahav*/שן של זהב). With such [a tooth of gold] she is not allowed to go out, since it is very expensive and she could [be tempted to] put it back when it has fallen out [from the mouth]". How is [the rule regarding] a [common] **artificial tooth** (*shen totevet*/שן תותבת)? Also [in this case], she would be too shy to ask the craftsman: "Make me another one!". Thus, when [the artificial tooth] has fallen out, she would most likely put it back [instead of waiting and asking for a replacement].[48]

The opinion voiced by R. Yosse stresses two aspects of the artificial teeth that disqualify them both from being 'worn', most likely for ornamental purposes, on Shabbat. First, the gold tooth is too expensive to get lost. Second, it is suggested that the woman would feel ashamed frequently approaching the craftsman, obviously no dentist, who produces artificial teeth. This procedure seems to have been rather uncomfortable, or even painful. Both arguments are supported by scholarly discussion of surviving dental prostheses. First, all artefacts indicate that artificial teeth were produced mostly for ornamental or cosmetic reasons, since despite their importance for human mastication no inserts for molar teeth were found. Second, findings have proven the accuracy and the elaborate production of the brands, wires and bridges, which were adjusted to the actual caveat of the lost teeth, often achieved by removing the roots and preparing the gums. This procedure, one can imagine, must have been rather painful and time-consuming.[49]

If we compare this explanation in the Western rabbinic tradition of the Yerushalmi with the discussion in the Babylonian Talmud we can notice as a major difference the brief, or rather lapidary, character of the latter:

> [Mishnah] "An artificial tooth, [or] a gold tooth – Rabbi permits but the sages forbid it". [Talmud-Gemara] R. Zera said: They taught this **only of a golden [tooth], but as for a silver [tooth], all agree that it is permitted**. Thus, it was taught: regarding silver [teeth] all agree to permit, [but] as for gold [teeth, only] Rabbi permits but the sages forbid.[50]

The text does not take any pains to reconstruct the arguments possibly underlying the two opinions in the earlier tradition of the Mishnah. In fact, R. Zera just states that the disagreement only pertained to teeth made of gold. As for a prosthetic tooth made of silver (or any other material) all the sages would surely permit the usage ('carrying' or 'wearing') on Shabbat. From this terse statement, it is not entirely clear if R. Zera (and 'all of the sages') allow the silver tooth because it is considerably less expensive or because it was the more common prosthetic device and the sages apply a lenient ruling on the matter.[51]

Be that as it may, we turn our attention to another reference to artificial and golden teeth in an entirely different context. In the Mishnah and both Talmudim on the tractate *Nedarim* ('Vows') we find an anecdote regarding some religious rulings which emphasises the aesthetic or cosmetic dimension inherent to the discourse on tooth implants. The Mishnah, in tractate Nedarim 9: 6–7 and 10, reads as follows:[52]

> [. . .] until Rabbi Akiva came and taught: a vow which is partially released is entirely released. How so? If one says, "*Konam* that I will not benefit from any of you," if one of them was released, they are all released. [. . .]

> "*Konam* that I will not marry that ugly woman (פלונית כעורה)," and she turns out to be beautiful (נאה); "That black-skinned woman," and she turns out to be light-skinned; "That short woman," and she turns out to be tall, he is permitted to marry her; not because she was ugly, and became beautiful, or black and became light-skinned, short and grew tall, but because the vow was in error (אלא שהנדר טעות). And it happened with one who vowed not to benefit (i.e., to marry) his sister's daughter [who was in need/poor].[53] **And she was taken into Rabbi Ishmael's house and they made her beautiful (והכניסוה לבית רבי ישמעאל ויפוה).** Rabbi Ishmael said to him, "My son! Did you vow not to marry his one?" He said, "No," and Rabbi Ishmael permitted her [to him]. In that hour Rabbi Ishmael wept and said, "The daughters of Israel are beautiful, but poverty disfigures them." And when Rabbi Ishmael died, the daughters of Israel raised a lament, saying, "Daughters of Israel weep for Rabbi Ishmael." And thus it is said too of Saul, "Daughters of Israel, weep for Saul" (II Samuel 1:24).[54]

This chapter of the tractate addresses the question of how vows can be released which are normally binding according to biblical rules and require a sometimes-complicated procedure of offerings and other ritual actions to be released. Such a self-imposed restrictive vow is especially delicate if it pertains to family or marital relations. The discussion about vows not to marry a woman with certain anatomical features or traits makes clear that vows cannot be released when the underlying premise has changed in the meantime but if the vow was regarded as having been made in error. In the Mishnah's case, a man vows not to marry his (poor and unattractive) niece – such a marriage was usually a step frequently taken in order to support orphaned girls who could not find a husband. The logic behind this vow seems to have been the destitution of the girl who supposedly was not regarded as a good match and might have not appeared very attractive to her uncle.[55] This is supported by R. Yishmael's complaint that the beauty of Jewish girls is veiled by their poverty. The last point was corrected by an intervention of R. Yishmael who lets her undergo a thorough beauty treatment in order to convince the man to rethink his decision. The Palestinian Talmud, in tractate Nedarim 9; 41c, enquires into the nature of this make-up procedure:

> "[Mishnah:] And thus it happened with one who vowed not to benefit from his sister's daughter. She was taken into R. Yishmael's house and they made her beautiful."

> R. Yishmael asked him: Did you take a vow regarding her? He answered: No! Thus he [R. Yishmael] annulled the man's vow. In the same hour, R. Yishmael started weeping [. . .]. [Talmud/Gemara] Thus, he made her an **[artificial] eye of gold and a tooth of gold** and said to him [the man] as follows: "benefit from what is upon her!"[56]

The version in the Babylonian Talmud, Nedarim 66b, takes a slightly different twist:

> R. Ishmael said: Even if she was ugly and became beautiful, black and turned pale, or short and grew tall. "[Mishnah:] And thus it happened with one who vowed not to benefit from his sister's daughter. She was taken into R. Yishmael's house and they made her beautiful."

> [Gemara/Talmud] A Tanna taught: She **had a [common artificial] false tooth, and R. Ishmael made her a gold tooth** at his own cost (של זהב שן משלו שן תותבת היתה לה ועשה לה רבי ישמעאל של זהב). 'When R. Ishmael died, a professional mourner commenced [the funeral eulogy] thus: "*You daughters of Israel, weep over R. Ishmael, who clothed you* etc".[57]

In these Talmudic discussions, one can see clearly the same line of thinking. The 'ugliness' of the girl is not understood metaphorically as being directly linked to her economic situation, i.e., not being regarded a 'good match', but is interpreted literally. According to the Palestinian tradition, R. Yishmael equipped her with an artificial eye and tooth made of gold as an adornment increasing her attractiveness. By contrast, the Babylonian Talmud reports that she already had a standard artificial tooth (probably made of wood) which was apparently not very appealing and R. Yishmael made her a golden one to make her more attractive for her future husband.[58] Both anecdotes support our previous observation and match also with Bliquez's interpretation of the material findings. The use of artificial dental and ocular prosthetics, especially if made of gold, was rather for ornamental than for functional purposes.

In terms of a rather clear gender bias it is, however, striking that in these narratives of 'prosthetic enabling' the trigger is not a discussion about the participation of women in religious duties. Rather, all accounts highlight the importance of beauty and the sheer adornment for the purpose of marriage. On the one hand, we should notice that the beautifying of the girl is initiated and authorised, in the context of vows, by a male rabbi in order to attract another male Jew to marry her. On the other hand, the procedure of this 'make-over' can be seen as enabling the girl to become a full member of Jewish society, albeit within the limits of her role as wife and mother as defined by a predominantly male, rabbinic discourse.[59]

Conclusion

In light of the previously discussed findings, one cannot but notice the very peculiar nature of the discourse on prostheses in Talmudic texts. Certainly, the rabbinic traditions mention technical aids for specific impairments only in passing. Already the earliest tradition of the Mishnah from the third century CE discusses walking aids and other types of prosthesis as entirely embedded within everyday culture. They seem to have been used by people with different mobility impairments, mainly due to congenital deformation or amputations of feet, legs or arms. However, these passages tell us hardly anything about the medical necessities involved or the surgical procedures applied. Moreover, relevant terms such as *qav ha-kite'a* (literally 'cavity of the amputee'), *beit qibbul ketutin/ketitin* (receptacles for pads), *samokhot/semukhot* (literally 'supports'), *kisse* (chair/stool), *anqatmin*, or artificial teeth and eyes are introduced and used in different discursive context throughout the Talmudic corpus. Still, one cannot learn much from these texts about the actual materials, production and producers of these prostheses. The discussions about them are mostly confined to permission or prohibition of usage on certain occasions (pilgrimage holidays, days of fasting and Shabbat), in a certain status (ritual impurity) or in different religious realms (Temple court/ritual of *halitza*). Those Talmudic elaborations stick quite tenaciously to their respective halakhic context with overtly technical discussions, while attesting to a familiarity of the sages with prosthetic devices of various kinds.

Despite the scanty sources, one may try to discern some of the ideas and discursive structures that surface in most of the discussed examples. We can observe often a twofold discursive strategy that is applied in discussions on impairments and prosthetic aids. These Talmudic discussions are simultaneously similar to and different from what has been described for biblical accounts by Rebecca Raphael as 'narrative prosthesis', based on modern literary studies by Snyder and Mitchell. Raphael summarises this approach as follows: 'the disabled character introduces the anomaly that sets the plot in motion, and the narrative then uses elimination of the disability, or of the disabled character, for resolution'.[60]

In order to be more precise, one has to slightly appropriate this idea for the topic under discussion here. Also, Talmudic texts use the impairment and prosthetic devices or procedures as a trigger for their Halakhic discussions. In many instances, this discursive representation and integration of prostheses makes them disappear, since they become just another item among many others in a long rabbinic discussion on Shabbat laws, purity issues or ritual aspects. However, one may indeed find two levels of 'discursive prosthetics' which help to enable the actual or allegedly disabled persons.

First, one finds the technical level of the prosthetic discourse. Here, we find the permission of wearing certain prostheses in several contexts (Shabbat/ Holidays/Temple court, etc.) and for various purposes (for example, the *halitzah*-ritual, or the pilgrimage to Jerusalem on the festivals). Although the details and description provided for those devices are limited, one gets a glimpse into a variety of prosthetic aids made of different materials for impairments of different kinds and degrees (teeth, hands, feet, legs, etc.).

Second, we can discern also a certain kind of discursive rehabilitation or relief of some of the people deemed otherwise disabled and excluded. This is in most cases accomplished through a minute discussion of all relevant details and the creation of exceptional cases. For example, the Palestinian Talmud assumes a person on wooden legs is considered as 'one unable to ascend'. While this discussion clearly broadens the number of people affected by the original category of exclusion, the discourse seems to aim at actually relieving the 'burden' of a commandment from someone who seems incapable of fulfilling it. In other religious contexts, we encounter the permissibility of prostheses for some ritual performances (e.g., *halitzah*) or in certain spatial or temporal frameworks (i.e., the question of impurity of prostheses in the Temple precinct, or the usage of such devices on Shabbat).

In both cases, the actual disability and the physical marker of it, namely the prosthetic device, function as the trigger for a rabbinic discussion that at times appears even theoretical or scholastic – prostheses are good to think with. However, through the Talmudic discussion the specific impairment and the prosthetic aids tend to disappear, either by an 'exclusion as relief' or through an inclusion of such prosthetic usage into the socio-religious world as one feature among others. On the one hand, we can certainly understand these Talmudic strategies as an inclusive approach of easing or erasing a burden of bodily imperfection. However, on the other hand, both the exclusion of certain persons, be it motivated by compassion or not, as well as the pattern of 'repair', focusing on attempts to correct or to rehabilitate the disabled, always remain workarounds in face of the grave physicality of many impairments and limited technical means in ancient times.

Notes

1 I am grateful to Dr Jane Draycott for inviting me to the 2015 workshop at the University of Wales Trinity Saint David, and for her meticulous editorial work and her helpful remarks on my chapter and on the volume as a whole. I also thank the anonymous reviewers whose comments and suggestions helped me to reshape some parts of my study. My research on this subject is funded by the German Research Foundation (DFG). Since 2013 I have been working on rabbinic knowledge of medicine and the body within the Collaborative Research Center SFB 980 'Episteme in Motion' at Freie Universität Berlin as part of the research project A03 'The Transfer of Medical Episteme in the "Encyclopaedic" Compilations of Late Antiquity'. I am indebted to the heads of project Prof. Markham J. Geller and Prof. Philip J. van der Eijk as well as to the whole A03-team, to my colleagues working on the ERC-funded project BabMed and the many colleagues at the CRC/SFB 980 for being always supportive and available for an inspiring exchange of thoughts. I worked on the final revision of this chapter as a Harry-Starr-Fellow in Judaica at Harvard University. I have benefited much from the resources available at Widener Library and from my conversations with faculty and co-fellows. Finally, I owe special thanks to Prof. Julia Watts Belser who has become an invaluable interlocutor regarding disability studies and rabbinic literature.
2 On Egyptian and Babylonian artefacts and depictions, see Reeves, 1999; Nerlich *et al.*, 2000; Dupras *et al.*, 2010; Blomstedt, 2014. For a positivistic approach to Graeco-Roman prostheses, see von Brunn, 1926; Fliegel and Feuer, 1966; Thurston, 2007. Those views have been re-evaluated by Bliquez, 1996 and most recently by Turfa and Becker, 2017.
3 I refer here to the ideas elaborated upon by Ilan, 2015.
4 Bliquez, 1996; Turfa and Becker, 2017, especially pp. 13–82.
5 For further studies and methodological aspects, see Miller, 2015; Fine, 2006 and 2014; Goodman, 1994; Hezser, 2010; Geller, 2015.
6 I will provide in the following a reference to the rabbinic texts, their source (print or manuscript) and the original texts in Hebrew/Aramaic. Unless indicated differently, the translations are my own, based at times and in parts on common translations in the Soncino or the Steinsaltz editions of the Babylonian Talmud. Stemberger, 1996 may serve as a thorough introduction to rabbinic literature. For the study of the Babylonian Talmud, see Friedman, 2010; Halivni, 2013; Vidas, 2014.
7 Moreover, the rabbinic movement in Late Antiquity is no longer understood as a uniform socio-religious and political elite exercising control over all Jews. Rather, scholars suggest a co-existence of rabbinic groups with other branches within a multifaceted Judaism. For different positions on this topic, see Hezser, 1997; Miller, 2006; Schwartz, 2007; Gafni, 2011; Lapin, 2012.
8 The *Sefer ha-refu'ot* ('Book of remedies'), attributed to a certain Asaph, is the first exclusively medical text in Hebrew and originated between the seventh and the ninth centuries CE, most likely in the Persian sphere rather than in the Byzantine West. On this work and its multiple sources in Greek, Persian, Indian and ancient Mesopotamian medical traditions, see Muntner, 1951; Lieber, 1984; Newmyer, 1992.
9 Most likely, the rabbis were not trained physicians but acquired their knowledge in different contexts and from various informants. Thus, the Talmud cannot be read either like the Hippocratic corpus or like Gray's Anatomy, since its medical information is deeply entrenched in the overarching Talmudic discourses. Geller, 2000 and 2004, Lehmhaus, 2015; Lehmhaus *et al.*, 2016.
10 At times, one can find explanations regarding the origins of certain disabilities, including some forms of teratology that try to systematise and explain congenital impairments. Talmudic traditions frequently explored such issues in further detail

with regard to Halakhic discussion on purity, marriage and family laws, or ritual fitness, while being aware of how disabilities affect the socio-religious life of these individuals *vis à vis* their community. For a more thorough discussion of the rabbinic discourse on disability, see Abrams, 1998, and most recently Belser and Lehmhaus, 2016. On the health care system in ancient Israel, see Avalos, 1995; Zucconi, 2010. On ancient Graeco-Roman ideas about disabilities, see Rose, 2003; Laes *et al.*, 2013.

11   The dominance of a 'technical' understanding holds true for specialised discourses but also for everyday language, when the heart is envisioned as the engine, the brain as the computer with sensorial experiences or cognition as its 'software'; or the limbs are depicted as 'tools' for certain work. See Seltzer, 1992; Morus, 2002; Johnson, 2007; Black, 2016; Bridgman, 1939; Budd, 2007. Another conception of the human body is strongly linked to spatial experiences. These approaches include techniques of mapping or projecting a body-landscape as well as ideas of the body as a house. See for example Nas and Brakus, 2004, pp. 27–56; Broome, 2007; Olwig, 2002; Davies, 2000.

12   See Wills, 1995. For disability in Jewish culture, see Abrams, 1998; Marx, 2001; Olyan, 2008.

13   For ancient Mesopotamian culture, scholars have pointed to interesting repre-sentations of the intestines as rivers and channels (in accordance with the landscape of ancient Babylonia and its sophisticated irrigation systems). These traditions also describe the female body, especially the reproductive organs, in analogy to buildings, landscapes or to some kind of container or vessel. An Old Babylonian belly incantation (CT 4, 8a), thus, reads: 'The sick belly is closed up like a basket, like the waters of a river it does not know where it should go, it has no flow like water of a well, its orifice is covered like (that of) a fermenting vat, no food and drink can enter it'. See also Steinert, 2013 and 2017.

14   For ancient Chinese medicine in comparison with Western (Greek) medical thought, Paul Unschuld has analysed how concepts of the body, especially anatomy and physiology, are based on the socio-political formations in their respective societies of origin. It is intriguing for our discussion that the Chinese medical discourse refers to the body and its parts as if they were forming a system of political administration, in which the organs and limbs serve as bureaucratic officials within a well-structured hierarchy. See Unschuld, 2009.

15   Some texts in biblical and later Jewish traditions dealing with certain impairments seem to confine to this concealing pattern. Discourses of blindness frequently revolve around metaphors of light and a compensatory perfection of all other senses, as noted by Abrams, 1998; Olyan, 2008; Gracer, 2003; Avalos *et al.*, 2007. Other rabbinic texts, in ways similar to ancient Mesopotamian traditions, depict the woman's body as a house with the womb as the most inner chambers mirroring the cultural confinements of the religious and social female sphere and space. See Fonrobert, 2000, especially pp. 40–67; Baker, 2002; Bordo, 2003, especially pp. 1–97.

16   See Rosen-Zvi, 2005/6; Belser, 2011 and 2015. This list of priestly blemishes, while making at times use of medical knowledge to clarify the biblical categories, includes also temporary impairments like *shever regel* ('a broken leg'), but mostly refers to different types of bodily blemishes, such as *pisseach* ('the limping'), one whose foot is either hollow, crooked or crescent-shaped; *qashan/qishan* (X- or O-legs), *iqal/iqlan* (distortion or contortion of the lower leg); *qulbon/qalban/qilban* (see Bek 45a; uncertain, possibly distorted or lopped thighs or legs); *ba'al ha-piqon/ha-piqa* is according to the Talmud someone who has lots of *qetzatzot* (possibly doubling of the knuckles/ankles, distinct amounts of subcutaneous fat); also all types of adhesion of fingers and toes; distortion or imbrications of toes (*murkabot*); any excess of limbs (fingers/toes). See the discussion in Babyonian

Talmud Bekhorot 45b. The catalogue in the Mishnah also mentions several uncommon appearances of the head, such as the *qilon* (wide below, pointed at the top); *liphtan* (wide at the top, pointed below); *maqaban/maqban* (head of malleus; i.e., 'hammerhead'); a bowed head (possibly adhesion between head and chest, or *seqipas/sheqiphas* (missing parts on the back part of the head/occiput; or a hunchbacked person), often combined with *aqmut* (like cyphosis or scoliosis, see BT Sanhedrin 91a); *ba'al ha-chatarot/ha-choteret* (literally 'the humped', possibly referring to some bulges of meat or skin in the neck). See Tosefta Bekhorot 5:2; Bab. Talmud Bekhorot 43b. For a kind of retrospective diagnosis approach to this list, see Preuss, 1992, pp. 237–270. Compare with Preuss, 1978; Wyszinski, 2001. Moreover, Talmudic texts report of other severe physical impairments, especially the ones related to a person's sexual organs. These injuries are either tied to accidents or were described as being congenital. See also Belser and Lehmhaus, 2016, pp. 443f. For other passages, see the references in Rosner, 2000, pp. 16–17.

17 Rabbinic texts as works that were crafted within a network of learned experts tend to use frequently an elliptic style and lots of abbreviations and technical terms. Thus, in this passage, as in all following passages, I will use square brackets to mark my own additions to the original text, which make the passages legible and understandable by providing information about the context, the actual speaker or the sources cited. Quotations from the Bible are marked by the use of italics and the respective reference is given in brackets following the quoted verse.

18 Mishnah Hagigah 1:1: הכל חייבין בראיה חוץ מחרש שוטה וקטן וטומטום ואנדרוגינוס ונשים ועבדים שאינם משוחררים החיגר והסומא והחולה והזקן ומי שאינו יכול לעלות ברגליו.

19 We find a frequently used triad of someone with hearing impairments (Heresh/ חרש), a mentally impaired person (*shote*/שוטה), and a minor (*qatan*/קטן). The following group of the person of unknown or undefined sex (*tumtum*/טומטום), the double-sexed (*androgynos*/אנדרוגינס) and women are excluded because of their obvious or uncertain sexual nature: none of them can be straightforwardly defined as male. See Lev, 2007 and 2010; Levinson, 2000. The slave is not allowed because of his social status. See Hezser, 2002.

20 See also Belser and Lehmhaus, 2016, p. 436, discussing Abrams, 1998.

21 Yerushalmi Hagiga 1:1, 76a: 'Our Mishnah has taught [this regarding the duty to] appear for an offering. [. . .] [Mishnah] "Except for the lame". As it is written: *walking pilgrimage/regalim* (Ex. 23:14). "Except for the sick". As it is written: *And you shall rejoice (Deut. 16:11).* "Except for the old". As it is written: *walking pilgrimage (Ex. 23:14).* R. Yosse said: Both [verses] are for alleviating [the duty of participation]. If one can rejoice, but is unable to walk, I will say: *walking pilgrimage* [and, thus, free him from the duty]. If one can walk, but cannot rejoice, I will say: *And you shall rejoice* [and, thus, free him from the duty]'.

22 The dual form [two] *legs/raglayim* is a homograph to a plural form with a slightly different meaning, i.e., *regalim* = walking *pilgrimage*.

23 Babylonian Talmud Chagiga 3a (Vilna edition/print): אמר רבי תנחום חיגר ברגלו אחת פטור. מן הראיה שנאמר רגלים והא רגלים מבעי ליה פרט לבעלי קבין ההוא מפעמים נפקא דתניא פעמים אין פעמים אלא רגלים וכן הוא אומר {ישעיהו כ"ו} תרמסנה רגל רגלי עני פעמי דלים ואומר {שיר השירים ז'} מה יפו פעמיך בנעלים בת נדיב דרש רבא מאי דכתיב מה יפו פעמיך בנעלים בת נדיב כמה נאין רגליהן של ישראל בשעה שעולין לרגל.

24 Belser and Lehmhaus, 2016, p. 438.

25 See MS Parma Biblioteca palatina De Rossi 138 (Cod. Parm. 3173), in which the first teaching is attributed to R. Yosse, while R. Meir states the stricter ruling.

26 The fragment New York – JTS ENA 2946.12 reads: 'one may go out with them on the Sabbath but one may not enter the Temple court while wearing them'. The ruling about the stool/chair and supports (*kisse wu-semukhot*/כסא וסמוכות) does not appear in this text.

27   Mishnah Shabbat 6:8: הקיטע יוצא בקב שלו דברי ר"מ ורבי יוסי אוסר ואם יש לו בית קיבול כתותים
טמא סמוכות שלו טמאין מדרס ויוצאין בהן בשבת ונכנסין בהן בעזרה כסא וסמוכות שלו טמאין מדרס
ואין יוצאין בהם בשבת ואין נכנסין בהן בעזרה אנקטמין טהורין ואין יוצאין בהן.

28   For some comprehensive explanations on the *niddah*-state of impurity and Jewish
laws regarding the menstruating woman, see Meacham, 1999; Fonrobert, 2000.

29   While direct contact by touch is the most common and intelligible form of transmitting impurity, rabbinic traditions also know indirect transmission by carriage
or 'shift' (i.e., moving or being moved by the source of impurity). In the later
rabbinic discourse, this maximal indirect mode of transferring impurity through
midras is elaborated into complicated discussions about pressure, weight and
time-spans of contacts. See Kazen, 2013, pp. 140–174; Balberg, 2014, pp. 17–47,
53–56.

30   See the references in Rosner, 2000, p. 258.

31   Usually scholars explain the issue of impurity regarding this prosthetic device as
follows: a wooden item is susceptible to impurity only when it has receptacles for
other objects, which are carried, thus, by the prosthesis. If a log is merely hollowed
out for the stump, it is not a receptacle in this sense.

32   Later Mishnah commentaries *ad loc.*, like the one by Obadiah ben Abraham
Bartenura (Venice, 1549), usually explain the *smukhot* as a leather cover for the
stumps of both legs.

33   The medieval commentator Rashi *ad loc.* explained that this refers to one who is
unable to walk on supports (*semukhot*) alone, since the muscles of the lower leg
were paralysed or simply not strong enough. A stool is made for such a person,
and also supports for the stumps, and one lifts and moves along by using the hands
and possibly also a little bit the feet, too. Bartenura *ad loc.*, obviously from an early
modern perspective, describes this device as used by people whose remaining limbs
are formed back and of reduced size so that one is unable to use one of the other
prostheses. In this case, a small chair or stool is fixed to a person's back who lifts
the body and moves along by using small (wooden) benches as 'supports', in a
way similar to crutches.

34   The fragment New York – JTS ENA 2946.12 has the variant spelling: *'nqtwmyn*[0]
/*anqatumin*/ אנקטומין. In MS Parma Biblioteca palatina De Rossi 138 (Cod. Parm.
3173) this term is vocalised as *'anaqtamin'*.

35   Tosefta Shabbat 5:1–2 (Edition Lieberman): ר' לעזר אומ' קב של קיטע אם יש בו בית קבול
כתיתין יוצאין בו ואם לאו אין יוצאין בו. הגדמין טמאין אין יוצאין בהן.

36   The text in Berlin – Staatsbibliothek (Preussischer Kulturbesitz) Ms. or. fol. 1220 reads
instead: 'the *nqtmyn* are ritually impure, one may not go out with them (הנקטמין
טמאין ואין יוצאין בהן').

37   Talmud Yerushalmi, in Shabbat 8:8, 8c (Venice edition/print): שמואל אמר יוצאין בו משום
סנדל ונכנסין בו לעזרה רבי ינאי מקשה יוצאין בו משום סנדל והוא סנדל נכנסין בו לעזרה ואינו סנדל
אמר רבי בעא עד די הוות מקשה לה על די לשמואל קשייתה על דמתניתין סמוכות שלו טמאין מדרס יוצאין
שלו טמאין 'בהן בשבת ונכנסין בהן בעזרה א"ר מנא אמור סופה דלית היא פליגא על דשמואל כסא סמוכו
מדרס אין יוצאין בהן בשבת ואין נכנסין בהן לעזרה אנקטמין טהורין ויוצאין בהן מהו אנקטמין טהורין
א"ר אבהו הונם קטמין חמרא דיי'.

38   See previous note. The reference to an 'ass on one's shoulder' (possibly a donkey
figure or mask) in Krauss, *Lehnwörter*, 224, *id.*, *Talmudische Archäologie* II, note 118
and III, 106 appears to be rather misleading. It might have been inspired by the
rather irritating guesses of some Babylonian rabbis cited in the Babylonian Talmud
Shabbat 66b (Vilna edition/print): "[Mishnah] *lwqtmyn* are (ritually clean). – What
is *lwqtmyn*? – Said R. Abbahu: a 'donkey on the shoulder'. Raba b. Papa said: stilts.
Raba son of R. Huna said: a mask." (לוקטמין טהורין. מאי לוקטמין? אמר רבי אבהו: חמרא
דאכפא.) Maimonides *ad loc.* describes רבא בר בר פפא אמר: קשירי. רבא בר רב הונא אמר: פרמי
the *anqatmin*, however, as similar to a shoe that does not contract *midras*-impurity.
In general, he sticks to the restrictive ruling by R. Yosse in the Mishnah.

39 Babylonian Talmud Shabbat 66a–b (Vilna edition/print): ‏ואם יש לו בית קיבול כתיתין טמא.‏
‏אמר אביי: טמא טומאת מת, ואין טמא מדרס. רבא אמר: אף טמא מדרס. אמר רבא: מנא אמינא לה -‏
‏דתנן: עגלה של קטן טמאה מדרס. ואביי אמר: התם - סמיך עילויה, הכא - לא סמיך עילויה. אמר אביי:‏
‏מנא אמינא לה - דתניא: מקל של זקנים - טהור מכלום. ורבא? – התם לתרוצי סוגיא עבידא, הכא -‏
‏לסמוך עילויה הוא דעבידא, וסמיך עליה.‏

40 Balberg, 2014, p. 72 (emphasis in the original text). For the whole concept of the human body and the importance of intentionality and the self, see Balberg, 2014, especially pp. 58–73 and 148–179; Fürstenberg, 2015.

41 Babylonian Talmud Yoma 78b (Vilna edition/print): ‏הקיטע יוצא בקב.‏ ‏מתיב רמי בר חמא:‏
‏שלו, דברי רבי מאיר. ורבי יוסי אוסר. ותני עלה: ושוין שאסור לצאת בו ביום הכפורים! אמר אביי: התם‏
‏דאית ביה כתיתין, ומשום תענוג. אמר ליה רבא: ואי לאו מנא הוא - כתיתין משוי ליה מנא? ועוד: כל‏
‏תענוג דלאו מנעל הוא, ביום הכפורים מי אסור? והא רבה בר רב הונא הוה כריך סודרא אכרעיה ונפיק.‏
‏ועוד: מדקתני סיפא אם יש לו בית קבול כתיתין טמא, מכלל דרישא לאו בדאית ליה כתיתין עסקינן! אלא‏
‏אמר רבא: לעולם דכולי עלמא מנעל הוא, ובשבת בהא פליגי; מר סבר: גזרינן דילמא משתמיט ואתי‏
‏לאתויי ארבע אמות, ומר סבר: לא גזרינן.‏

42 Babylonian Talmud Yebamot 102b–103a (Vilna edition/print): ‏חלצה‏ ‏תניא כוותיה דרבא:‏
‏במנעל הנפרם שחופה את רוב הרגל, בסנדל הנפחת שמקבל את רוב הרגל, בסנדל של שעם ושל סיב,‏
‏בקב הקיטע, במוק, בסמיכת הרגלים, באנפיליא של עור, והחולצת מן הגדול בין עומד בין יושב בין מוטה,‏
‏והחולצת מן הסומא - חליצתה כשרה; אבל במנעל הנפרם שאין חופה את רוב הרגל, בסנדל הנפחת שאינו‏
‏מקבל את רוב הרגל, ובסמיכת הידים, ובאנפיליא של בגד, וחולצת מן הקטן - חליצתה פסולה.‏

43 In the following, this Talmudic passage discusses the material qualities of the permissible prosthesis, which should be covered by leather in order to resemble a proper shoe. See also Babylonian Talmjud Yebamot 103a:
   "Whose [opinion is reflected in the first teaching regarding] the prosthesis? [The opinion of] R. Meir, for we learned [in the Mishnah]: 'An amputee may go out [on Sabbath] with a [wooden] leg/[hollowed out] prosthesis; according to R. Meir, but R. Jose forbids it'. So [the latter teaching]: 'with a cloth-sock' represents the view of the sages. Abaye answered: Since the latter teaching [represents the opinion of] the sages, the first also [must represent the opinion of] the sages; the first [then refers to a prosthesis] covered with leather. Said Raba to him: What, however, [if it was] not covered with leather? Is it then unfit? If it is so, instead of teaching in the latter statement, 'With a cloth sock', a distinction should have been drawn [regarding the prosthesis resembling a shoe]: only where it was covered with leather it is permissible, but if it was not covered with leather it is unfit!"

44 See also Babylonian Talmud, Shabbat 66b: [Mishnah] "One's stool/chair and supports (*kisse u-semukhot*/‏כסא וסמוכות‏) are ritually impure as *midras*, and one may not go out with them on the Sabbath, and one may not enter the Temple precinct with them." [Talmud/Gemara] A reciter (tanna) recited before R. Johanan: "One may enter the Temple precinct with them". Said to him: "I learn: a woman can perform *halizah* therewith [as if it is a shoe] – nevertheless you say [that] they may enter [the Temple precinct, which is forbidden with shoes]! Recite [now rather): One may not enter the Temple court with them".

45 Mishnah Shabbat 6:5: ‏יוצאה אשה בחוטי שער בין משלה בין משל חברתה בין משל בהמה‏, ‏ובטוטפת, ובסנבוטין בזמן שהן תפורין, בכבול ובפאה נכרית לחצר, במוך שבאזנה, ובמוך שבסנדלה, ובמוך שהתקינה לנדתה, בפלפל, ובגרגיר מלח, ובכל דבר שתתן לתוך פיה, ובלבד שלא תתן לכתחלה בשבת. ואם נפל, לא תחזיר. שן תותבת ושן של זהב - רבי מתיר, וחכמים אוסרים.‏
   For all references discussed in the following, see Rosner, 2000, p. 31.

46 See Bliquez, 1996; and most recently Turfa and Becker, 2017.

47 Preuss, 1911, pp. 332–333.

48 Palestinian Talmud Shabbat 6,5 (Vilna edition): ‏א"ר מנא שמעית טעם מן ר' שמואל בשם ר'‏
‏ועירא ולא אנא ידע מה שמעית. מיי כדון. אמר רבי יוסי מסתברא בשן של זהב שעמדה לה ביוקר לא‏
‏תצא די נפלה ומחזרה ליה. שן תותבת מה אית לך. עוד היא מבהתתה מימור לנגרא עבד לי חורי היא נפלה‏
‏ליה ומחזרה ליה.‏

120   *Lennart Lehmhaus*

49 Bliquez, 1996.

50 Babylonian Talmud Shabbat 65a (Vilna edition/print): שן תותבת שן של זהב רבי מתיר
    וחכמים אוסרין: אמר רבי זירא לא שנו אלא של זהב אבל בשל כסף דברי הכל מותר תניא נמי הכי בשל
    כסף דברי הכל מותר של זהב רבי מתיר וחכמים אוסרין.

51 The medieval commentary of Rashi (eleventh century CE, France) argues that a
    gold tooth was precious. Thus, the woman may take it out of her mouth for
    display, and meanwhile carry it in the street, while this does not apply to a silver
    tooth.

52 Mishnah Nedarim 9:6–7 and 10: פותחין בימים טובים ובשבתות בראשונה היו אומרים אותן הימים
    מותרין ושאר כל הימים אסורין עד שבא רבי עקיבא ולימד שהנדר שהותר מקצתו הותר כולו . כיצד אמר
    קונם שאיני נהנה לכולכם הותר אחד מהן הותרו כולן (..) קונם שאיני נושא את פלונית כעורה והרי היא
    נאה שחורה והרי היא לבנה קצרה והרי היא ארוכה מותר בה לא מפני שהיא כעורה ונעשית נאה שחורה
    ונעשית לבנה קצרה ונעשית ארוכה אלא שהנדר טעות ומעשה באחד שנדר מבת אחותו הנייה\עניה
    והכניסוה לבית רבי ישמעאל ויפוה אמר לו רבי ישמעאל בני לזו נדרת אמר לו לאו והתירו רבי ישמעאל
    באותה שעה בכה רבי ישמעאל ואמר בנות ישראל נאות הן אלא שהעניות מנוולתן וכשמת רבי ישמעאל
    היו בנות ישראל נושאות קינה ואומרות בנות ישראל אל רבי ישמעאל בכינה וכן הוא אומר בשאול: בנות
    ישראל אל שאול בכינה (שמואל ב' א') .

53 The manuscript commonly regarded as the earliest and best textual witness (MS
    Kaufmann) reads: הניה /*hanayah* = benefit, while other variants provide the reading
    as עניה /*oniyah* = poor/needy. The latter actually might be influenced already by
    the statement of R. Yishmael that 'poverty disfigures the daughters of Israel'.

54 The choice of the biblical proof text to support the anecdote is only compelling,
    if one knows also the second half of the verse not cited here: 'Daughters of Israel,
    weep for Saul, who clothed you in scarlet and finery, who adorned your garments
    with ornaments of gold'.

55 Note the list of blemishes or defects of a future husband in case of which a woman
    is allowed to ask for divorce in Mishnah Kettuboth 7:9–10.

56 Palestinian Talmud/Yerushalmi Nedarim 9,8 (41c) (Venice edition/print): קונם שאיני?
    וכשמת עשה לה עין של זהב שן של זהב בלשון הזה אמר לו זכה במה שעליה נושא את פלנית כעורה כו
    'כתיב בנות ישראל על שאול בכינה וגו 'רבי ישמעאל כו

57 Babylonian Talmud Nedarim 66a–b (Vilna edition/print): מעשה לסתור חסורי מחסרא והכי:
    קתני ר' ישמעאל אומר אפילו כעורה נאה שחורה ונעשת ונעשת לבנה קצרה ונעשת ארוכה מעשה באחד
    שנדר מבת אחותו והכניסוה לבית ר' ישמעאל ויפוה וכו. תנא שן תותבת היתה לה ועשה לה ר' ישמעאל
    שן של זהב משלו כי שכיב רבי ישמעאל פתח עליה ההוא ספדנא הכי בנות ישראל על ר' ישמעאל בכינה
    ' מלבישכן וכו.

58 While this is the common explanation in medieval commentaries to the Talmud
    like Rashi, the text does not address the 'ugliness' of the common dentures expli-
    citly.

59 On the ambiguous approach of the rabbis to female beauty as desirable and
    dangerous for men, see Ilan, 1997, pp. 174–183; and Ilan, 2006, especially
    pp. 200–213. For women's beauty as causing distraction and destruction in a man's
    life, see in addition Palestinian Talmud Avoda Zara 2,2 (40d); ibid Sanhedrin 10,2
    (28d).

60 See in general, Raphael, 2008; for the quote, see p. 53 (with a reference to
    Mitchell and Snyder, 2000, pp. 53–54). For a similar strategy and the biblical figure
    of the suffering servant, see Schipper, 2001.

Bibliography

Abrams, J. (1998) *Judaism and Disability: Portrayals in Ancient Texts from the Tanach
through the Bavli*. Washington, DC: Gallaudet University Press.

Avalos, H. (1995) *Illness and Health Care in the Ancient Near East: The Role of the Temple
in Greece, Mesopotamia, and Israel*. Atlanta, GA: Scholars Press.

Avalos, H., Melcher, S. J. and Schipper, J. (2007) *This Abled Body: Rethinking Disabilities in Biblical Studies*. Atlanta, GA: Society of Biblical Literature.

Baker, C. (2002) *Re-building the House of Israel. Architectures of Gender in Jewish Antiquity*. Stanford, CA: Stanford University Press.

Balberg, M. (2014) *Purity, Body, and Self in Early Rabbinic Literature*. Berkeley, CA: University of California Press.

Becker, M. J. and Turfa, J. M. (2017) *The Etruscans and the History of Dentistry: The Golden Smile through the Ages*. Abingdon and New York, NY: Routledge.

Belser, J. W. (2011) 'Reading Talmudic Bodies: Disability, Narrative, and the Gaze in Rabbinic Judaism', in Schumm, D. and Stolzfus, M. (edd.) *Disability in Judaism, Christianity and Islam: Sacred Texts, Historical Traditions and Social Analysis*. New York, NY: Palgrave Macmillan, pp. 5–27.

Belser, J. W. (2016) 'Brides and Blemishes: Queering Women's Disability in Rabbinic Marriage Law', *Journal of the American Academy of Religion* 84.2, pp. 401–429.

Belser, J. W. and Lehmhaus, L. (2016). 'Disability in Rabbinic Traditions', in Laes, C. (ed.) *Disability in Antiquity*. Abingdon and New York, NY: Routledge, pp. 434–451.

Black, D. (2016) *Embodiment and Mechanisation: Reciprocal Understandings of Body and Machine from the Renaissance to the Present*. London and New York, NY: Routledge.

Bliquez, L. (1996) 'Prosthetics in Classical Antiquity: Greek, Etruscan, and Roman Prosthetics', *ANRW* II 37.3, pp. 2640–2676.

Blomstedt, P. (2014). 'Orthopedic Surgery in Ancient Egypt', *Acta Orthopaedica* 85.6, pp. 670–676.

Bordo, S. (2003) *Unbearable Weight: Feminism, Western Culture, and the Body*. Berkeley, CA: University of California Press.

Bridgman, G. B. (1939) *The Human Machine: The Anatomical Structure & Mechanism of the Human Body*. New York, NY: Dover Publications.

Broome, J. (2007) *Fictive Domains: Body, Landscape, and Nostalgia, 1717–1770*. Lewisburg, PA: Bucknell University Press.

Budd, M. A. (2007) *The Sculpture Machine: Physical Culture and Body Politics in the Age of Empire*. New York, NY: New York University Press.

Davies, B. (2000) *(In)scribing Body/landscape Relations*. Oxford: Rowman & Littlefield.

Dupras, T. L., Williams, L. J., De Meyer, M., Peeters, C., Depraetere, D., Vanthuyne, B. and Willems, H. (2010) 'Evidence of Amputation as Medical Treatment in Ancient Egypt', *IJO* 20, pp. 405–423.

Fliegel, O. and Feuer, S. G. (1966) 'Historical Development of Lower-Extremity Prostheses', *Archives of Physical Medicine and Rehabilitation* 47, pp. 275–285.

Fine, S. (2006) 'Archaeology and the Interpretation of Rabbinic Literature: Some Thoughts', in Kraus, M. A. (ed.) *How Should Rabbinic Literature Be Read in the Modern World?* Piscataway, NJ: Gorgias, pp. 199–217.

Fine, S. (2014) *Art, History and the Historiography of Judaism in Roman Antiquity*. Leiden: Brill.

Fonrobert, C. (2000) *Menstrual Purity; Rabbinic and Christian Reconstruction of Biblical Gender*. Stanford, CA: Stanford University Press.

Fonrobert, C. (2006) 'The Semiotics of the Sexed Body in Early Halakhic Discourse', in Kraus, M. A. (ed.) *Closed and Open: Readings of Rabbinic Texts*, Piscataway, NJ: Gorgias Press, pp. 69–96.

Fonrobert, C. (2007) 'Regulating the Human Body: Rabbinic Legal Discourse and the Making of Jewish Gender', in Fonrobert, C. and Jaffee, M. (edd.) *Cambridge Companion to Rabbinic Literature*. Cambridge: Cambridge University Press, pp. 270–294.

Friedman, S. (2010) *Talmudic Studies: Investigating the Sugya, Variant Readings, and Aggada*. New York, NY and Jerusalem: The Jewish Theological Seminary [Hebrew].

Fürstenberg, Y. (2015) 'Outsider Impurity: Trajectories of Second Temple Separations Traditions in Tannaitic Literature', in Kister, M. *et al.* (edd.) *Tradition, Transmission, and Transformation from Second Temple Literature through Judaism and Christianity in Late Antiquity*. Leiden: Brill, pp. 40–68.

Gafni, I. (2011) 'Rethinking Talmudic History: The Challenge of Literary and Redaction Criticism', *Jewish History* 25, pp. 355–375.

Garland, R. (2010) *The Eye of the Beholder. Deformity and Disability in the Graeco-Roman World*. Second edition. London: Bristol Classical Press.

Geller, M. J. (2000) 'An Akkadian Vademecum in the Babylonian Talmud', in Kottek, S. and Horstmannshoff, M. (edd.) *From Athens to Jerusalem: Medicine in Hellenized Jewish Lore and in Early Christian Literature*. Rotterdam: Erasmus Press, pp. 13–32.

Geller, M. J. (2004) *Akkadian Healing Therapies in the Babylonian Talmud*. Berlin: Max Planck Institute for the History of Science [Preprint 259].

Geller, M. J. (ed.) (2015) *The Archaeology and Material Culture of the Babylonian Talmud*. Leiden: Brill.

Goodman, M. (1994) 'Jews and Judaism in the Mediterranean Diaspora in the Late-Roman Period: The Limitations of Evidence', *Journal of Mediterranean Studies* 4, pp. 208–224.

Gracer, B. (2003) 'What the Rabbis Heard: Deafness in the Mishnah', *Disability Studies Quarterly* 23.2, pp. 192–205.

Halivni, D. (2013) *The Formation of the Babylonian Talmud. Introduced, Translated and Annotated by Jeffrey L. Rubenstein*. New York, NY: Oxford University Press.

Hezser, C. (1997) *The Social Structure of the Rabbinic Movement in Roman Palestine*. Tübingen: Mohr Siebeck.

Hezser, C. (2002) 'The Social Status of Slaves in the Talmud Yerushalmi and in Graeco-Roman society', in Schäfer, P. (ed.) *The Talmud Yerushalmi and Graeco-Roman Culture*. Tübingen: Mohr Siebeck, pp. 91–138.

Hezser, C. (2010) 'Material Culture and Daily Life', in Goodman, M. and Alexander, P. (edd.) *Rabbinic Texts and the History of Late-Roman Palestine*. Oxford: Oxford University Press, pp. 301–317.

Ilan, T. (1997) *Mine and Yours Are Hers: Retrieving Women's History from Rabbinic Literature*. Leiden: Brill.

Ilan, T. (2006) *Silencing the Queen: The Literary Histories of Shelamzion and Other Jewish Women*. Tübingen: Mohr Siebeck.

Ilan, T. (2015) 'A Menstruant "Forced and Immersed": "Women to Think With" about Intention in the Performance of the Commandments · BT Ḥulin 31a–b', *Nashim: A Journal of Jewish Women's Studies & Gender Issues* 28, (Special issue: Feminist Interpretations of the Talmud), pp. 51–60.

Johnson, M. (2007) *The Meaning of the Body. Aesthetics of Human Understanding*. Chicago, IL: Chicago University Press.

Kazen, T. (2013) *Scripture, Interpretation, or Authority?: Motives and Arguments in Jesus' Halakic Conflicts*. Tübingen: Mohr Siebeck.

Klawans, J. (2000) *Impurity and Sin in Ancient Judaism*. New York, NY: Oxford University Press.

Krauss, S. (1898–1899) *Griechische und lateinische Lehnwörter im Talmud, Midrasch und Targum: preisgekrönte Lösung der Lattes'schen Preisfrage*. 2 Volumes. Berlin: Calvary.

Laes, C., Goodey, C., and Rose, M. (edd.) (2013) *Disabilities in Roman Antiquity: Disparate Bodies* a Capite ad Calcem. Leiden: Brill.

Lapin, H. (2012) *Rabbis as Romans. The Rabbinic Movement in Palestine, 100–400 CE.* Oxford: Oxford University Press.

Lehmhaus, L. (2015) 'Listenwissenschaft and the Encyclopedic Hermeneutics of Knowledge in Talmud and Midrash', in Cale Johnson, J. (ed.) *In the Wake of the Compendia: Infrastructural Contexts and the Licensing of Empiricism in Ancient and Medieval Mesopotamia.* Berlin and Boston, MA: de Gruyter, pp. 59–100.

Lehmhaus, L. *et al.* (2016) 'Canon and Authority in Greek and Talmudic Medicine', in Wissen in Bewegung. Institution – Iteration – Transfer (Episteme in Bewegung. Beiträge zur einer transdisziplinären Wissensgeschichte, Bd. 1), Wiesbaden: Harrassowitz, pp. 195–221. (with Geller, M. J., van der Eijk, P. J., Martelli, M. and Salazar, C. F.).

Lev, S. (2007) 'How the 'Aylonit Got Her Sex', *AJS Review* 31.2, pp. 297–316.

Lev, S. (2010) 'They Treat Him As a Man and See Him As a Woman: The Tannaitic Understanding of the Congenital Eunuch', *Jewish Studies Quarterly* 17.3, pp. 213–243.

Levinson, J. (2000) 'Cultural Androgyny in Rabbinic Literature', in Kottek, S. and Horstmanshoff, M. (edd.) *From Athens to Jerusalem: Medicine in Hellenized Jewish Lore and in Early Christian Literature.* Rotterdam: Erasmus Publishing, pp. 119–140.

Lieber, E. (1984) 'Asaf's Book of Medicines: a Hebrew Encyclopedia of Greek and Jewish Medicine, possibly compiled in Byzantium on an Indian Model', *Dumbarton Oaks Papers* 38, pp. 233–249.

Marx, T. C. (2002) *Disability in Jewish Law.* New York, NY: Routledge.

Meacham, T. (1999) 'An Abbreviated History of the Development of the Jewish Menstrual Laws', in Wasserfall, R. (ed.) *Women and Water: Menstruation in Jewish Life and Law.* Hanover: Brandeis University Press/University Press of New England, pp. 23–39.

Miller, S. S. (2006) *Sages and Commoners in Late Antique Erez Israel: A Philological Inquiry into Local Traditions in Talmud Yerushalmi.* Tübingen: Mohr Siebeck.

Miller, S. S. (2015) *At the Intersection of Texts and Material Finds: Stepped Pools, Stone Vessels, and Ritual Purity among the Jews of Roman Galilee.* Göttingen: Vandenhoeck & Ruprecht.

Mitchell, D. T. and Snyder, S. L. (2000) *Narrative Prosthesis: Disability and the Dependencies of Discourse.* Ann Arbor, MI: University of Michigan Press.

Morus, I. R. (ed.) (2002) *Bodies/Machines.* London and New York, NY: Bloomsbury.

Muntner, S. (1951) 'The Antiquity of Asaph the Physician and His Editorship of the Earliest Hebrew Book of Medicine', *Bulletin of the History of Medicine* 25, pp. 101–131.

Nas, P. J. M. and Brakus, C. (2004) 'The Dancing House – Instances of the Human Body in City and Architecture', in Shahshahani, S. (ed.) *Body as Medium of Meaning.* Münster: LIT–Verlag, pp. 27–56.

Nerlich, A. G., Zink, A., Szeimies, U. and Hagedorn, H. G. (2000) 'Ancient Egyptian Prosthesis of the Big Toe', *Lancet* 356.9248.23–30, pp. 2176–2179.

Neumann, J. N. (1992) 'Die Mißgestalt des Menschen – ihre Deutung im Weltbild von Antike und Frühmittelalter', *Sudhoffs Archiv* 76. 2, pp. 214–231.

Newmyer, S. T. (1992) 'Asaph's "Book of Remedies": Greek Science and Jewish Apologetics', *Sudhoffs Archiv* 76, pp. 28–36.

Nunn, J. (2002) *Ancient Egyptian Medicine.* Norman, OK: University of Oklahoma Press.

Olwig, K. R. (2002) *Landscape, Nature, and the Body Politic. From Britain's Renaissance to America's New World*. Madison, WI: The University of Wisconsin Press.

Olyan, S. (2008) *Disability in the Hebrew Bible: Interpreting Mental and Physical Differences*. New York, NY: Cambridge University Press.

Preuss, J. (1978) *Biblical and Talmudic Medicine*. Edited and Translated by Fred Rosner. New York, NY: Sanhedrin Press/Hebrew Publishing Company.

Preuss, J. (1992) *Biblisch Talmudische Medizin. Beiträge zur Geschichte der Heilkunde und der Kultur überhaupt*. Wiesbaden: Fourier (Reprint of the original edition Berlin: Karger, 1911).

Raphael, R. (2008) *Biblical Corpora: Representations of Disability in Hebrew Biblical Literature*. New York, NY: T & T Clark.

Reeves, N. (1999) 'New Light on Ancient Egyptian Prosthetic Medicine', *Studies in Egyptian Antiquities. A Tribute to T.G.H. James*. London: British Museum Press, pp. 73–77.

Rose, M. L. (2003) *The Staff of Oedipus: Transforming Disability in Ancient Greece*. Ann Arbor, MI: University of Michigan Press.

Rosen-Zvi, I. (2005/6) 'The Body and the Book: The List of Blemishes in Mishnah Tractate Bekhorot and the Place of the Temple and Its Worship in the Tannaitic Beit Ha-Midrash [Hebrew]', *Mada'ei Hayahadut/Jewish Studies* 43, pp. 49–87.

Rosner, F. (2000) *Encyclopedia of Medicine in the Bible and The Talmud*. Northvale, NJ and Jerusalem: Jason Aronson.

Schipper, J. (2001) *Disability and Isaiah's Suffering Servant*. Oxford and New York, NY: Oxford University Press.

Schwartz, S. (2007) 'The Political Geography of Rabbinic Texts', in Fonrobert, C. E. and Jaffe, M. (edd.) *The Cambridge Companion to the Talmud and Rabbinic Literature*. Cambridge: Cambridge University Press, pp. 75–96.

Seltzer, M. (1992) *Bodies and Machines*. Abingdon and New York, NY: Routledge.

Steinert, U. (2013) 'Fluids, Rivers, and Vessels: Metaphors and Body Concepts in Mesopotamian Gynaecological Texts', *Journal des Médecines Cunéiformes* 22, pp. 1–23.

Steinert, U. (2017) 'Concepts of the Female Body in Mesopotamian Texts on Women's Healthcare', in Wee, J. (ed.) *The Comparable Body: Imagination and Analogy in Ancient Anatomy and Physiology*. Berlin: De Gruyter.

Stemberger, G. (1996) *Introduction to the Talmud and Midrash*. London: Bloomsbury T & T Clark.

Thurston, A. J. (2007) 'Paré and Prosthetics: The Early History of Artificial Limbs', *ANZ Journal of Surgery* 77, pp. 1114–1119.

Unschuld, P. (2009) *What Is Medicine?: Western and Eastern Approaches to Healing*. Berkeley, CA: University of California Press.

Vidas, M. (2014) *Tradition and the Formation of the Talmud*. Princeton, NJ: Princeton University Press.

Von Brunn, W. (1926) 'Der Stelzfuß von Capua und die antiken Prothesen', *Archiv für Geschichte der Medizin* 18.4, pp. 351–360.

Wills, D. (1995) *Prosthesis*. Stanford, CA: Stanford University Press.

Zucconi, L. M. (2010) *Can No Physician be Found?: The Influence of Religion on Medical Pluralism in Ancient Egypt, Mesopotamia and Israel*. Piscataway, NJ: Gorgias Press.

5 Evidence of a Late Antique amputation in a skeleton from Hemmaberg

Josef Eitler and Michaela Binder

Introduction

Despite a host of iconographic and written sources attesting to the knowledge of replacing severed body parts through prosthetic devices, archaeological evidence has unambiguously proved the existence of this practice and allows further insights into its technological and medical practicalities that has so far been mostly absent in Europe prior to the Medieval Period. Here we present the new discovery of a middle-aged man with an amputated left foot replaced by a wooden prosthesis recovered at the Hemmaberg excavation in southern Austria in 2009. Dated to the sixth century CE, it represents one of the earliest examples of a functional prosthetic device in Europe recovered up until the present day. Combining archaeological and palaeopathological evidence, this significant new find will be examined within its historical, cultural and medical context in order to explore the technological and functional details and to discuss the potential reasons for the amputation, as well as the social implications that emerged from this physical impairment.

The archaeological site of Hemmaberg

Hemmaberg is a foothill of the Karawanks in southern Carinthia near the Austrian border with Slovenia. Due to its striking rock faces to the north, the 842 m high Hemmaberg is an impressive and widely visible landmark of Jauntal, which is the regional name for this part of the wide valley of the river Drava. The sheltered position of the hilltop and a spring not far from the summit made it a favourable location for settlement from prehistoric times onwards.[1] Even if some finds might date to the Neolithic period, the earliest reliable indications for a settlement are from the Middle Bronze Age (1500/1450–1250 BCE).[2] Although nearly all buildings of this period were at the latest destroyed during Late Antiquity, the amount of early ceramic material gives clear evidence of the inhabitation of Hemmaberg in the Middle Bronze Age. A sanctuary from the beginning of the Roman period led to a fundamental redesign of the hilltop plateau.[3] The area was levelled during its construction, but the name of the deity *Iuenat*,[4] which is pre-Roman, refers rather to a transformation of a sacred location than to a new foundation.[5]

Nevertheless, the archaeological site of Hemmaberg is famous for its Late Antique remains.[6] With the increasing insecurity during the later Roman Empire, the protective aspects of the hilltop again became important. With the spread of Christianity, a first church was built around 400 CE.[7] This building is typical for the size of the settlement as well as for the period and comparable to many other sites in the alpine region.[8] Much more exceptional are the two major double church complexes following at the beginning of the sixth century CE. Both were constructed at the same time with identical mortar for the masonry[9] and also one workshop laid the mosaics in both ensembles.[10] Their much larger dimensions and furnishings illustrate a prestigious claim when the churches at Hemmaberg became of supra-regional importance. The duplication of the facilities led to an extensive scientific discussion of religious and political structures in Late Antiquity.[11] In the context of Hemmaberg the best explanation seems to be found in the theory of two competing Christian communities.[12] Between 493 and 536 CE, the province of Noricum Mediterraneum was part of the Ostrogoth realm.[13] The presence of an Ostrogothic community in the valley below Hemmaberg is indicated by an extensive cemetery in Globasnitz, where the Roman way station Iuenna was located.[14] The Ostrogoths were of Arianic denomination, while the local Late Antique Roman population was Catholic.[15] Research on these churches and associated guesthouses at Hemmaberg pointed out its far-reaching importance and has made it a model study of a Late Antique centre of early Christian pilgrimage in the alpine region.[16]

The church and graveyard at the hilltop plateau

As the widely known double church complexes were set to the slope of the hill, research was shifted to the centre of the summit plateau since 2009. Excavations started in the north of the post-medieval church dedicated to St. Hemma and St. Dorothea in the area of the assumed Roman sanctuary. It was a surprise, therefore, to unearth not only the remains of the Roman period but also a small cemetery of twenty-nine graves. The burials discovered during the first excavation campaign were in close proximity to the aforementioned Church of St. Hemma and St. Dorothea. They had the same deviation in the orientation to the east as the late Gothic church first mentioned between 1498 and 1512 CE.[17] Due to historical considerations, the burials could not be associated with this building. There had never been a parish at Hemmaberg since the construction of the late Gothic church and regular burials took place in the churchyard of Globasnitz, the village at the foot of Hemmaberg.[18] The first impression of the graves also suggested that they were from an earlier period.[19] This led to the discovery of an earlier building below the foundations of the late Gothic church. This newly discovered church was approximately of the same size (19.5 x 9.5–11 m) with a wide apse in the east, which was clearly to distinguish from the later choir.[20] A small sondage in the middle of the apse just in front of the high altar of the later church uncovered a pit cut into the bedrock with remains of a shrine for relics in form of two large stones originally containing a now lost reliquary casket.[21] Here, the altar of the first church has to be assumed right above the relic of a martyr.

The cemetery has to be seen in the context of this earlier church. According to Christian beliefs, the deceased were buried in a supine position facing to the east awaiting the Second Coming of the Lord and the resurrection of the dead.[22] The orientation is not exact but the cemetery was aligned to the church.[23] Due to the geological situation at the hilltop, the graves were only shallow and sometimes carved into the bedrock. Despite the fact that the corpses were not deeply buried, even the skeletons of small children were preserved because of the favourable soil conditions.[24] Of the twenty-nine burials recovered in the cemetery, only seven individuals reached adult age. All the deceased were buried in single graves, which is typical for Late Antique and early medieval cemeteries. Nevertheless, the graveyard gives the impression that the cemetery was reserved for a certain group of the population buried together at the hilltop plateau.[25]

As in many early Christian cemeteries there were no grave goods; even personal property of the deceased was rare. One of the children was bearing a little ring with ring-and-dot ornament on a finger of the right hand. Another grave contained a bronze needle. An exception could be found in only one grave.

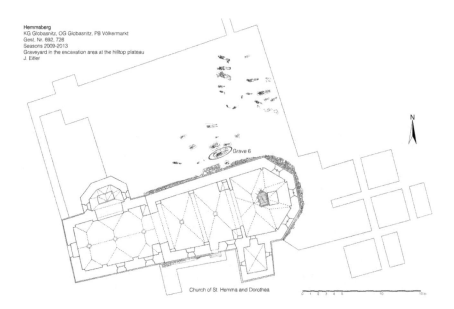

Figure 5.1 Plan of the Frankish Cemetery adjacent to the church of St. Hemma and St. Dorothea. Image courtesy of J. Eitler.

The grave of the amputee

In proximity to the church, an adult man was buried in a grave aligned to the northern wall of the building. A 2.10 m long pit was carved into the bedrock. Apart from the fact that the deceased was buried with some personal property, especially objects of clothing and a weapon, the amputation of the left foot and remains of a prosthesis made the individual of particular interest for research as there are only three other amputees known from the Early Medieval Period: a man from Bonaduz,[26] another man from Aesch,[27] both Switzerland, and an old adult male burial at Griesheim,[28] Germany.

The remains of the prosthesis

In this burial, the lower end of the left leg and the entire left foot of the deceased were missing, but the remnants of a prosthesis could be found slightly to the east of the absent limb. An iron band was bent to form a slightly oval ring with a diameter of 6.8–7.3 cm. The overlapping ends of this band (1.5–1.8 cm wide and 0.3–0.4 cm thick) were closed with two small rivets. A wooden bottom was fixed in the ring by three nails. The function of another iron rivet with an elevated head on the outer side of the ring could not be determined, though perhaps it could have been used for fixing some leather parts of the prosthesis. Small residues of wood were preserved in the corrosion of the iron ring. During the excavation, it was also possible to document wooden imprints in the loam showing that there were slats forming a kind of cup held together by the iron ring. Its presumed function was to cover and protect the amputation site and resultant stump and to provide sufficient stability to strain it at least for a certain degree. In terms of usability, the prosthesis also had to compensate for the difference in length between the legs. This could have been achieved by the addition of a short wooden stilt, which was fixed into the iron ring by the documented nails, or, what is more likely according to the situation of the remnants in the grave, by extending

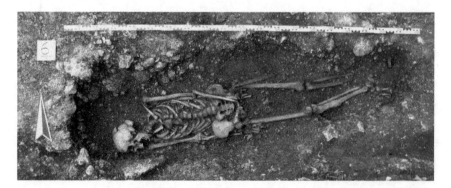

Figure 5.2 Grave 6 containing the burial of the man with the prosthetic leg. Image courtesy of J. Eitler.

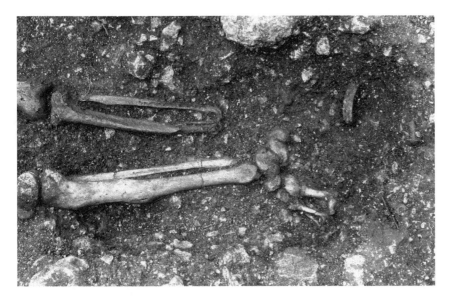

Figure 5.3 The prosthesis in situ. Image courtesy of J. Eitler.

the cup-shaped part. In this case, the iron ring was the lower end of the device. The resulting cavity between the stump and the bottom of the cup may have been filled with padding, thus reducing the pressure on the end of the leg. It is not clear how the prosthesis was fixed to the leg, but according to its construction it was most likely by some organic materials, possibly leather straps bound around the stump. In order to maintain the movability of the knee and still ensure adequate stability, a kind of shaft would have had to reach above the calf. Decomposition of these components attached to the left leg might also have led to the dark discoloration of the bones in the grave.

Finds and social status of the deceased

Of the twenty-nine excavated burials at the hilltop plateau, this is the only grave that allows us to gain further information about the deceased by studying the objects of clothing and personal belongings. A buckle lying next to the waist of the skeleton was part of a belt. This indicates that the individual was buried wearing a tunic.[29] A short scramasax was found immediately above the left femur. Its approximately 20 cm long blade with ring-and-dot decoration was recovered and is well preserved. The tang with a length of 7 cm is heavily corroded but shows remains of the weapon's wooden handle. Due to its find position in the grave and the presence of another small buckle, it can be assumed that this kind of combat knife was hung on a thin belt and was worn diagonally across the chest of the deceased. This is typical for saxes in contrast to swords, which were usually placed as grave goods alongside the deceased.[30]

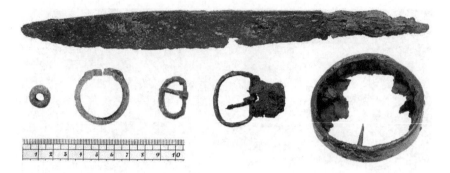

Figure 5.4 Finds from the grave of the man with the prosthetic leg. Image courtesy of K. Allesch with permission from Landesmuseum Kärnten.

A penannular brooch with stylised animal heads at the terminals was located between the femora. It also indicates a folded cloak was laid over the man's legs.[31] A single glass bead associated with the deceased was probably a kind of amulet.

In comparison to the other burial garments, most probably a shroud, the clothing of this individual is remarkable. Together with a short sax, which can be seen as a status symbol,[32] the finds indicate that the man was a person of importance in the community and was bestowed the privilege to be buried next to the church in the cemetery at the hilltop. Although weapons are usually common finds in male burials in early medieval times,[33] this is an exception at Hemmaberg as there are no similar finds from other regional cemeteries of this period.[34]

The position of the grave points to the social status of the deceased as well.[35] The space within or close to the church was a very desirable location for burials wishing to rest as near as possible to the relic of a martyr who was thought to be a great help at the Resurrection and the Day of Judgement.[36] Therefore, these locations were reserved for persons of high standing. The grave of the amputee is one of the closest to the church and the place of the relic in the middle of the apse, even if it has to be assumed that the local leader had his burial place inside the church.

Dating the grave in the context of the church

Although reliable radiocarbon dating of the cemetery and church has not yet been carried out, it is possible to date the graves rather precisely based on burial customs, finds associated with the skeletons and the historic framework. The buckles are of common types and not helpful in this attempt and so is the finger ring with ring-and-dot decoration from a child's grave which is also a widespread style during Late Antiquity and the Early Medieval Period. Even though ordinary ring fibulae that were found in the context of burials are common from the pre-Roman Iron Age to the Medieval Period,[37] the brooch from the grave at Hemmaberg allows us to draw some conclusions about the owner. A similar find from the Wallis in Switzerland is dated only generally as Late Antique,[38] but in northern Italy the earliest penannular brooches of this type do not appear before the late sixth century CE.[39] The spread of these fibulae with terminals in the form of stylised animal heads make it possible to set it at least in the context of Germanic influence expanding continuously from the periphery to the centre of the Roman world.

The short scramasax of the amputee points this out even more precisely.[40] Saxes are familiar within the sphere of Frankish culture but they are not common among Ostrogoths or Romans. So, it is not surprising that no comparable weapon could be found in the Ostrogothic burial ground in Globasnitz[41] and the cemetery of the Roman population of the Late Antique settlement at Hemmaberg.[42]

The burials here therefore likely represent a group settling on the Hemmaberg during the period when the region was part of the Frankish kingdom between 536 and the beginning of the seventh century CE.

The small cemetery located in the centre of the hilltop settlement also shows an obvious change in customs. The hilltop plateau in the centre of the settlement became a burial place for a certain group of the population. In contrast, all the earlier Late Antique tombs at Hemmaberg are individuals gaining privileged burial places in or next to churches most likely according to donations and their social status[43] when the common burial grounds are outside the settlement at the slope of the hilltop[44] or even down in the valley next to Globasnitz.[45] It is the transition from a single person in the context of a church to a group obtaining the possibility to bury at the hilltop plateau pointing out the transformation, particularly as the common cemetery outside the settlement was still in use.

This conforms to the interpretation of the church which the graves are associated with. The building was constructed with a wide apse in the east following the Late Antique tradition. But being the first church set into the former Roman sanctuary at Hemmaberg, it marks a turning point in history. After the prohibition of non-Christian religious customs under Emperor Theodosius in 392 CE,[46] pagan sanctuaries became state property.[47] This seems also to be the reason for building both major double church complexes at the slope of the hill at the beginning of the sixth century CE as none of the Christian communities could acquire ownership of the hilltop plateau.[48] The historical context of this period makes it even more comprehensible. The former Roman province Noricum Mediterraneum was part of the Ostrogothic kingdom from 493 to 536 CE.[49] Although Theodoric the Great himself was of Arian belief in his authority as king he did not favour any Christian denomination and represented a policy of tolerance.[50] Therefore, Roman legislation was highly respected even during the Ostrogothic reign.[51] But when King Witigis handed over the Noricum Mediterraneum for tactical reasons to the Frankish realm in 536 CE in an attempt to avoid a second theatre of war during the conflict with the Byzantine Empire,[52] interest in Roman traditions were lost. Due to this change, the newly built church at the hilltop has to be seen as an early proprietary church of the new ruling class.

According to the finds and the context of the church, the amputee was a person of higher rank in a community that was part of the Frankish cultural sphere, allowing us to date the grave to a short period between 536 CE and the Slavic appropriation of the region at the beginning of the seventh century CE, when the settlement at Hemmaberg was abandoned.[53] It is also remarkable that the church at the hilltop plateau is the only known example in Carinthia where an early Christian church has a succeeding building of a later period built in exactly the same place, when the Christian tradition usually was interrupted by the immigration of pagan Slavic populations for at least 150 years.[54]

Anthropological aspects

In order to elucidate the nature of the amputation and shed light on possible causes that led to the loss of the foot, the skeleton of the man was submitted to the bioarchaeology lab of the Austrian Archaeological Institute at the Austrian Academy of Science for further study. Osteological analysis[55] confirmed the biological sex to be male. Based on morphological features it can be assumed that he died between 35 and 50 years of age. Advanced degeneration of the hip joints and the spine together with strongly developed attachment sites of the muscles stabilising the hip and knee suggests that the man was involved in habitual horseback riding prior to the amputation.

The left tibia and fibula where the amputation occurred were studied in more detail, both macroscopically applying CT scanning and X-ray. On the surface, both skeletal elements displayed a small amount of new bone formation surrounding the ends where the amputation had occurred. Supported by the radiographic and CT examination, these changes could be identified as indicators of an osteomyelitis, an infection and consecutive inflammation of the bone and bone marrow which had already healed at the time of death. However, whether this arose as a consequence of the amputation wound or by an injury or infection that necessitated the amputation will remain unknown. Equally unclear remains the cause of the amputation or the tools with which it was carried out.

In general, three possible causes have to be taken into account: medical treatment, trauma (accidental or violent) and punishment.[56] As a medical intervention, it may have been used as a consequence of an infection arising from an open wound or a severe compound fracture. While written sources suggest that such a form of surgical procedure was known to the Romans, it remains unclear to what degree this knowledge persisted into the Early Medieval Period. As a form of punishment, removal of limbs was an accepted practice in the Frankish judicial system,[57] even though this was restricted to

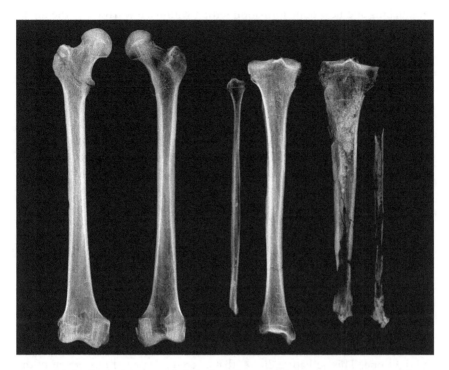

Figure 5.5 Radiographic images of the long bones of the lower extremities of the man with the prosthetic leg. Image courtesy of M. Binder.

lower social classes until the beginning of the seventh century CE. Thus, the high social rank of the man from Hemmaberg, indicated through his grave goods and burial position, strongly argues against the cause of the amputation being punitive. More likely is the cause of amputation being trauma, either violent or by accident. Widespread warfare during the Early Medieval Period is well evidenced in the historic record. The location of the cut in the lower portion of the tibia is a common site of sharp force trauma and interpreted as being inflicted by men on foot to mounted men.[58] Given the other indicators of habitual horse riding in the skeleton of the man, this certainly seems plausible. On the other hand, the most common form of loss of limbs through crushing or severing of the limb reported in clinical studies in less developed and non-industrialised countries are accidents related to farming, involving vehicles or falls from great heights.[59] Trans-tibial amputations similar to the lesion in the man from the Hemmaberg are by far the most common site affected by accidental traumatic amputation. Consequently, accidental trauma serves as possible explanation for the lesion seen in the man from the Hemmaberg as well.

The amputation edges on the bones themselves do not hold any further clues as to their origin. The natural repair process of bone tissue involves remodelling and new bone formation setting within a few days after the injury occurs. After several weeks, the edges of the cut or break would have been completely grown over by new bone, obscuring any traces of possible tool marks or other signs that may have allowed for an identification of the original cause of the amputation. Regardless of the cause, the amount of remodelling surrounding the edges shows that the man survived the injury for at least several months.

Radiographic examination of the long bones of both legs of the man revealed further information with regard to the time the injury was survived but also the functionality of the prosthesis. It is a well-established fact that if a limb is immobilised for a long time a marked imbalance between bone formation and resorption occurs which further results in decreased bone density and structural weakness.[60] Consequently, bone density serves as a useful indicator of survival time and functionality of amputated limbs and prostheses in archaeological human remains,[61] even though this has to be viewed with caution due to fact that there is also a wide range of unknown parameters potentially influencing the recovery process such as health, environment, social status or genetic background.

Comparing the femora, tibiae and fibulae of the man from the Hemmaberg, there are marked differences between both legs, attesting an immobilisation of the amputated left leg for at least one to two years. However, there are also advanced degenerative changes in the left knee which are not present in the right one. This perhaps indicates that a certain degree of movement of the amputated leg was still possible, though an altered strain on the joint due to changes in the stability, distribution of pressure and orientation of the joint and leg together with the prosthesis may have led to the osteoarthritis in the knee. This potentially indicates that the prosthesis was actually usable and did not simply serve as a cosmetic device. In addition, there are discernible differences in the amount of osteoarthritis in the shoulder joints, with a markedly higher degree on the left side. This may point towards the use of a crutch to aid walking with the prosthesis.

Conclusion

The deceased with the amputation has to be considered in the complex context of Hemmaberg during the transition from the Late Antique Period to the Early Medieval Period. Due to the major double church complexes of the beginning of the sixth century CE, the site had been a destination of pilgrimage at the time.[62] Only a few decades later the western double church complex was abandoned and some parts were reused for secular purposes.[63] Nevertheless, the site itself still must have been of great importance as a new church was built in the spared area of a former Roman sanctuary at the hilltop plateau. This does not only point to the transformation process at the beginning of the Medieval Period but also a prestigious claim of its founders. The small cemetery reflects this transition at an intermediate level as well: burials were no longer restricted to single tombs of donors next to a church but to a certain group of the population despite the fact that the common cemetery was still outside the settlement at the slope of the hill. As part of this outstanding group, the grave of the amputee fits within this general context. The proximity of his tomb to the church and the grave goods attest to the deceased's higher rank in a community which was part of the Frankish cultural sphere. Therefore, he could be considered to have had a leadership position in the community we have evidence of in the small cemetery. This is also congruent with the results of the anthropological analysis attesting that he was a horseman. It has yet to be established whether these burials belong to the inhabitants of Hemmaberg or whether they were there for prestigious purposes at the hilltop. Although we know nearly nothing about the relation of the amputee to Hemmaberg in detail, it seems very unlikely that in death he was buried at a place he had never been in life. As pathology shows, he regained a certain degree of mobility after the amputation and was at least able to walk with a crutch. The prosthesis itself has to be seen above all as a practical device which aimed to improve the ability of the man to use what remained of his left leg after the amputation. There is also no indication that he could not have ridden after the procedure, as he was a horseman before. In view of this possibility, Hemmaberg would not have been a more difficult destination for him to reach than any other location.

Evidence of the amputation is an outstanding find. The amputee from Hemmaberg was obviously of high social status, which can be considered an advantage for acquiring this level of medical care. Nevertheless, the fact that amputations could be carried out successfully during the Early Medieval Period indicates that this kind of medical treatment was not that uncommon at the time as reflected in the confirmed archaeological finds in the current state of research.

Notes

1 Glaser, 1982, p. 11.
2 Glaser, 1984, pp. 31–33.
3 Eitler and Reiter, 2009/10, pp. 70–71.
4 Iouenat is addressed on a Roman votive altar from Hemmaberg: *CIL* 3 14366/3; Glaser, 1982, p. 42.
5 Detailed analyses of the finds from latest the excavations at the hilltop plateau (2009–2013) have been started within the research project *Cult Continuity at the Summit of Hemmaberg* funded by the Austrian Science Fund (FWF) Project Number P 29542–G25 in October 2016.
6 Glaser, 1991; Ladstätter, 2000.
7 Glaser, 1991, pp. 65–69.
8 See Sennhauser, 2003.
9 Ladstätter and Sauer, 1998, pp. 327–328.
10 Glaser, 1992, p. 28.
11 The scientific dispute was mostly carried out between F. Glaser and V. Bierbrauer, who had different theories concerning the necessity of building two major double church complexes at the same time. For a compilation of the different theories see Glaser, 2004a, pp. 85–89.

12 Glaser, 1996, pp. 90–95; Wolfram, 2003, p. 63.

13 Wolfram, 2003, pp. 58–65.

14 Glaser, 2002, p. 129.

15 Wolfram, 2003, pp. 62–63.

16 Glaser, 1996, pp. 90–95; Ladstätter, 2000.

17 Glaser, 2006, p. 9.

18 The parish of Globasnitz was first mentioned in 1296 CE, see Schroll, 2001, pp. 197–198.

19 Eitler and Reiter, 2011, p. 71.

20 Eitler, 2012, pp. 79–80.

21 Eitler, 2014, p. 95. For comparable sites: Glaser, 1997, pp. 235–246; Glaser, 2003, pp. 420–424.

22 For the orientation of Christian burials in general, see Deichman, 1983, p. 90. For orienting Christian churches and graves to the east and the garden of Eden following the Book of Genesis 2.8: Basil of Caesarea, *Book of the Holy Spirit* 27.66 (PG 32, pp. 189–192); Gregory of Nyssa, *On the Lord's Prayer* 5 (PG 44, p. 1184).

23 Only two newborn babies were not orientated to the east.

24 Eitler and Reiter, 2009/2010, p. 71.

25 Genetic testing would be desirable but has not been possible yet.

26 Baumgartner, 1982.

27 Cueni, 2009, pp. 115–118.

28 Keil, 1977/1978.

29 Glaser, 2009/2010, pp. 61–62.

30 Siegmund, 1997, p. 701.

31 Glaser, 2009/2010, p. 62.

32 Koch, 1997, pp. 729–730; Siegmund, 1997, pp. 705–706.

33 Siegmund, 1997, p. 700.

34 Glaser, 2009/2010, p. 62.

35 Koch, 1997, pp. 734–735.

36 Glaser, 1982, pp. 52–55; Glaser, 1996, p. 93; Glaser, 1997, pp. 232–233.

37 Heynowski, 2012, p. 46.

38 Ettlinger, 1973, p. 132. Taf. 15.13.

39 Riemer, 2000, pp. 123–124.

40 For the type of sax: Grünzweig, 2009, pp. 183–184; Szameit, 1997, pp. 56–57, p. 59, pp. 61–62.

41 Eitler, 2008, p. 89.

42 Glaser, 1985, pp. 85–89; Glaser, 1986, pp. 132–134; Kersting, 1994, pp. 124–125.

43 Glaser, 1982, pp. 52–55; Glaser, 1996, p. 93; Glaser, 1997, pp. 232–233.

44 Glaser, 1985, pp. 85–89; Glaser, 1986, pp. 132–134; Kersting, 1994, pp. 124–125.

45 Glaser, 2004a, pp. 89–100; Glaser, 2004b, pp. 129–134; Eitler, 2005, pp. 79–82; Eitler, 2008, pp. 89–91.

46 *Theodosian Code* 16, 10, 12; Leppin, 2003, pp. 175–176.

47 Demandt, 2007, pp. 496–497, p. 542.

48 Glaser, 1996, p. 94.

49 Ladstätter, 2002, pp. 344–348.

50 For example, the Roman Senate in a letter to the Emperor Justinian in Constantinople, at Cassiodorus, *Variae* 11.13.3: *Quid enim pro me [i.e. Roma] nitaris amplius agree, cuius region, quae tua est, cognoscitur sic florere.*

51 According to H. Wolfram, Late Antiquity ceased in Noricum Mediterraneum with the end of the Ostrogothic domination, see Wolfram, 2003, p. 65; Wolfram, 2001, pp. 315–324.

52 The Gothic war lasted from 535 to 554 CE, see Demandt, 2007, pp. 243–246.

53 Ladstätter, 2000, pp. 205–207.

54 Gleirscher, 2000, pp. 128–129.

55 The osteological examination was carried out macroscopically following standard procedures in bioarchaeology according to the following guidelines: Brickley and McKinley, 2004; Buikstra and Ubelaker, 1994.
56 Mays, 1996.
57 Radbruch, 2001, p. 360.
58 Kjellström, 2005; Slaus *et al.*, 2010.
59 Al-Turaiki and Al-Falahi, 1993.
60 Minaire, 1989.
61 Czarnetzki *et al.*, 1983; Mays, 1996.
62 Glaser, 1996, pp. 90–95; Ladstätter, 2000.
63 Ladstätter, 2000, pp. 54–56, p. 204.

Bibliography

Al-Turaiki, H. S. and Al-Falahi, L. A. A. (1993) 'Amputee Population in the Kingdom of Saudi Arabia', *Prosthetics and Orthotics International* 17, pp. 147–156.

Baumgartner, R. (1982) 'Fussprothese aus einem frühmittlealterlichen Grab aus Bonaduz', *Helvetia Archaeologica Zürich* 13, pp. 155–162.

Brickley, M. and McKinley, J. I. (2004) 'Guidelines to the Standards for Recording Human Remains', *Institute of Field Archaeologists Technical Paper* 7. Southampton: University of Southampton.

Buikstra, J. E. and Ubelaker, D. H. (1994) *Standard for Data Collection from Human Skeletal Remains*. Fayetteville AR: Arkansas Archeological Survey Research Series 44.

Cueni, A. (2009) 'Die frühmittelalterlichen Menschen von Aesch (Anthropologische Untersuchungen)', in Hartmann, C., Cueni, A. and Rast-Eicher, A. (edd.) *Aesch: ein frühmittelalterliches Gräberfeld*, Archäologische Schriften Luzern 11. Bildungs und Kulturdepartement des Kantons Luzern, Kantonsarchäologie Luzern, pp. 83–126.

Czarnetzki, A., Uhlig, C. and Wolf, R. (1985) *Menschen des Frühen Mittelalters im Spiegel der Anthropologie und Medizin*. Stuttgart: Wurttembergisches Landesmuseum.

Demandt, A. (2007) *Die Spätantike: Römische Geschichte von Diocletian bis Justinian 284–565 n. Chr.* Handbuch der Altertumswissenschaft 3, 6. Munich: Verlag C. H. Beck.

Eitler, J. (2005) 'Neue Ergebnisse aus dem ostgotischen Gräberfeld in Iuenna', Rudolfinum *Jahrbuch des Landesmuseums Kärnten*, pp. 79–82.

Eitler, J. (2008) 'Ausgrabungen im ostgotischen Gräberfeld von Globasnitz abgeschlossen', Rudolfinum *Jahrbuch des Landesmuseums Kärnten*, pp. 89–92.

Eitler, J. (2012) 'Ausgrabung Hemmaberg 2012', Rudolfinum *Jahrbuch des Landesmuseums Kärnten*, pp. 75–83.

Eitler, J. (2014) 'Eine weitere Kirche des 6. Jahrhunderts am Gipfel des Hemmabergs', in Trinkl, E. (ed.) *Akten des 14. Österreichischen Archäologentages am Institut für Archäologie der Universität Gaz vom 19. bis 21. April 2012*. Wien: Phobos Verlag, pp. 93–98.

Eitler, J. and Reiter, J. (2009/2010) 'Neue Forschungen am Hemmaberg – überraschende Ergebnisse der Grabung am Gipfelplateau', Rudolfinum *Jahrbuch des Landesmuseums Kärnten*, pp. 69–72.

Ettlinger, E. (1973) *Die römischen Fibeln in der Schweiz*. Bern: Franke.

Gassner, V., Jilek, S. and Ladstätter, S. (edd.) *Am Rande des Reiches, Die Römer in Österreich*. Wien: Ueberreuter.

Glaser, F. (1982) *Die römische Siedlung Iuenna und die frühchristlichen Kirchen am Hemmaberg.* Klagenfurt: Verlag.

Glaser, F. (1984) 'Der älteste Fund von Hemmaberg: Ein mittelbronzezeitliches Grab', *Carinthia I* 174, pp. 31–33.

Glaser, F. (1985) 'Das spätantike Gräberfeld auf dem Hemmaberg', *Carinthia I* 175, pp. 85–89.

Glaser, F. (1986) 'Die Ausgrabung Hemmaberg 1985', *Carinthia I* 176, pp. 131–134.

Glaser, F. (1991) 'Das frühchristliche Pilgerheiligtum auf dem Hemmaberg', *Aus Forschung und Kunst* 26. Klagenfurt: Verlag.

Glaser, F. (1992) 'Die Ausgrabung der vierten und Entdeckung der fünften Kirche auf dem Hemmaberg', *Carinthia I* 182, pp. 19–45.

Glaser, F. (1993) 'Eine weitere Doppelkirche auf dem Hemmaberg und die Frage ihrer Interpretation', *Carinthia I* 183, pp. 165–186.

Glaser, F. (1996) 'Kirchenbau und Gotenherschaft, Auf den Spuren des Arianismus in Binnennorikum und in Rätien II', *Der Schlem* 70, pp. 83–100.

Glaser, F. (1997) 'Reliquiengräber – Sonderbestattungen der Spätantike', *Arheološki vestnik* 48, pp. 231–246.

Glaser, F. (2002) 'Iuenna – Hemmaberg', in Šašel Kos, M. and Scherrer, P. (edd.) *The Autonomous Towns of Noricum and Pannonia: Noricum*, Situla 40. Ljubljana: Narodni muzej Slovenije, pp. 129–132.

Glaser, F. (2003) 'Der frühchristliche Kirchenbau in der nordöstlichen Region (Kärnten/Osttirol)', in Sennhauser, H. R. (ed.) *Frühe Kirchen im östlichen Alpengebiet von der Spätantike bis in ottonische Zeit*. Munich: Verlag der Bayerischen Akademie der Wissenschaften, pp. 413–437.

Glaser, F. (2004a) 'Christentum zur Ostgotenzeit in Noricum (493–536): Die Kirchen auf dem Hemmaberg und das Gräberfeld im Tal', *Mitteilungen zur Christlichen Archäologie* 10, pp. 80–101.

Glaser, F. (2004b) 'Frühchristliche Kirche im Gräberfeld der Ostgotenzeit (493–536) am Fuße des Hemmaberges', Rudolfinum *Jahrbuch des Landesmuseums Kärnten*, pp. 129–134.

Glaser, F. (2006) *Die Wahlfahrtskirche auf dem Hemmaberg*. Passau: Kunstverlag Peda.

Glaser, F. (2009/2010) 'Ausgrabungen Hemmaberg in Iuenna/Globasnitz', Rudolfinum *Jahrbuch des Landesmuseums Kärnten*, pp. 61–62.

Gleirscher, P. (2000) *Karantanien: Das slawische Kärnten*. Klagenfurt: Verlag Carinthia.

Grünzweig, F. E. (2009) *Das Schwert bei den "Germanen": Kulturgeschichtliche Studien zu seinem "Wesen" vom Altertum bis ins Hochmittelalter*. Wien: Philologica Germanica 20.

Hartmann, C., Cueni, A. and Rast-Eicher, A. (edd.) (2009) *Aesch: ein frühmittelalterliches Gräberfeld*, Archäologische Schriften Luzern 11. Bildungs und Kulturdepartement des Kantons Luzern, Kantonsarchäologie Luzern.

Heynowski, R. (2012) *Fibeln: erkennen, bestimmen, beschreiben*. Berlin and Munich: Deutscher Kunstverlag.

Keil, B. (1977/78) 'Eine Prothese aus einem fränkischen Grab von Griesheim, Kreis Darmstadt-Dieburg'. Anthropologische und medizinhistorische Befunde, *Fundberichte aus Hessen* 17.18, pp. 195–211.

Kersting, U. (1994) *Spätantike und Frühmittelalter in Kärnten*. Berlin: Ulrike Kersting.

Kjellström, A. (2005) 'A Sixteenth-Century Warrior Grave from Uppsala, Sweden: The Battle of Good Friday', *IJO* 15, pp. 23–50.

Koch, U. (1997) 'Stätten der Totenruhe – Grabformen und Bestattungssitten der Franken', in Wieczorek, A. (ed.) *Die Franken – Wegbereiter Europas vor 1500 Jahren: König Chlodwig und seine Erben 2*. Mainz am Rhein: Verlag P. von Zabern, pp. 723–737.

Ladstätter, S. (2000) *Die materille Kultur der Spätantike in den Ostalpen. Eine Fallstudie am Beispiel der westlichen Doppelkirchenanlage auf dem Hemmaberg.* Wien: Österreichische Akademie der Wissenschaften.

Ladstätter, S. (2002) 'Die Spätantike', in Gassner, V., Jilek, S. and Ladstätter, S. (edd.) *Am Rande des Reiches, Die Römer in Österreich.* Wien: Ueberreuter, pp. 285–368.

Ladstätter, S. and Sauer, R. (1998) 'Ergebnisse petrographischer Untersuchungen von Mörtelproben aus dem frühchristlichen Pilgerheiligtum und der spätantiken Siedlung vom Hemmaberg/Kärnten', *Arheolški vestnik* 49, pp. 315–328.

Leppin, H. (2003) *Theodosius der Große.* Darmstadt: Wissenschaftliche Buchgesellschaft.

Mays, S. A. (1996) 'Healed Limb Amputations in Human Osteoarchaeology and Their Causes: A Case Study from Ipswich, UK', *IJO* 6, pp. 101–113.

Minaire, P. (1989) 'Immobilization Osteoporosis: A Review', *Clinical Rheumatology* 8, pp. 95–103.

Radbruch, G. (2001) *Strafrechtsgeschichte.* Heidelberg: C.F. Müller.

Riemer, E. (2000) 'Romanische Grabfunde des 5.–8. Jahrhunderts in Italien', *Internationale Archäologie* 57, Leidorf.

Šašel Kos, M. and Scherrer, P. (edd.) (2002) *The Autonomous Towns of Noricum and Pannonia: Noricum, Situla* 40. Ljubljana: Narodni muzej Slovenije.

Schroll, A. (2001) *Dehio-Handbuch. Die Kunstdenkmäler Österreichs. Kärnten.* Berlin: Wien.

Sennhauser, H. R. (ed.) (2003) *Frühe Kirchen im östlichen Alpengebiet: von der Spätantike bis in ottonische Zeit.* Munich: Verlag der Bayerischen Akademie der Wissenschaften.

Siegmund, F. (1997) 'Kleidung und Bewaffnung der Männer im östlichen Frankenreich', in Wieczorek, A. (ed.) *Die Franken: Wegbereiter Europas vor 1500 Jahren: König Chlodwig und seine Erben.* Mainz am Rhein: Verlag P. von Zabern, pp. 691–706.

Šlaus, M., Novak, M., Vyroubal, V. and Bedić, Z. (2010) 'The Harsh Life on the 15th Century Croatia-Ottoman Empire Military Border: Analyzing and Identifying the Reasons for the Massacre in Čepin', *American Journal of Physical Anthropology* 141, pp. 358–372.

Szameit, E. (1997) 'Frühmittelalterliche Waffen in Niederösterreich', in Windl, H. J. (ed.) *Waffen und deren Wirkung in Ur- und Frühgeschichte, gegeneinander – nebeneinander – miteinander, Ausstellung im Niederösterreichischen Landesmuseum für Frühgeschichte im Schloß Traismauer vom 2. Mai bis 1. November 1997.* St. Pölten: Amt d. NÖ Landesregierung Abt. K1-Kulturabt, pp. 47–68.

Wieczorek, A. (ed.) (1997) *Die Franken: Wegbereiter Europas vor 1500 Jahren: König Chlodwig und seine Erben.* Mainz am Rhein: Verlag P. von Zabern.

Wieczorek, A. (ed.) (2009) *Die Franken – Wegbereiter Europas vor 1500 Jahren: König Chlodwig und seine Erben 2.* Mainz am Rhein: Verlag P. von Zabern.

Windl, H. J. (ed.) (1997) *Waffen und deren Wirkung in Ur- und Frühgeschichte, gegeneinander – nebeneinander – miteinander, Ausstellung im Niederösterreichischen Landesmuseum für Frühgeschichte im Schloß Traismauer vom 2. Mai bis 1. November 1997.* St. Pölten: Amt d. NÖ Landesregierung Abt. K1-Kulturabt.

Wolfram, H. (2001) *Die Goten: von den Anfängen bis zur Mitte des sechsten Jahrhunderts: Entwurf einer historischen Ethnographie.* Munich: C. H. Beck.

Wolfram, H. (2003) *Grenzen und Räume: Geschichte Österreichs vor seiner Entstehung.* Wien: Ueberreuter.

6   Living prostheses[1]

Katherine D. van Schaik

Introduction

Stephen Hawking, renowned physicist and, until his passing in 2018, Professor of Mathematics at the University of Cambridge, suffered from extensive paralysis secondary to amyotrophic lateral sclerosis. Since 2005, he had been incapable of moving his wheelchair independently. Before he passed away, his muscle activity was limited to the single cheek muscle he used for communication, as the movements of this muscle provided the inputs for a speech-generating device. Concerns about locked-in syndrome, the condition in which an individual retains mental capacity and sensation yet lacks any ability to move, prompted researchers to seek methods of communication that relied directly on Hawking's brain waves.[2] He had been hospitalised several times, on many of these occasions requiring the assistance of a ventilator to breathe, and his paralysis rendered him reliant upon these functional prostheses even as he retained all of his limbs and organs.[3] The ventilator that breathed for him, the computer devices that turned the contractions of his cheek muscle into speech, even the glasses that helped him to see: all of these may be understood as functional prostheses. These prostheses replaced lost function: his legs, arms, eyes, and internal organs were all present, but the disease process of amyotrophic lateral sclerosis meant that Hawking had no conscious motor control over most of his body.

Professor Hawking is an extreme example of one aspect of prostheses that I seek to address in this chapter. Many chapters in this volume discuss how prostheses – artificial attachments – replace a missing part of the body. But 'replacement' is a deceptively simple term. Does the replacement occur in order to create the appearance of an intact foot with all five toes, for example?[4] Or is the replacement functional, that is, does it play a role previously carried out by a limb or organ that has become less effective because of weakness, sickness or injury? Of course, the aesthetic and functional aspects of a prosthesis are sometimes, but do not have to be, mutually exclusive.[5] Focusing on the functional aspect of prostheses, this chapter will discuss the medical problems of paralysis and blindness as extreme examples of lost function in order to draw out questions – and, hopefully, to suggest some answers – about how we might define prostheses in ancient and modern contexts.

The medical problem of paralysis, which we will define here, in broad terms, as an individual's inability to control voluntary motor function consciously, is notable in that it necessitates the use of functional prostheses even as limbs remain fully sensitive and firmly attached to the body. Fitting a prosthetic leg or toe to an individual who lacks one is a different matter – clinically, socially, psychologically and mechanically – from the situation in which a prosthetic device is needed to restore functionality to an individual with a present but paralysed leg or toe. Study of ancient cases of paralysis, and of the methods paralysed individuals used to restore function in their lives, provides an expanded understanding of the nature and goals of prostheses, and of insight into the importance of caregiving in antiquity. The same can be said for blindness. The first part of this paper will present descriptions of paralysis from ancient Mediterranean medical texts, highlighting the recognised fatality, intractability and incurability of this condition. An additional kind of often-intractable loss of function, blindness, will also be discussed to illustrate my argument about the functional component of prostheses. The second part of the paper explores how function could be restored through reliance on a particular type of functional prosthesis: other people. Examples of human assistance provided in the setting of lost physical function will be discussed, and the paper will conclude with a reflection on the role of caregiving.

Paralysis in medical texts from *circa* 1600 BCE to the second century CE: an overview

Early descriptions of paralysis are found in the Edwin Smith Surgical Papyrus, an Egyptian medical text from the mid-second millennium BCE. Often praised for being more 'scientific' than other Egyptian medical texts because of its diminished focus on spells and prayers to gods and its clear descriptions of pathological conditions and their associated treatment, the papyrus is organised anatomically, from head to toe.[6] Forty-eight cases, most of which are brief descriptions of trauma, are presented alongside one of three verdicts of 'an ailment which I shall treat' (twenty-nine cases), 'an ailment with which I shall contend' (six cases), and 'an ailment which I shall not treat' (twelve cases). A treatment decision for case #9 is not given. Sometimes, the cases include glosses on the language. The translations and case numbering used here derive from Sanchez and Meltzer's thorough new edition of the text.[7]

Cases 31 and 33 describe injuries to the vertebrae of the neck and the resultant alterations in motor function, sensory function, and control of other bodily functions. In both cases, the patient is described as being 'unaware (or unconscious) of both his arms and legs', and this problem is explicitly designated as 'a medical condition that cannot be handled/dealt with' (Cases 31 and 33). Sanchez and Meltzer's comments on the text suggest that the syntax of the verb form of being 'unaware' implies the permanence of this state, and that the patient's condition is a consequence of a previous action – in this case, the injury.[8] One possible implication of this suggestion is that the syntax reflects the writer's knowledge that the patient's lack of awareness of his arms and legs in this setting is permanent and a consequence of injury to the neck. Based on the specific constellation of symptoms given in Case 31, it is possible to make a reasonable conjecture that 'unware of both his arms and legs' could mean both motor and sensory paraplegia:[9] that is, the injured individual can neither move his or her limbs independently, nor feel any stimulus applied to the arms and legs.[10] In addition, Case 31 describes priapism, a persistent erection, immediately following an injury to the neck (and by implication, we may assume, to the spinal cord). Modern medical literature describes how priapism immediately follows spinal cord injury and is accompanied by complete motor and sensory paraplegia.[11] The author also describes fluid emerging from the urethral meatus: though efforts to determine the nature and extent of the injuries recorded in ancient sources should be undertaken with caution, one potential interpretation is that this reference to involuntary urethral discharge could be the author's attempt to characterise the urinary incontinence that can result from injury at any level of the cord (that is, from cervical to sacral). Case 33 preserves less detail though uses the same language regarding the lack of awareness of the arms and legs. These case descriptions provide evidence that paralysis secondary to neck injury was known in pharaonic Egypt, and that the author of the Edwin Smith Papyrus knew the seriousness of such an injury.

Shifting time and place from pharaonic Egypt to Greece in the middle of the first millennium BCE, we discover that the Hippocratic Corpus, too, describes patients who are incapable of voluntary motor control as a consequence of spinal injury. The author of the surgical treatise *On Joints*, in the section of the text discussing spinal pathologies, graphically describes symptoms associated with these injuries and the impossibility of treating them:

> Even if they survive, they are more liable to incontinence of urine, and have more weakness and torpor of the legs; while if the incurvation occurs higher up, they have loss of power and complete torpor of the whole body.[12]

Similarly to the Edwin Smith Papyrus, this Hippocratic text mentions problems with incontinence or retention of urine and faeces and a loss of voluntary motor control, the extent of which depends on the level at which the spinal cord is injured. This author, too, laments the impossibility of treatment (οὐ γὰρ οἷόν). We may note that in this passage the terms ἀποπληξία (*apoplexy*) or παράλυσις (*paralysis*) do not appear, though they are used elsewhere in the Corpus to indicate disorders of movement (more about this below). Instead, the author of *On Joints* describes the lack of control experienced by the injured patient as a state of becoming powerless to control the body (παντὸς τοῦ σώματος ἀκρατέες, and subsequently in the same section, σκελέων τε καὶ χειρῶν ἀκρατέες γίνονται).[13] Like the author of the Edwin Smith Papyrus, the Hippocratic author of *On Joints* links vertebral injury, lack of voluntary motor control of the extremities, anomalies of the urinary and gastrointestinal systems, and intractability or futility of treatment.[14] The Hippocratic author, too, acknowledges the lethality of these kinds of injuries.

If we seek descriptions of paralysis (here using the term in its modern medical sense) in the sections of the Corpus that use ἀποπληξία (*apoplexy*) or παράλυσις (*paralysis*), we find that these two words are used in many different contexts and are linked to what appear to be variable pathological conditions, among them the lack of voluntary motor control over limbs. *Aphorisms* connects the state of becoming powerless to control (ἀκρατής) the tongue with ἀποπληξία, sometimes translated into English as 'stroke'.[15] The author of *Epidemics* 4 seems to suggest that παράλυσις is reversible,[16] and the author of *Prorrhetic* 1 says convulsions (σπάσμα) can occur in the context of παράλυσις.[17] The *Coan Prenotions* links complete παράλυσις with imminent death, though again it is difficult to determine the nature of παράλυσις in this context.[18] The texts of the Corpus often connect groups of symptoms as a way of arriving at a prognosis: in the examples I have given here, the Hippocratic authors provide associated symptoms (which do not necessarily have to do with compromised movement) and give prognoses about the extent of the reversibility of the paralysis, but they do not suggest treatment. Indeed, the passage in the *Coan Prenotions* suggests the futility of treatment or intervention, and this is the important point. Though the descriptions of patients suffering from an inability to move use different words, the intractability of this problem is frequently emphasised.

These references to loss of motor control do not offer suggestions of how patients might achieve even limited functionality, though the Corpus is not without references to assistive devices, especially for restoring mobility. *On Joints* 52 describes how a support may be required for a patient who struggles to walk because of a hip dislocation that was never properly put back into place. Individuals who suffered from dislocated hips as children, writes the author, can effectively learn to walk with one or two crutches (σκίπων), and do so into adulthood.[19] Additional references to crutches or assisted locomotion appear in 55 and in 58, where the author describes how crutches of different lengths affect gait. These references do not discuss prostheses as we typically understand them today, that is, as artificial devices that replace lost limbs, thereby restoring functionality, though they can be understood as a type of prosthesis in that they enhance compromised functionality for patients who have a baseline level of physical capability. The author of *On Joints* provides evidence that in cases of compromised movement resulting from dysfunctional hip joints, patients could and did use assistive devices – which we might understand as a type of prosthesis – to enhance their mobility and stability. These patients are unlike those suffering from paralysis, however, in that they still clearly maintain nerve function and the ability to move most of their limbs, even if their mobility is limited.

Moving forward in time from the world of the Hippocratic Corpus to Hellenistic Alexandria, we see that the anatomists Herophilus and Erasistratus explicitly noted the anatomical relationship between nerves, motor function and sensation.[20] Their writings are preserved for us through quotations from other, later medical authors, and it is therefore difficult to appreciate the full extent of their ideas and observations; however, even from these fragments, we can appreciate their understanding of the relationship between nerves and motor control. A fragment potentially attributable to Rufus of Ephesus records that Herophilus and Erasistratus noted a relationship between nerves, sensation and motion.[21] Galen, too, wrote that Herophilus believed the nerves to play a role in voluntary motion,[22] and that he demonstrated that injury to nerves could cause alterations in motion or sensation, or a combination of the two.[23] The Hellenistic Alexandrian anatomists, through their dissections, strengthened the understanding of the relationship between nerves and movement. While this contributed to clarification of the aetiology of paralysis, and potentially, knowledge of how it might be treated, sources subsequent to the Alexandrians still acknowledge the intractability of problems related to nerve injury.

Writing in Latin during the century before Galen, the Roman encyclopaedist Celsus presents a description of paralysis secondary to spinal injury that demonstrates anatomical knowledge and close observation of signs and symptoms. Like the writers of the Edwin Smith Papyrus and the Hippocratic Corpus, he describes alterations of continence and a lack of control of the extremities (*resolvuntur*) that vary depending upon the vertebral level at which the injury occurs. Besides describing the same symptoms as those his predecessors did, he adds difficulty breathing, vomiting, diminished hearing and pain. He concludes his discussion in terms already familiar to us, conceding that the problem is permanent and intractable and that this is no fault of the physician. It is, rather, the nature of the injury.[24] In this section, Celsus applies the issue of incurability to an aspect of medical practice, cautioning that healers are sometimes wrongly blamed for being unable to solve the problem. It is better for the physician to stand back, he says, and to avoid accusations than to risk helping a lost cause.

Galen certainly knew that paralysis was a consequence of spinal cord transection, and that the level at which the transection occurred determined the extent of the paralysis. Lower transections resulted in paralysis only in the lower limbs, and higher transections led to more extensive paralysis. Transection at the thoracic level compromised respiration. Galen furthermore identified that partial transections in different parts of the spinal cord could differentially affect sensation and motion. In one instance of spinal cord injury resulting in nerve-related symptoms in the extremities, he chided rival physicians for treating the extremity, instead of treating the spinal cord directly: he applied a remedy to skin over the vertebral column and, he writes, cured the patient.[25] But this case, while it demonstrates how Galen was able to translate the knowledge of nerves and paralysis he acquired in the dissection laboratory into his clinical practice, is an anomaly among the spinal injury cases that he describes. He records several cases of paralysis, some of which he cures, most of which he merely mentions: he liked to record his successful cures, but paralysis – then and today – rarely provides such stories of successful treatment and complete rehabilitation. In *On Affected Parts* 1.6, Galen mentions two men with conditions of paralysis: paralysis of the hand and paralysis after a fall. The extent of Galen's involvement in these cases is difficult to determine. He mentions them to comment upon the issue of nerve damage but does not describe a particular treatment procedure. In some instances, as was discussed previously, Galen notes that a cure can be brought about by paying attention to the spinal cord region associated with the nerves animating the affected limb, but in other cases, he is curiously silent about specific cures for these patients.[26]

Later in the same work,[27] Galen mentions two patients whom he saw and diagnosed with spinal cord disease: one with paralysis below the head and incontinence, and another with paralysis throughout his body except for his hands. Again, no treatment is mentioned, only observation. Like the author of the Edwin Smith Papyrus, Hippocrates and Celsus, he notes a relationship between spinal injury and incontinence when he describes a patient who injured his spine after a fall. He says that he managed to help this patient through treating the spinal cord directly.[28] Similarly, he treats a man with a neck injury and urinary retention, but he notes that his treatment is specifically for the bladder in this case. For a second patient with the same problem, a remedy is applied to the spinal cord, and for a third case, no specific treatment is mentioned.[29] Galen was an outstanding anatomist, a good physician, and a skilled rhetorician: he is not always so forthcoming when he is unable to bring about a cure consistently, and we especially observe this tendency in his descriptions of cases of spinal cord injury and paralysis.

The experiments of Galen and his Alexandrian predecessors revealed many of the nuances of permanent nerve damage, but in cases of severe paralysis, these experiments only emphasised the permanence of the disability. Galen – always proud of his ability to treat what others could not – records his observations of these cases while often remaining silent on issues of treatment. Indeed, as Celsus cautioned earlier, physicians should not intervene in these cases, lest the physician be accused of inflicting the problem upon the patient. In the rare cases that patients survived the trauma that led to paralysis, they were left with intractable disabilities characterised by a devastating loss of function. Limbs remained yet were devoid of movement and, in some cases, sensation. The patient was unaware of his arms and legs, and the arms and legs were irrevocably unaware of the control signals sent by the brain via the spinal cord. What kind of prosthesis, if any, could restore function in this setting?

Divine healing and living prostheses

To find a potential answer to this question, we turn to sources that do not provide the perspective of the physician or medical writer, whose words we have read up to this point. Instead, our sources here represent a lay perspective, or perhaps even a patient perspective: they are Epidaurean miracle inscriptions and the Gospel texts of the Bible.[30]

In cases of intractable illness, it is understandable that patients – in the past as in the present – would seek divine aid. The Epidaurean miracle inscriptions contain collected descriptions of Asclepius' intervention in the lives of suppliants who came to his temple in Epidaurus. Inscribed on stone around the fourth century BCE but representing stories that could be much older, the words describe how Asclepius cured blindness, barrenness and dumbness; alleviated women of years-long pregnancies; healed wounds and other internal afflictions; and even repaired broken cups and helped suppliants find lost wealth. Interpretation of these inscriptions is problematic. Though they provide descriptions of the god's intervention in specific individuals' lives, their ultimate collation was likely carried out by temple priests, with reference to variable stock material that could have included votives deposited by the sick.[31] However, despite the questions surrounding their composition, and the possibilities of metaphorical interpretations of the afflictions they describe, the inscriptions still constitute an important source of information about health and disease in classical antiquity precisely because they are not a 'medical' text like those written by the Hippocratic authors, Herophilus, Erasistratus, or Galen. Their existence attests to the variable options that a sick person could have pursued in search of health,[32] and the words used to describe their afflictions share some similarities with those used in the Hippocratic Corpus. As was discussed above, ἀκρατής is used in parts of the Hippocratic Corpus to denote paralysis, and this word appears at least two times, and possibly five, in the Epidaurean miracle inscriptions from the healing sanctuary to describe paralysis of some or all of the body.[33] Asclepius is reported to have healed all of these individuals. In one case, the inscription seems to say that the suppliant was carried into the sanctuary, and he is described as ἀπερειδόμενος, supporting himself on a crutch.[34] We will return to this point about the patient being carried into the sanctuary once we have discussed paralytics in the Gospels.

In these stories, descriptions of healing miracles abound, as is typical for texts seeking to present examples of divine power. The Gospels, like the Epidaurean miracle inscriptions from half a millennium before, describe restoration of the ability to see and to speak, as well as the healing of paralysis. In the Synoptic Gospels, we read, καὶ δύναμις κυρίου ἦν εἰς τὸ ἰᾶσθαι αὐτόν ('. . . the power of the Lord was with [Jesus] to heal [him] . . .').[35] Immediately following this verse, we read that men arrive carrying a paralysed (παραλελυμένος) man on a bed, seeking to place the man before Jesus so that Jesus would heal him. Thwarted in their task by the crowd, they climb onto the roof with their paralysed friend, remove the roof tiles, and lower him down through the ceiling. Jesus heals the man, and he picks up his mat and walks. In the Gospel of John, we likewise read of a man who suffered from a disability that hindered his ability to walk.[36] The man tells Jesus that he is unable to reach the healing pool beside which he lies, specifically because he has no one to put him into the pool . . . (Κύριε, ἄνθρωπον οὐκ ἔχω ἵνα ὅταν ταραχθῇ τὸ ὕδωρ βάλῃ με εἰς τὴν κολυμβήθραν . . .).[37] Jesus instructs this man, in language similar to that found in the Synoptic Gospels, to stand up, pick up his mat and walk.

As we have read, paralysis was widely acknowledged to be an intractable medical problem. This is precisely why it is an excellent illness for a divinity to cure – treatment is impossible for human physicians, as they themselves repeatedly acknowledged in their texts. I think it is even possible to suggest, based on the comments from Celsus' text, that paralytics were a kind of outcast to the medical profession because of the incurability of their condition. Physicians shied away from intervening in these cases because they feared accusations of having inflicted permanent harm: paralytics were, from the perspective of the physicians, the irredeemable. From the perspective of the writers and audiences of religious texts such as the miracle inscriptions and the Gospels, one who could cure this disease would surely be perceived as greater than human.

These religious texts, by emphasising that individuals in Graeco-Roman antiquity appreciated that paralysis was incurable, lead us to the argument I seek to make about the relationship between paralysis and prostheses. These texts show us a paralysed patient's prostheses in action – and those prostheses are other caring people. In the *Gospel of Mark*, the paralytic's friends carry him to Jesus and then lower him through the roof. In the *Gospel of John*, the man by the pool of Siloam laments that he has no one – ἄνθρωπον οὐκ ἔχω – to carry him to the water at the appropriate time. Others, either because they have greater physical capabilities than this man, or because they have friends, family or slaves who will carry them to the pool, reach the water before he does. The paralytic at Epidaurus, too, seems to have been carried to the sanctuary.[38] If we understand a prosthesis to be that which affords function, we see in these texts the prosthesis of antiquity for those whose limbs, while present, lacked function, and that prosthesis is another human being. As Horn stresses, visitors to the healing shrines of antiquity do not seem to have been concerned with whether or not their particular ailment could be considered, in our terms, a 'disability'.[39] Rather, they were worried about the curability of their problems. In this context of concern about curability, physicians' repeated and explicit acknowledgement, throughout centuries of medical literature, of the incurability of paralysis makes this condition a particularly dramatic example of one that would have required permanent adaptation. Yet, as we have seen, paralysis differs from the loss of a limb (another situation necessitating permanent adaptation), in that the 'replacement' of a lost limb is more straightforward. In the case of paralysis, functionality could be restored through resorting to the abilities of others.

Blindness: a parallel case of permanent loss of function with intact anatomy

Though the central focus of this paper is on paralysis and loss of mobility, blindness – another kind of loss of function – merits a brief mention as a parallel case study in an analysis about the loss of physical function. Unlike paralysis, the topic of blindness in the ancient Mediterranean has been discussed more extensively and will therefore be treated cursorily in this paper.[40] For the purposes of our study, blindness, or even severely diminished vision, differs from the kind of paralysis we have considered in three significant ways: its causes are multi-factorial (i.e., it can be a result not only of trauma, but also of cataracts, glaucoma or infection), its onset is generally not provoked by sudden trauma, and, in certain cases, physicians felt competent to treat it (or at least they were more willing to try). Blindness shares one important attribute with paralysis that makes it useful for our analysis of the role of human prostheses: like a paralysed individual whose legs and arms are still present but permanently nonfunctional, a blind individual's eyes, too, are present but permanently nonfunctional.[41]

Discussions of eye pathology in ancient medical texts have been well examined in modern secondary literature.[42] Hippocratic authors,[43] the Alexandrian anatomists,[44] Celsus[45] and Galen[46] all describe pathologies of the eye, offer various explanations of the mechanism of the problem and suggest methods of treatment. Particular diets, specific ointments, surgical tools adapted for operative management of eye problems and even specialists in eye diseases were available for those suffering from eye troubles.[47] Source material outside of medical texts makes it clear that eye problems were not uncommon in the ancient Mediterranean and were a significant source of disability, to varying degrees.[48] Yet, although discussion of eye diseases appears not infrequently in ancient medical texts, descriptions of the successful treatment of *blindness* are rare in these texts. Authors seem to know that certain problems, if untreated, could progress to blindness, which was then irreversible. Though its onset was often less instantaneous than paralysis secondary to trauma, blindness, too, was in many ways a medical lost cause: an assertion supported by the dedicatory inscription of a public slave who describes how his physicians gave up trying to treat his blindness.[49]

This dedicatory inscription, suggesting physicians' unwillingness to treat blindness, highlights a similarity between blindness and paralysis. The slave has given this inscription in thanks to Bona Dea, who healed him of his ten-month blindness. As was the case for paralysis, the intractability of blindness, and the ostensible unwillingness of physicians to deal with a problem they likely considered untreatable, meant it was a problem especially suitable for divine healing. Indeed, each canonical Gospel records at least one instance of Jesus healing the blind,[50] and multiple examples are also found in the miracle inscriptions from Epidaurus.[51] In sum, blindness, like paralysis, was recognised as being both debilitating and difficult to cure. The next section will examine how those suffering from paralysis and blindness lived with these challenges to their physical capabilities.

Human prostheses and the restoration of function

As we have seen, the medical practitioners of antiquity have much to say on the topics of paralysis and blindness, even if their statements are (especially in the case of paralysis) a disavowal of responsibility for treatment. While physicians and anatomists debated their understanding of paralysis and blindness, those with these afflictions, and their caregivers, confronted the pragmatic reality of permanently lost functionality. If these individuals survived the onset of their disability, they would have needed to depend on others for their day-to-day functioning and survival. Evidence for these 'human prostheses' is less immediately obvious because our medical writers are generally less concerned with the mundane, repetitive, less glamorous details of daily caregiving than they are with their own theory and practice. We have already seen how, in the Gospels, one paralysed man's friends assisted in bringing him before Jesus to be healed, while another paralysed man laments that he has no friends to carry him to the nearby healing waters of the pool. This section will present more examples of what we might consider 'human prostheses', focusing also on the role of slaves in enhancing human functionality.

Greek tragedy and epic provide notable examples of the blind being helped by those around them: blind bards and seers are led by slaves.[52] One of the most infamous blind men of Greek myth, Oedipus, laments his own disability, saying that others must perform a sacrifice for him since he lacks physical capability and sight.[53] In telling statements about his dependence upon his daughter's sight, Oedipus refers to Antigone's eyes as his eyes.[54] The importance of the human agent in restoring functionality is especially highlighted by the action of the play just prior to Oedipus' statement about Antigone's role in helping him see. Creon, having just sent Antigone away, has said that Oedipus will never walk again with his crutches (σκήπτροιν). The context suggests a layered meaning to 'crutches': they are not only the physical object that Oedipus, in his blindness, uses to assess the ground at his feet, but also Oedipus' daughter, who has been guiding his steps.[55] In his response to Creon, Oedipus emphasises this latter aspect of σκῆπτρον, stating that *his daughter* helps him to walk. Her eyes are his eyes: she restores functionality to him. The parallel drawn between objects, and the person who fulfills the role that the object would normally occupy, underscores the importance of the physical assistance of others in the lives of people with altered functional capabilities.

Additional examples from outside the realms of epic and tragedy underscore the role that others played in restoring lost mobility. A papyrus from Oxyrhynchus records a request from a sick man to his sister: having become ill from a riding accident, he says that he cannot turn on to his other side without two additional people to help move him, and he asks his sister to return home to nurse him.[56] Pliny describes in detail the poor health of Domitius Tullus, and how he was cared for by both his wife and his slaves:

> In fact he was gnarled and crippled in every limb. He attended to his massive wealth only by eyeing it, and even in bed he could change his posture only by help from others; disgusting and pitiful to relate, he had even to have his teeth washed and brushed for him. He was often heard to say, when he was complaining about the indignities of his weakened

state, that every day he licked the fingers of his slaves. Yet he continued to live on, and wanted to live on, sustained above all by his wife, who by her perseverance had transformed the obloquy incurred at the beginning of their marriage into good repute.[57]

The nature of Domitius Tullus' illness is uncertain, though the limitations it placed upon his own functionality are clearly described. He survived through the caregiving of his wife and, especially, his slaves.

The example of Domitius Tullus shows that while devoted family or friends were often involved in caring for the disabled, this was not necessarily the case. Those who could afford slaves, like Domitius Tullus, had access to a source of labour that provided enhanced functionality for many in the ancient Mediterranean world, not just those with compromised physical capabilities. Slaves were litter-bearers, for example, performing the work of walking;[58] they could pre-chew children's food to make it easier for them to eat; they were wet-nurses, even for women who were physically able to nurse their own infants; they could read aloud to their masters, a service that would have been vital for those with failing eyesight; educated slaves could also take dictation, writing when their masters could not or did not wish to write.[59] Extending Garnsey's definition of slavery, which emphasises masters' property rights over their slaves' bodies,[60] to the idea of prostheses, we might even see how slaves' bodies could become replacements for masters' nonfunctional bodies. The importance of a slave's physical functionality is revealed in Gellius' comments about the difference between a *morbus* and a *vitium* in the context of purchasing a slave: 'the ability to perform work' determines how a slave's health problem should be classified.[61] Two examples from classical Greece suggest similar awareness of a slave's physical capabilities (and limitations): Pericles, upon observing a slave break his leg, reportedly remarked that the slave would now have to become a *paedagogus*, and Alcibiades' tutor became such because of physical infirmity.[62] Physical fitness was (obviously) an important attribute for a slave to have, and this physical capability was leveraged by masters not only to enhance what a single man was able to do (e.g., large groups of slaves working on a landowner's estate), but also to perform the work that a master was unwilling or unable to do. This included, for example, providing their bodies as a means of walking (litter-bearing), seeing (reading, leading the blind), and even chewing.

The idea of a 'living prosthesis' – that is, of a human who (freely or under compulsion) uses his or her body to carry out the functions of another person's body – raises questions not encountered in considerations of other kinds of prostheses. Chiefly, a human prosthesis has primary agency. A freely serving 'human prosthesis' can decide when and how he or she would like to carry out his or her task, and there is consequently a particular relationship between the individual without function, and the individual with it. Love, duty, devotion and other emotions and social obligations inform this relationship in ways that are irrelevant for a peg leg, a crutch or a wheelchair, and we are therefore confronted with the questions involving the issues of independence and self-sufficiency. In a chapter about slave labour and Roman society, John Bodel explores these concepts of self-sufficiency and the labour of others particularly as they relate to the idea of the gentleman farmer, though they are also applicable to our discussion of 'human prostheses':

> It was the transparency of the slave as a surrogate that made slave labour essential to the ideology of self-sufficiency, since it allowed the slave-owner to reap the material and social benefits of labour (revenue, prestige, autonomy) without incurring the physical and social costs (fatigue, toil, dishonour). The advantages of this personal transparency can be seen throughout the system.[63]

This 'personal transparency' – especially pronounced for slaves, who were, in many respects, socially invisible – is perhaps a fundamental part of living prostheses. The barrier between the one who permanently lacks function, and the one who can restore it, is particularly diaphanous. Yet, unlike the estate slave labour that Bodel is describing, in the case of those with incurable disability, attainment of enhanced functionality through the 'surrogate' does not equate to 'self-sufficiency'. Rather, it is a reminder of dependence on others.

Caregiving and conclusions

This chapter has sought to expand our understanding of 'prostheses' by focusing on the role of a prosthesis in restoring functionality when it has been irrevocably lost. Using paralysis (especially that occurring secondary to spinal injury) and blindness as case studies for exploring the issues surrounding permanent loss of function, we first observed, in broad strokes, how the medical texts of the ancient Mediterranean described these problems and their treatment. The physicians of the past recognised that these patients, if they survived the trauma or illness that precipitated their condition, would be permanently disabled. Texts encourage physicians not to treat those with paralysis, and reference to assistive walking devices, for example, is not common in the passages describing the symptoms and anatomical mechanism of paralysis. Additional literary evidence reveals physicians' reticence to treat patients who suffered from prolonged blindness. Descriptions of the miraculous healing of patients whom the medical profession hesitated to treat yielded evidence of the particular importance of other people in these patients' lives.

Focusing on ways in which people could restore or enhance the functionality of others led to consideration of the role of slaves in these tasks. Slaves could and did serve as replacements of physical capabilities when their masters were lacking them or simply did not wish to exert themselves in a particular task. Although it cannot be emphasised enough that slave labour is fundamentally not equivalent to the freely given services of family and friends who took care of their incapacitated loved ones, both scenarios do share a reliance upon another individual to provide a physical function (e.g., locomotion). The idea that one would rely on slaves to engage in these tasks of carrying an individual who could not walk, or acting as eyes for one who could not read, or chewing a child's food, underscores their difficulty and, in a certain sense, their undesirability. Lending one's physical capabilities to another who lacks or does not want to use them can be mentally, emotionally and physically exhausting. It can also involve feelings of frustration and indignity for the individual who has lost the capabilities he or she once had.[64]

It is this dynamic – the relationship between a disabled person and his or her carer – that I seek to highlight in this chapter. Studies focusing on the medical treatments of antiquity – instruments, devices, medicaments and regimens – run the risk of overlooking two important facts. First, as has already been discussed in existing literature, patients with medical problems more often than not relied on their own devices (and the goodwill of their families and friends) for help. Firsthand accounts of the lives of the patients who lived and died in the world of the ancient Mediterranean are sadly rare,[65] and we more often hear their stories from the physicians who preserve them, in their own carefully crafted form, in medical case histories. These stories are less likely to contain details of day-to-day caregiving by slaves or family members, and more likely to record, for example, physicians' observations of bodily fluids or efforts at intervention. The second important fact to remember is perhaps somewhat obvious but bears noting explicitly: the ancient Mediterranean was a physically dangerous place. Institutions providing medical care were rather non-existent; there were no physician licensing procedures; average life expectancy was significantly lower than in today's developed world; child mortality was high; there was little in the way of 'disability insurance';[66] and the idea of a sophisticated prosthesis of the kind used today (or even one that could afford functionality beyond what is possible today) was utterly unthinkable outside the realm of dreams and mythology.[67] Awareness of these two facts leads us to a conclusion hopefully highlighted by this study. In the setting of disability, reliance upon one's family, friends, and community was of vital importance in the past, as it is today. Our ancient medical sources could lead us, inadvertently, to overlook this reality.

Modern research in the field of medical anthropology has in recent years begun to focus on what the field has called 'caregiving'. In a moving *Lancet* article, physician and anthropologist Arthur Kleinman wrote of his practice of caregiving for his wife of forty-three years, who was diagnosed in her 60s with a severe and rapidly progressing from of Alzheimer's Disease which brought with it blindness. Kleinman describes how he led his wife around the home in which she had lived for over twenty years; how he fed and dressed her; how he reminded her of her surroundings when she was lost. He became her eyes and her memory, restoring functionality and ensuring that she could remain living at home with him until her illness became too severe.[68]

I mention Dr Kleinman and his wife, who passed away in 2010, to broaden our understanding of 'prosthesis'. It has been mentioned in this volume that a prosthesis is, literally, 'that which is set to'.[69] In modern parlance, the term is commonly understood to refer to an artificial limb or organ, one which replaces what was lost and takes over its function. The cases of paralysis and blindness that we have explored provide extreme examples of situations in which much functionality has been lost. As we have seen, in antiquity, the prostheses – 'those which are set to' – in these settings are, in fact, other caring people. We speak of caregiving now as though it is a dying art. Perhaps, in a modern Western culture in which the sick are taken to hospital, approximately 98.4 per cent of individuals are born in hospital[70] and approximately 78 per cent of individuals die in hospital or in professional care settings,[71] 'non-professional' caregiving is more rare and unexpected today than it was in antiquity. This chapter has been wide-ranging, and I hope that it has served to broaden our concept of 'prosthesis' to recognise the value of caregiving, thereby helping us to glimpse the way in which people helped one another in antiquity, and the way they help each other today.

To return to the example with which we began, perhaps the idea of caregiving as a kind of prosthesis is precisely what makes the story of Stephen Hawking, especially as dramatised in the associated film *The Theory of Everything*, so compelling.[72] The might of his agile mind comprehended the universe to an extent that few ever have or ever will know, yet the frailty of his paralysed body necessitated his utter dependence upon others – namely his first wife, Jane – for continued survival. The story of Stephen and Jane Hawking fascinates us, I believe, because it shows how a man so reliant upon highly developed, highly functional mechanical and electronic prostheses, depends upon the love, fortitude (physical and otherwise) and patience of those around him. Mechanical devices and the physical assistance of others certainly restore physical functionality – but perhaps *functionality* is not purely physical. Perhaps, when we think of disease and disability, we should also think of the strength of the heart and the mind. Stephen and Jane Hawking's story, like the stories of those preserved for us in these case histories and texts, reminds us that, in many ways, the most powerful and most effective prostheses – that is, those restoratives of function and of ability – are the people who care for us in our infirmity.

Notes

1 The author thanks Jane Draycott for her thoughtfulness, creativity and rigour in organising the conference on prostheses that led to this volume, and for her help in the revision process; the anonymous reviewer whose comments improved the strength of the argument; and James L. Zainaldin, whose careful eye and incisive mind greatly enhanced the arguments and evidence presented.

2 'Start-up attempts to convert Prof Hawking's brainwaves into speech.' BBC News, 7 July 2012. Available <http://www.bbc.com/news/technology-18749963> (accessed January 2018).

3 For the full, remarkable story of Professor Hawking's life, see Hawking, 2013, and Hawking, 2010.
4 For discussion of prosthetic toes, see Finch, this volume.
5 Consider, for example, the prosthetic legs that competitive runners use: generally 'blades', these do not resemble 'real legs' but in the setting of competitive running, these blades function as well as, or better than, biological human legs. See the Introduction, this volume, on combination cosmetic and functional prostheses.
6 Sanchez and Meltzer, 2012.
7 Sanchez and Meltzer, 2012.
8 Sanchez and Meltzer, 2012, pp. 202–203.
9 See Sanchez and Meltzer, 2012, p. 206 for arguments supporting the claim that 'non-awareness would then encompass absence of both motion and sensation, in other words, nonexistence of that bodily entity'. See also Walker, 1993, p. 83.
10 The concept of 'retrospective diagnosis' is controversial, and it should be acknowledged that any attempt to identify the nature of injuries recorded in the case histories of the past is neither certain nor, without the ability to examine and speak with the patient him- or herself, verifiable. However, I believe that a careful, informed attempt to provide multiple possible explanations of what is described can be a fruitful exercise. It is in this spirit that I discuss this and subsequent cases.
11 Todd, 2011.
12 Hippocrates, *On Joints* 48 (trans. E. T. Withington): καὶ ἢν περιγένωνται δὲ, ῥυώδεες τὰ οὖρα μᾶλλον οὗτοι, καὶ τῶν σκελέων ἀκρατέστεροι καὶ ναρκωδέστεροι: ἢν δὲ καὶ ἐν τῷ ἄνω μέρεϊ μᾶλλον τὸ λόρδωμα γένηται, παντὸς τοῦ σώματος ἀκρατέες καὶ καταναρκωμένοι γίνονται.
13 ἀκρατής also appears at least twice, and as many as five times (depending on how one restores the text), in the miracle inscriptions from the healing sanctuary at Epidaurus. See LiDonnici, 1995: for paralysis of the fingers, p. 87, inscription A3, and the entire body, p. 113, inscription B17. For the third, fourth and fifth references (which are less certain), see B18, p. 113; C14, p. 125; and C21, p. 129.
14 Spinal cord injury can cause urinary incontinence and/or retention, as well as bowel incontinence and/or retention. The precise nature of the incontinence/ retention depends upon many factors, including the level and severity of the spinal cord injury. This Hippocratic author's description of urinary and bowel retention secondary to vertebral injury, and the Edwin Smith Papyrus author's description of urinary incontinence secondary to vertebral injury, are both plausible descriptions of spinal injury sequelae.
15 Hippocrates, *Aphorisms* 7.40.
16 Hippocrates, *Epidemics* 4.50; see also Hippocrates, *Epidemics* 2.2.8.
17 Hippocrates, *Prorrhetic* 1.118.
18 Hippocrates, *Coan Prenotions* 395.
19 Hippocrates, *On Joints* 52. σκίπων is also the word used for 'crutch' in inscription A16 from Epidaurus; LiDonnici, 1995, p. 97.
20 See von Staden, 1989, p. 159; also Solmsen, 1961, p. 185.
21 (?) Rufus of Ephesus, *On the Anatomy of the Parts of the Body* 71–75; see also von Staden, 1989, pp. 200–201 and p. 250.
22 Galen, *On Tremor, Palpitation, Spasm, and Rigor* 4 (7.605 Kühn); see also von Staden, 1989, pp. 255–256.
23 Galen, *On the Affected Parts* 3.14 (8.212 Kühn); see also von Staden, 1989, p. 200.
24 Celsus, *On Medicine*, 8.13–14.
25 Galen, *On Anatomical Procedures* 3.1 (2.343–345 Kühn).
26 Galen, *On the Affected Parts* 1.6 (8.56–61 Kühn) for examples of therapy directed toward the spinal cord, and of Galen's silence about cures for certain types of paralysis.

27 Galen, *On the Affected Parts* 3.14 (8.211–213 Kühn).

28 Galen, *On the Affected Parts* 6.4 (8.407 Kühn).

29 *Ibid.*

30 A recent comparison of the Epidaurean miracle inscriptions and the Gospel texts of the Bible, in the context of disability studies, has been made by Horn, 2013.

31 LiDonnici, 1995. The entire introduction explains the origins of the text of the inscriptions in detail; see especially pp. 65–67.

32 Nutton, 1992; Nutton, 2013; and Israelowich, 2015 are just a few of the many sources that describe the options available to patients regarding care and treatment.

33 See note 13.

34 LiDonnici, 1995, p. 129, inscription C21. See Plato, *Symposium* 190a and *Timaeus* 44e, as well as Aristotle, *Posterior Analytics* 684a3 for how this word seems to describe weight-bearing on an external object.

35 *Luke* 5:17. See *Luke* 5:17–26 for the full excerpt; see also *Matthew* 9:1–8 and *Mark* 1:1–12. This and subsequent biblical texts are from *The Greek New Testament*, 3rd edition, United Bible Societies, 1975. Translations are from the Oxford Annotated Bible, 2007. On mobility impairments in the Jewish tradition, see Lehmhaus, this volume.

36 While the language here implies an inability to walk, it should be noted that it is not the same as the language typically used to describe paralysis in medical texts of the time. *John* 5:2–5.

37 *John* 5:7.

38 See note 34.

39 Horn, 2013, p. 116.

40 See, for example, Buxton, 1980; Bernidaki-Aldous, 1990; Vlahogiannis, 1998; Rose, 2003; Kelley, 2007; Létoublon, 2010; and Trentin, 2013.

41 Note also the opening lines of Hippocrates, *Prorrhetic* 2, which discuss how physicians make fantastic prognoses: the first two afflictions listed as examples of these awe-inspiring prognoses are weakness of the upper extremity (which Nutton, 2013, p. 88, considers to be paralysis), and blindness. Perhaps it was the incurable and disabling nature of both paralysis and blindness that made prognosis of their future occurrence particularly impressive.

42 In addition to the sources mentioned in n. 41, see Jackson, 1996.

43 Hippocrates, *On Sight*; see also Craik, 2005 and Craik, 2006.

44 von Staden, 1989, T85–89, T140, T260; and pp. 570–578.

45 Celsus, *On Medicine* 6.6, 7.7.6 and 7.7.9.

46 Galen's descriptions of patients with eye problems include *On Hippocrates' Aphorisms* 6.31 (18A.45–49 Kühn) and *On Examinations by which the Best Physicians are Recognized* 3.12 (58–60 Iskandar).

47 Jackson, 1996.

48 A duty roster from Vindolanda, *T. Vindol.* 154, provides one illustrative example: of the 752 men listed present at a particular auxiliary fort, 31 are reported as unfit for duty: eye problems were the source of disability for 10 of these 31 men; Bowman and Thomas, 1991.

49 *ILS* 3513 (*derelictus a medicis*).

50 *Matthew* 9:27–31 and 20:29–34; *Mark* 8:22–26 and 10:46–52; *Luke* 18:35–43; *John* 9:1–11. 'Blindness' has obvious metaphorical significance in religious contexts, though its practical significance should not be overlooked, especially in the setting of additional evidence which demonstrates the prevalence of eye afflictions in antiquity (see discussion and notes, above).

51 LiDonnici, 1995, inscriptions A4 (pp. 88–89); A9 (pp. 92–93).; A18 (pp. 98–99); A20 (pp. 98–99); B2 (pp. 100–101); B12 (pp. 108–109); C22 (pp. 128–129).

52 Homer, *Odyssey* 8.62, 106. See also Rose, 2003, pp. 79–94; Noel, this volume.

53 Sophocles, *Oedipus at Colonus*, 496.

54   Sophocles, *Oedipus at Colonus*, 864–867. See also 1–31, where Antigone guides Oedipus and describes what she sees.
55   Sophocles, *Oedipus at Colonus*, 848–849.
56   *P. Oxy.* 3314.5–17; see Draycott, 2016, pp. 442–443.
57   Pliny the Younger, *Letters* 8.18.9–10 (trans. P. G. Walsh): *Quippe omnibus membris extortus et fractus, tantas opes solis oculis obibat, ac ne in lectulo quidem nisi ab aliis movebatur; quin etiam – foedum miserandumque dictu – dentes lavandos fricandosque praebebat. Auditum frequenter ex ipso, cum quereretur de contumeliis debilitatis suae, digitos se servorum suorum cotidie lingere. Vivebat tamen et vivere volebat, sustentante maxime uxore, quae culpam incohati matrimonii in gloriam perseverantia verterat.*
58   Seneca, *Moral Letters* 55. Note that he highlights the physical functions of walking and seeing.
59   Golden, 2010, p. 141; for slaves and literacy, see Harris, 1989, p. 111.
60   Garnsey, 1996, p. I.
61   Gellius, *Attic Nights* 4.2; see also Laes *et al.*, 2013, p. 7. The *Digest*, too, discusses slaves' bodies in terms of the extent to which injuries or 'defects' of particular parts of the body affect their ability to perform work: *Digest* 21.1.12.1–4; see also Bradley 1994, p. 52, and Weiler, 2002, pp. 22–23.
62   Hieronymus of Rhodes in Stobaeus, *Florilegium* 31.121; Plato, *Alcibiades* 1 122b. See also Golden, 2010, p. 141.
63   Bodel, 2010, p. 316.
64   Refer again to Pliny's words of praise of Domitius Tullus' wife in note 57, and Tullus' lament of his total dependence on others for completion of even simple tasks of self-care.
65   An exception to this is the extensive autobiographical writings of Aelius Aristides, though he is an atypical patient for many reasons, not least because of his wealth and social privilege. Recent work about health and disease in the ancient Mediterranean has increasingly focused on reconstructing the patient experience independently of what ancient physicians tell us about it. See, for example, Petridou and Thumiger, 2016, and Israelowich, 2015.
66   Nutton, 2013, pp. 19–36.
67   Consider the replacement of Pelops' shoulder (Ovid, *Metamorphoses* 6.405); Hephaestus' *automata* (Homer, *Iliad* 18.371); and even Daedalus' wings that were to help him and Icarus escape their Cretan prison (Ovid, *Metamorphoses* 8.183–235).
68   Kleinman, 2009.
69   For discussion of this, see the Introduction, this volume.
70   US Centers for Disease Control, *Trends in Out-of-Hospital Births in the United States, 1990–2012*, NCHS Data Brief No. 144, March, 2014. This statistic refers to the United States alone.
71   NCHS Data, Worktable 309. Deaths by place of death, age, race, and sex: United States, 2005. Available http://www.cdc.gov/nchs/data/dvs/Mortfinal2005_worktable_309.pdf (accessed 30 January 2016).
72   This film is based on the memoir written by Stephen Hawking's first wife; see Hawking, 2010.

Bibliography

BBC. 'Start-up attempts to convert Prof Hawking's brainwaves into speech'. Last modified 7 July 2012. Available <http://www.bbc.com/news/technology-1874 9963> (accessed January 2018).

Bernidaki-Aldous, E. (1990) *Blindness in a Culture of Light: Especially in the Case of Oedipus at Colonus of Sophocles*. New York, NY: Peter Lang.

Bodel, J. (2010) 'Slave Labour and Roman Society', in Bradley, K. and Cartledge, P. (edd.) *The Cambridge World History of Slavery*. Cambridge: Cambridge University Press, pp. 311–336.

Bowman, A. K. and Thomas, J. D. (1991) 'A Military Strength Report from Vindolanda', *JRS* 81, pp. 62–73.

Bradley, K. (1994) *Slavery and Society at Rome*. Cambridge: Cambridge University Press.

Bradley, K. and Cartledge, P. (edd.) (2010) *The Cambridge World History of Slavery*. Cambridge: Cambridge University Press.

Buxton, R. G. A. (1980) 'Blindness and Limits: Sophokles and the Logic of Myth', *JHS* 100, pp. 22–37.

Craik, E. (2005) 'The Hippocratic Treatise περὶ ὄψιος (*de vivendi acie, On the Organ of Sight*)'. *Studies in Ancient Medicine* 31, pp. 191–207.

Craik, E. (2006) *Two Hippocratic Treatises*, On Sight *and* On Anatomy. Leiden: Brill.

Draycott, J. (2016) 'Literary and Documentary Evidence for Lay Medical Practice in the Roman Republic and Empire', in Petridou, G. and Thumiger, C. (edd.) Homo Patiens: *Approaches to the Patient in the Ancient World*. Leiden: Brill, pp. 432–450.

Garnsey, P. D. A. (1996) *Ideas of Slavery from Aristotle to Augustine*. Cambridge: Cambridge University Press.

Golden, M. (2010) 'Slavery and the Greek Family', in Bradley, K. and Cartledge, P. (edd.) *The Cambridge World History of Slavery*. Cambridge: Cambridge University Press, pp. 134–152.

Harris, W. (1989) *Ancient Literacy*. Cambridge, MA: Harvard University Press.

Hawking, J. (2010) *Traveling to Infinity: My Life with Stephen*. London: Alma Books Ltd.

Hawking, S. (2013) *My Brief History*. London: Bantam Books.

Horn, C. (2013) 'A Nexus of Disability in Ancient Greek Miracle Stories: A Comparison of Accounts of Blindness from the Asklepieion in Epidauros and the Shrine of Thecla in Seleucia', in Laes, C., Goodey, C. F. and Rose, M. L. (edd.) *Disabilities in Roman Antiquity: Disparate Bodies* a Capite ad Calcem. Leiden: Brill, pp. 115–144.

Israelowich, I. (2015) *Patients and Healers in the High Roman Empire*. Baltimore, MD: Johns Hopkins University Press.

Jackson, R. (1996) 'Eye Medicine in the Roman Empire', *ANRW* II 37. 3, pp. 228–251.

Kelley, N. (2007) 'Deformity and Disability in Greece and Rome', in Avalos, H., Melcher, S. J. and Schipper, J. (edd.) *This Abled Body: Rethinking Disabilities in Biblical Studies*. Atlanta, GA: Society for Biblical Literature, pp. 31–45.

Kleinman, A. (2009) 'Caregiving: The Odyssey of Becoming More Human', *The Lancet* 373, pp. 292–293.

Laes, C., Goodey, C. F. and Rose, M. L. (2013) *Disabilities in Roman Antiquity: Disparate Bodies* a Capite ad Calcem. Leiden: Brill.

Létoublon, F. (2010) 'To See or Not to See: Blind People and Blindness in Ancient Greek Myths', in Christopoulos, M., Karakantza, E. D. and Levaniouk, O. (edd.) *Light and Darkness in Ancient Greek Myth and Religion*. Lanham, MD: Lexington Books, pp. 167–180.

LiDonnici, L. R. (1995) *The Epidaurian Miracle Inscriptions*. Atlanta, GA: Scholars Press.

Nutton, V. (1992) 'Healers in the Medical Market Place: Towards a Social History of Graeco-Roman Medicine', in Wear, A. (ed.) *Medicine in Society*. Cambridge: Cambridge University Press, pp. 1–58.

Nutton, V. (2013) *Ancient Medicine*. New York, NY: Routledge.

Petridou, G. and Thumiger, C. (edd.) (2016) Homo Patiens: *Approaches to the Patient in the Ancient World*. Leiden: Brill.

Rose, M. (2003) *The Staff of Oedipus*. Ann Arbor, MI: University of Michigan Press.

Sanchez, G. M. and Meltzer, E. S. (2012) *The Edwin Smith Papyrus: Updated Translation of the Trauma Treatise and Modern Medical Commentaries*. Atlanta, GA: Lockwood Press.

Solmsen, F. (1961) 'Greek Philosophy and the Discovery of the Nerves', *Museum Helveticum* 18, pp. 150–197.

Todd, N. V. (2011) 'Priapism in Acute Spinal Cord Injury', *Spinal Cord* 49, pp. 1033–1035.

Trentin, L. (2013) 'Exploring Visual Impairment in Ancient Rome', in Laes, C., Goodey, C. F. and Rose, M. L. (edd.) *Disabilities in Roman Antiquity: Disparate Bodies* a Capite ad Calcem. Leiden: Brill, pp. 89–114.

United States Centers for Disease Control (2014) *Trends in Out-of-Hospital Births in the United States, 1990–2012*. NCHS Data Brief No. 144.

United States National Center for Health Statistics. NCHS Data, Worktable 309. Deaths by place of death, age, race, and sex. 2005. Available http://www.cdc.gov/nchs/data/dvs/Mortfinal2005_worktable_309.pdf. (accessed 30 January 2016).

Vlahogiannis, N. (1998) 'Disabling Bodies', in Montserrat, D. (ed.) *Changing Bodies, Changing Meanings: Studies on the Human Body in Antiquity*. London and New York, NY: Routledge, pp. 13–35.

von Staden, H. (1989) *Herophilus: The Art of Medicine in Early Alexandria*. Cambridge: Cambridge University Press.

Walker, J. H. (1993) 'Egyptian Medicine and the Gods'. *The Bulletin of the Australian Centre for Egyptology* 4, pp. 83–101.

Weiler, I. (2013) 'Inverted *Kalokagathia*', in Wiedemann, T. and Gardner, J. (edd.) *Representing the Body of the Slave*. London: Routledge, pp. 11–28.

7 'Prosthetic imagination' in Greek literature[1]

Anne-Sophie Noel

Introduction

If 'prostheses are discursive frameworks, as well as material artefacts', this chapter will deliberately focus on the discursive side.[2] My aim is to investigate the 'prosthetic imagination', e.g., the ways in which 'the prosthetic' may be used as a metaphor to think about the boundaries between objects and bodies in ancient Greek literature.

'Prosthetic imagination' in modern times has been well analysed and criticised by scholars reflecting on disabilities. According to Jain and Sobchack, the trope of prosthesis has been used since the 1990s as an improper tool for reflecting upon human–technology relationships: after the 'cyborg' trend tarnished by 'academic overuse', writes Sobchack, 'the prosthetic' is the 'new, sexy metaphor' that 'has become tropological currency for describing a vague and shifting constellation of relationships among bodies, technologies and subjectivities'.[3] In her ironical critique of the trope, Sobchack draws from her own experience of a prosthetic leg to contradict fantasies that attribute to prostheses a status of quasi-living and autonomous being ('I know intimately my prosthetic leg's essential inertia and lack of motivating volition').[4] In 1999, Jain had criticised the use of this idealised metaphor as one that often masked the fact that prostheses could create rather than supply alienation and deficiency.[5] In 2006 Serlin adds that this techno-animist account of human–prosthesis relationship is perhaps another way to discriminate against disabled people, by excessively emphasising the object agency rather than the human one.[6] These convergent critiques are then based on methodological and ethical grounds. In this very volume, Adams points out that 'the metaphorical use of the term [prosthesis] is somewhat confusing', spanning not only artificial body parts, but also any machine or technology 'that intervenes in human subjectivity', like a telephone or a computer.[7] For the theorists of embodied and extended cognition for example, a pen that allows thinking in writing, or a notebook that acts as somebody's artificial memory, can be conceived in terms of 'bodily and cognitive prosthetic'.[8]

If the prosthetic metaphor has become a trite one, which conveys an inaccurate and deformed image of the reality of prostheses, is it really wise to search for it in ancient Greek literature? Firstly, part of the methodological issue can be avoided by acknowledging the fact that although I am trying to document the existence of a metaphor in Greek poetry, I do not pretend to say anything about the actual prostheses that existed in ancient Greece. I easily admit that if a 'prosthetic imagination' impregnated ancient authors' ways of describing relationships between human body and inanimate implements, this was probably detached from the prosthetic experience of Greek individuals in their daily life. That being said, what urges me to ask the question of the applicability of the prosthesis trope to ancient literature is that the oldest extant mention of a prosthesis (Pindar's first *Olympian Ode*) describes a symbiotic relationship between human and prosthesis. The aforementioned scholars assumed that this was characteristic of a modern 'prosthetic imagination' strongly associated with contemporary high-tech improvements, which they strive to deconstruct. The belief that a prosthesis can be a living implement enhancing the body is indeed perhaps easier to conceive at a time when double-amputee Aimee Mullins can build her fame on her rich set of prosthetic legs that allow her to be, in turn, a record-breaking sprinter (with her 'Cheetah legs'), a model (with her 'Barbie legs') or an intriguing hybrid creature in a contemporary art performance (with her 'glass legs' featured in a movie by Matthew Barney).[9]

Nevertheless, I will question the explicit assumption that 'prosthetic imagination' is a topical, fashionable metaphor of our time, whose birth and flourishing are anchored in modernity and *high-technophilia*. The first claim that will be made in this chapter is that it may be traced back to ancient 'low-tech' societies. Secondly, I will argue that in this first literary testimony of a mythological prosthesis (the ivory shoulder of Pelops), Pindar draws his inspiration from what I call the 'man–weapon compound': the striking representation of weapons as animated body-incorporations in Homer. Pindar's vibrant prosthesis is, in my view, a reworking of the Homeric human–weapon relationship, also reinterpreted on stage by Greek tragedians about the same time. Going back to this first extant mention of prosthesis and to what I consider as its counterparts in Greek tragedy – and thus, hoping to avoid the risk of vagueness pointed out by Adams – I will defend the relevance of the 'prosthetic imagination' to ancient Greek literature. Finally, this cultural 'fantasy' will be reassessed in light of its meaning and importance in Greek epic and tragedy: a response, be it ethical or not, to an irrepressible need to imagine and to stage *sympathetic* relationships between human beings and the things they live with.

On the very first prosthesis: Pindar's φαίδιμον ὦμον

Fame shines for him in the colony of brave men founded by Lydian Pelops, with whom mighty Earthholder Poseidon fell in love, after Klotho pulled him from the pure cauldron, adorned with his shoulder gleaming with ivory.[10]

Pindar's first *Olympian Ode* contains the oldest mention of a prosthesis in the whole of classical literature, the mythical ivory shoulder of Pelops. This refers to the famous story of Tantalus' banquet: Tantalus cut his own son Pelops into pieces and offered this perverted meal to the gods. Only Demeter, distracted by her grief for her daughter Persephone, eats the left shoulder of Pelops while the other gods refuse this abominable meat. Tantalus is then precipitated to the underworld and Pelops revived, plunged into the cauldron of Klotho. The interpretation of this passage from *Olympian* 1 is much debated: after having recalled the story of this mythical prosthesis, Pindar denies the authenticity of this traditional story just a few lines further, and proposes an alternative version, reflecting on the relationship between marvel and speech. Numerous scholars have commented about the choice Pindar made between co-existing and sometimes contradictory aetiological myths linked with Pelops and the foundation of the Olympic Games.[11] However, the nature of the prosthesis itself may be explored further. Indeed, Pindar describes a fascinating continuity between the hero's body and the ivory device that replaces the shoulder eaten by the grieving Demeter. As a gift supplied by the gods, the prosthesis is Pelops' special *arétè*, the mark that makes visible a particular divine favour and destiny. The 'prosthetic imagination' may well start as early as in this first literary mention of a prosthetic device.

The prosthesis is not called by a specific noun but by the name of the missing body part (ὦμον, 'shoulder'); the dative ἐλέφαντι ('ivory') indicates its material. This formulation is close to that of Herodotus, narrating the story of the diviner Hegesistratos who chose to cut off a part of his foot in order to escape from a Spartan prison and then replaced it with a prosthetic 'wooden foot' (ξύλινον πόδα, at *Histories* 9.37.4).[12] This way of naming the prosthetic device may suggest that it really becomes a part of the body, although carved in a hard and strong material. What is even more interesting in the Pindaric *Ode* is that the prosthesis is qualified by the adjective φαίδιμος, 'shining, radiant, gleaming': this radiance comes from the white and smooth ivory, material of the gods, as is suggested by the grammatical dependence of the dative ἐλέφαντι ('ivory') upon the adjective φαίδιμον.[13] Yet there is more than that: φαίδιμος is an epic adjective also applied to the body of the warriors in the works of Homer and Hesiod. In the *Iliad* (6.27) and in Hesiod's *Theogony* (492) warriors have 'glistening limbs' (φαίδιμα γυῖα); in the *Odyssey* (11.128), Odysseus' heroic stature is made visible through his 'glistening shoulder' (φαιδίμῳ ὤμῳ), a very close denomination to Pindar's one. Sophocles also imitates this epic designation in a fragment (453) that mentions the 'glistening shoulders' (φαιδίμοις ὤμοις) of Odysseus.[14] In epics, this shining appearance reveals the beauty and energy (μένος) circulating in the heroes' bodies: in the same way, the 'gleaming shoulder' of Pelops, although made of ivory, seems to be conceived as an animated part of his body.[15]

It is also noticeable that Pindar seems to suggest that this exceptional prosthesis enhances Pelops' beauty and seductive power.[16] The participle κεκαδμένον means both 'adorned with' and 'conspicuous', 'excelling' because of his divine prosthesis; moreover, the regenerative experience that Pelops enjoys in the 'pure cauldron' of Klotho, one of the Fates that assists at birth, can be interpreted as a second birth rejuvenating his beauty.[17] And according to whether one reads ἐπεί as temporal ('after') or causal ('since'), Poseidon is said to fall in love with Pelops either *after* his body has been reintegrated or *because* he was taken out of the cauldron with an ivory shoulder.[18] The latter version is at least as acceptable as the former, and it does very much emphasise the magnifying effect of Pelops' prosthesis.[19]

Just after this passage, Pindar introduces the controversial verses that hint at a recantation of the traditional story: 'indeed there are many wondrous things. And yet, the words that men tell, myths embellished by varying falsehoods, beyond wording that is true, are deceptive'.[20] Is this a way to discard this prosthetic fantasy? Is this specific passage erased by the ostentatious replacement of the dismemberment story by another narrative that starts with Pelops' abduction by Poseidon (63 sq.)?

Griffith and Nagy presented good evidence that Pindar could not discard Pelops' prosthesis, which stays a fixed element of the myth, be it at the cost of the narrative's logical coherence.[21] The artificial shoulder was indeed not only a literary artefact but also a real object, a Bronze Age relic (perhaps a ram shoulder-blade) that was probably on display in Olympia during Pindar's lifetime.[22] In Pausanias' account, the shoulder blade (simply called 'bone') was said to have travelled to Troy, as a token ensuring victory for the Greeks along with Philoctetes' bow and arrows.[23] Several symbolic explanations of the ivory shoulder have been proposed and they led to the downplaying of its prosthetic nature: instead of an external implement, it would be a birthmark or a trace of a failed transmutation of Pelops' body into the divine substance – on the model of Demeter's scheme to immortalise Demophon, Tantalus would have only managed to transform his son's shoulder.[24] And yet, writes Nagy, 'just as the ivory shoulder of Pelops was on display as a centerpiece in the ritual complex of the Olympics, so also it occupies primacy of place in the aetiological complex of Pindar's *Olympian* 1'.[25] The materiality of this prosthetic relic prevents us from thinking of it only in metaphorical and symbolic terms. Ironically, the hero who founded the Olympics, and was himself the paradigm of the victorious charioteer, was a prosthesis wearer, however divine and exceptional this prosthesis was. The Pindaric description seems to have left its trace on a tradition: five centuries later, Ovid follows the first *Olympian* closely when writing that Pelops' ivory device replaces the part of his body that was missing (*ebur impositum est in usum partis non comparentis*), thus completing the body of the hero, so that it becomes again *integer*, 'intact' and 'full' at the same time (*Metamorphoses* 4. 405).

Pindar and the epic heritage: body and arms in Homer

The 'gleaming shoulder' of Pelops (φαίδιμον ὦμον) has great chance to be Homeric in its wording (*Od.*, 11.23, quoted above). Yet, Pindar injects a new meaning in this formulaic phrasing by associating this gleaming aspect with the brilliance of ivory. Moreover, in my view, the Homeric influence is probably larger than the borrowing of these two words: the body–weapon relationship may have been a model for elaborating this 'super-prosthesis' that enhances Pelops' body. The radiance of the shoulder resembles that of the weapons in the *Iliad*: the δαίδαλα made of bronze, silver or gold that flash in the sun. These weapons are animated by the same vitality (μένος) that invigorates the heroes' bodies.[26] Some of them, like the arms of Achilles, possess a glistening radiance that raises a paralysing fear in the heart of his enemies.[27] A recurrent phrasing also attributes vitality (μένος) to spears on the battle-field, a force infused into the weapons by the warriors who manipulate them or by a divine intervention.[28]

This exchange of energy between the body and its 'integrated' weapon is reciprocal. The bronze of weapons can also take possession of the human body: the fantasy of a 'man of bronze', entirely merged with the metal of his weapons, permeates the *Iliad*. In book 20, according to Aeneas, the great Achilles pretends to be 'wholly made of bronze' (παγχάλκεος, 20.102). This allusion to a metallic superhuman being (maybe the first cyborg in literature) is unique in the *Iliad*, and in the mouth of Achilles, it is sheer boasting.[29] Nevertheless, we can note that in a general way, armour and weapons enjoy an intimate relationship with the warrior's body: 'Ni armure sans corps, (. . .) ni corps sans armure', as Oddone Longo sums up nicely.[30] Even the regular soldiers have well-adjusted weapons, which perfectly match their bodies as well as their value in war: in book 14, the commanders of the Greek army exchange the soldiers' panoplies so that each of them receives the weapons fitting to his qualities.[31] The defensive weapons that protect the body are like a second skin for the warrior: greaves (κνημίδες) for example, conform to the shape of the calf and ankle.[32] This poetic description finds a perfect material illustration in excavated objects, like the greaves from one of the Macedonian tombs at Vergina, which were adapted to fit an impaired leg.[33] In the *Iliad*, divine intervention also occurs, to adjust the weapons to the anatomy of their new possessors: when Hector spoils Patroclos' armour, Zeus blames him for usurping the immortal weapons of Achilles, but nevertheless adapts the armour to the size of Hector, literally to 'his skin' (Ἕκτορι δ᾽ ἥρμοσε τεύχε᾽ ἐπὶ χροΐ, *Iliad* 17.210). This solidarity between men and weapons is also expressed when heroes are shown sleeping, with their shield, spears and helmet lying just next to them (*Iliad* 10.75-6) or even sleeping with their armour on (*Iliad* 11.731): this is a protective measure but also proof of the inseparable relationship a warrior has with his panoply.[34] Scholars analyse it in terms of a *sympatheia*, a 'fellow-feeling' and strong 'affinity', which has reversible effects.[35] If the weapons become animated and 'attack' or 'rage' like the men who hold them,[36] the men can also acquire the metal qualities of their weapons: Achilles calls himself 'wholly made of bronze' (παγχάλκεος), but is also described as having 'men-slaying hands' (χεῖρας ἀνδροφόνους), as if the body parts in contact with the offensive sword melted with it.[37] The arm becomes the extension of the body, but the body might reciprocally be seen as the prolongation of the weapon. As Vernant put it:

> the hero's accoutrements, the prestigious arms that represent his career, his exploits, and his personal value, are a direct extension of his body. They adhere to him, form an alliance with him, are integrated into his remarkable figure like every other trait of his body armour.[38]

Greek tragedy and the 'prosthetic imagination'

In extant tragic dramas, there is not any character wearing a prosthesis: 'for the mutilated limbs of tragedy, no supplement is possible', wrote Robert Drew Griffith rightly in his article 'Corporality in the Ancient Greek Theatre'.[39] Characters who would today be considered as physically impaired are lacking any kind of prosthetic aid. In Sophocles' *Oedipus at Colonus*, the blind and weak Oedipus wanders on the paths from Thebes to Athens, deprived of any artificial device helping him on his way, not even a simple stick.[40] Filial love alone supplements the weaknesses of Oedipus' body: Antigone lends him her eyes (34) and she and her sister are objectified when called 'walking sticks' by Oedipus (σκῆπτρα, 848, 1109).

In Sophocles' *Philoctetes*, the lame hero, bitten by a snake, drags his swollen and festering foot along the ground. Critics have argued that the precision used by Sophocles to describe the wound derived from direct observation of a real wounded limb.[41] Building on the symptoms detailed in the theatrical text, modern physicians have diagnosed an acute gout arthritis,[42] which occurred at a relatively high frequency in the general ancient Greek population according to Martha Rose's research.[43] She suggested that the pathetic spectacle of the abandoned hero must have been rather familiar to the fifth-century BCE Athenian spectators, used to seeing in their daily life a variety of irregular gaits caused by war wounds, congenital deformities or illnesses.[44] In spite of this, Philoctetes does not have any brace, crutch, cane or staff to help him walk.

However, the prosthetic dimension of his weapon, the famous bow inherited from Heracles, is notably reinforced, inasmuch as it could be used as an implement for his impaired leg. Of course, the bow is not a device that replaces his swollen and purulent foot: the destiny of Philoctetes is to be cured by the divine Asklepios on the field of Troy.[45] However, it is conceived as a vital prolongation of Philoctetes' hands, which is his only means for survival on the desert island of Lemnos. The spectacular effect of Philoctetes' gait is indicated by verbal cues: when he first enters on stage, the chorus hears a noise made by a 'mortal oppressed by pain' (203 sq.), whose walk is very tiresome and difficult.[46] Philoctetes himself says that he crawls in pain and drags his throbbing foot behind him (290–291). It seems a reasonable hypothesis to assume that the bow was most probably an aid to help him walk and this was the choice made in a recent French production of the Sophoclean tragedy.

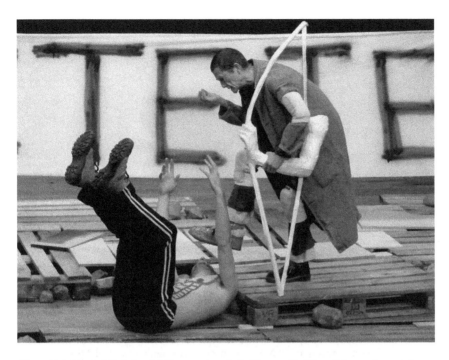

Figure 7.1 Marief Guittier (Philoctetes) and Guillaume Bailliart (Neoptolemus) in the *Philoctète d'après Philoctète de Sophocle*, directed by Gwenaël Morin. Image courtesy of © DR/ Compagnie Gwenaël Morin.

In this production, which took place in Paris (Aubervilliers) and Lyon in 2006 and 2007, Gwenaël Morin managed to make visible not only the wounded foot, but also the prosthetic relationship of Philoctetes to his bow, which was staged as an unprecedented 'crutch-bow'. The prop used for the bow is a poetic, unrealistic object, which brings out the peculiarity of Philoctetes' theatrical bow. Made in wood and plaster cast, painted in white, it features a dummy arm, attached to the limb and to the string of the bow.

Bent over it, the character holds this dummy arm and uses this extraordinary bow as a crutch to facilitate his walk. When deprived of it by Odysseus, Philoctetes is effectively, though metaphorically, deprived of a part of his body.

The director Gwenaël Morin thus managed to materialise in a prop the vital continuity existing between Philoctetes' hands and bow, as it is suggested by the very precise wording of the dramatic text. The object really becomes a metaphorical prosthesis: an arm, fixed to a bow, which complements the diminished body of the hero, though not in the way that we would expect.

The example of Philoctetes shows well how the prosthetic relationship with weapons can be reinforced in Greek tragedy. In her recent book, Melissa

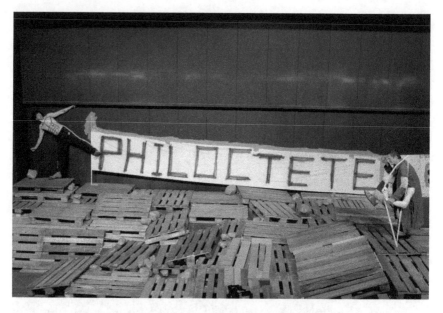

Figure 7.2 Marief Guittier (Philoctetes) and Guillaume Bailliart (Neoptolemus) in the *Philoctète d'après Philoctète de Sophocle*, directed by Gwenaël Morin. Image courtesy of © Marc Domage/Compagnie Gwenaël Morin.

Mueller affirms the relevance of this metaphor for another weapon, Ajax's shield:

> Prosthesis is an apt metaphor, in the sense that the shield is represented as being almost a part of Ajax's body, so closely identified it is with his physical self, and with his identity as the best of the Greek defenders.[47]

Here, the prosthesis is not considered literally as a replacement of a missing part of a human body with an artificial one. Underlying this statement is the metaphorical conception of prosthesis as a living extension of the body and of the self – the precise idea that modern scholars in Disability Studies have disapproved of, but that may be still relevant to think about the relationships between individuals and objects in ancient Greece. I will show now that tragic poets staged many 'body-integrated' weapons, beyond Philoctetes' bow or Ajax's shield, which can be seen as responses to the Homeric warrior–weapon compounds, and parallels to the Pindaric description of Pelops' shoulder. Yet, the dialogical nature of theatre creates a tension between the representation of the weapon as an extension of the self, and that of a weapon perceived as an independent being that can act as a friend.

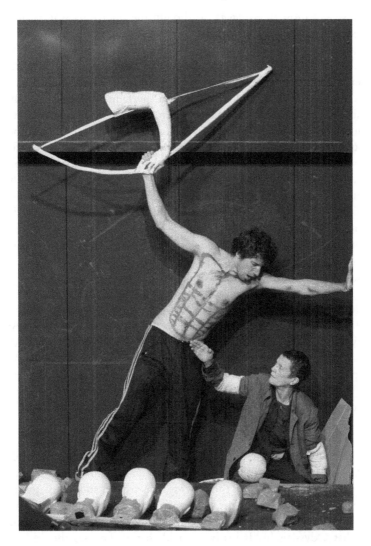

Figure 7.3 Marief Guittier (Philoctetes) and Guillaume Bailliart (Neoptolemus) in
the *Philoctète d'après Philoctète de Sophocle*, directed by Gwenaël Morin.
Image courtesy of © Marc Domage/Compagnie Gwenaël Morin.

Hybrid weapons as body parts

Tragic weapons are not only designated by their expected names (e.g., shield,
spear or sword) but also by compounds underlining their proximity to the
human body – just as Pindar and Herodotus used body part denominations to
refer to the 'ivory shoulder' and the 'wooden foot' mentioned at the beginning
of this chapter. These compounds are all the more remarkable in that they are

rather few and most often *hapax*, as though the dramatists wanted to use all the plasticity of language to suggest an exceptional intimacy between body and object. The lexical compound seems to be the direct verbal translation of the material blending of human and thing happening in this special relationship between men and weapons.

In Sophocles' *Ajax*, the plot is based on the famous struggle for the arms of Achilles. For the Salaminian hero, it is inconceivable to live without these weapons, and his failure to obtain them is the source of an unbearable dishonour. Ajax is still, and maybe even more than ever, a warrior defined by his weapons. In the prologue pronounced by Athena, the continuity between him and his sword is suggested by the wording ξιφοκτόνους χέρας (10), 'sword-killer hands', responsible for the slaughter of the cattle that has just been perpetrated. This *hapax* sounds undoubtedly Homeric – I commented earlier on Achilles' 'men-slaying hands' (χεῖρας ἀνδροφόνους). The comparison of the two compounds reveals that Sophocles stresses even more the intimate association of arm and weapon, by explicitly alluding to the sword. Later on, the same adjective, αἴθων, 'blazing', is successively applied to the sword (αἴθωνι σιδήρῳ, 147) and to Ajax himself (ἀνέρος αἴθωνος, 222), who thus seem to share the same aspect and nature.[48]

In *Alcestis*, Euripides uses a comparable coinage, when qualifying Apollo's hand by the compound τοξήρη (χέρα τοξήρη, 39), also a *hapax* rather difficult to translate: between Apollo *toxophoros* and his emblematic weapon, the relationship is so tight that the bow is always (αἰεὶ, 40) closely adjusted to his hand (-ήρης is a suffix deriving from the verb ἀραρίσκω), whatever use the god makes of it.[49]

In Sophocles' *Philoctetes*, the bow is obviously a very important and famous object; however, it has not been stressed that it is once called φίλης νευρᾶς (1005–1006) by Philoctetes, at a time when he has just been deprived of his bow by Odysseus.[50] The substantives νεῦρον and νευρά appear several times in epic poetry for the string of the bow: it is an archaic and poetic term whose first meaning, 'sinew', underlines the organic quality of the bow, made of a bull or sheep's sinew.[51] A bit later in the play, when Philoctetes thinks with horror that Odysseus holds his bow in his hands, he uses the verb ἐρέσσω (1135), which means 'to bend'; however, in tragedy, the verb can also be used for a part of the body put in quick motion – for instance a foot in Euripides' *Iphigeneia in Aulis* (138). All these brief notations contribute to presenting the bow as an organic instrument, which can be thought as a body part.[52]

In *Trojan Women*, Euripides also builds up a strong relationship between Hector and his shield, an object that appears twice on stage – it is first exhibited in the chariot of war spoils, next to Andromache (568–576). It finally serves as an impromptu recipient for the dead body of Astyanax (1136 sq.). The dramatic importance of this weapon is all the more remarkable since in the *Iliad*, the shield is not the focus of great attention in Hector's panoply. Once only, the shield is mentioned among his other weapons, and in book 7, Hector answers Ajax's provocations by saying that he also knows very 'well how to wield to right, and well how to wield to left [his] shield of seasoned hide'.[53] But these are the only fugitive allusions to Hector's shield, which may imply that Euripides has deliberately chosen to highlight the use of this weapon in an innovative way. The anthropomorphic status of the shield may have been translated visually if in Andromache's chariot, the weapons were arranged as a trophy, as has been argued convincingly.[54] Vase paintings offer us a useful visual testimony of these trophies, which consisted of the somewhat gruesome arrangement of weapons vertically, with the aid of a cruciform pole, as if they were still on the body of the warrior.[55] The poetic language also points towards this anthropomorphism of weapons: Euripides twice uses a compound (χαλκόνωτος), which literally means 'with a back of bronze' (χαλκόνωτον ἀσπίδα, 1136; χαλκόνωτον ἰτέαν, 1193). If this *hapax* firstly refers to the bronze cladding covering the wooden shield, it also suggests that the shield is like a protective cover, assimilated to a body part: this coinage is placed in the mouth of Hector's mother, Hecuba, who invests the object with strong feelings of affection, after the deaths of his son and her grandson Astyanax.

'Prosthetic objects' and physical continuity

To highlight the relationship of continuity between weapon and body, the tragic poets also insist on the haptic contact. The sword is firmly held in Ajax's hand, as we have already seen with the wording ξιφοκτόνος χέρας (10). This close association started when Ajax received 'in his hand' (χειρί, 661) the present of the hostile Hector – this substantive being underlined by its central position in the hexameter. In his *Philoctetes*, Sophocles develops drastically this association between weapon and hand: to Neoptolemus, Philoctetes presents the bow as the one he is 'carrying in his hands' (ἃ βαστάζω χεροῖν, 655) – χεροῖν intensifying pleonastically the verb βαστάζω, which already implies a physical contact.[56] When the hero is then deprived of his weapon, he longs for the bow and arrows (ἐμῶν ὅπλων) that he held in his 'strong hands' (κραταιαῖς μετὰ χερσὶν ἴσχων, 1110). The climax of his despair occurs when he formally addresses his hands and his bow, as though they formed a unity, a single section of his body that had been tragically separated by Odysseus' theft:

> O hands, what things you suffer in the lack of my dear bow, forced together by this man's order![57]

> Beloved bow, out of my loving hands, you were forced![58]

The address to his hands (ὦ χεῖρες) is an original kind of tragic lament: Philoctetes designates them as particularly outraged and spoiled by Odysseus – it is not him but his hands that 'need the beloved string-bow' (ἐν χρείᾳ φίλης νευρᾶς) and which are deprived of their possession (συνθηρώμεναι). The second formal address is directed to the bow itself, the 'beloved bow' violently snatched (ἐκβεβιασμένον) from Philoctetes' 'beloved hands' (φίλων χειρῶν, 1128–1129). It is all as if Philoctetes wanted to reunite hand and bow by his lament song, notably by the repeated use of the adjective φίλον/φίλων.

In Euripidean plays, we do not find this intense and exclusive relationship between hand and weapon: instead of it, Euripides is prone to emphasising the haptic contact of the object with several parts of the body. In his *Heracles*, the intimacy between Heracles and his emblematic weapons – his famous club and the bow (which, by the way, becomes Philoctetes' bow after his death) – is first expressed by physical contact with his arms (ἐμοῖς βραχίοσιν, 1099) and sides (πλευρά, mentioned twice, 1100 and 1379). His bow and arrows protect his arms and dangle against his sides, gently beating him when in motion (ἃ πλευρὰ τἀμὰ προσπίτνοντ᾽, 1379). But after the slaughter of his family, committed with these very weapons, Heracles legitimately wonders if he can keep them with him, or more precisely keep holding them 'in his arms' (εἶτ᾽ ἐγὼ τάδ᾽ ὠλέναις οἴσω, 1381). The substantive ὠλένη is rarely well translated: ὠλένη does not mean hand or shoulder, but the part of the arm going from the elbow downwards.[59] It is recurrently used by Euripides about mothers holding their children in their arms, which suggests its affective value. Applied to Heracles and his bow, it really stresses the haptic contact and affective relationship between man and weapons.[60]

Euripides also highlights the physical contact between the shield and Hector's body in *Trojan Women*: Hecuba pronounces a real funeral oration for both her grandson Astyanax and the shield that holds his broken body.

> O you that Hector's fair arm preserved, you have lost your best guardian! How lovely is the mark of his body upon your strap and the sweat on your well-turned rim, sweat which from his forehead Hector often in his toil dripped as he pressed you against his chin![61]

When Hecuba starts addressing the shield, we believe first that she is starting an encomiastic lament on her son Hector – σῴζουσ᾽, agreed with the feminine substantive ἰτέα, the 'wicker shield' found in l. 1193, is indeed rejected to the following line. But, in fact, she addresses the shield in a tragic lament that recalls that of Philoctetes mourning his lost bow. She builds a synesthetic reminiscence of Hector's intimate contact with his shield: the weapon covered his arm and leaned on his chin, so closely that it has kept the traces (τύπος) of his hand and of the sweat dripping from his forehead. By using the word τύπος, 'imprint', and mentioning the rim, part of the shield that was usually covered by a blazon, Euripides seems to allude to this traditional art of ornamentation.[62] But there is nothing engraved on Hector's shield: nothing but the physical and sensuous traces of his body, attesting once again a symbiotic relationship between the man and his weapon.

Reciprocal protection

As I have already suggested, the weapon that extends the body of the warrior is not an inert artefact, a simple instrument used passively. If it does not really have a life of its own, it is perceived as giving back to its possessor energy and protection.[63]

The bow of Philoctetes is not only assimilated with a part of his body, but is also his only means for surviving on the hostile Lemnos: the bow *is* his food (τροφή, 953 and 1126) and his life – Sophocles plays on the homophony in the Greek language between the words βίος, 'life' and βιός, 'bow' (930–932).[64]

In Euripides' *Heracles* and *Trojan Women*, the interaction between men and weapons is expressed in terms of reciprocal protection. Heracles describes in such a way his bow and arrows, scattered over the ground after the killing of his family:

> My winged arrows and bow are scattered on the ground, those which before, standing by my arms, both kept my sides safe and were kept safe by me.[65]

This reciprocal protection is stressed by the circularity of the line 1100, where the infinitive verb σῴζειν starts and finishes the line, applied first to the objects, then to the man. The verb παρασπίζειν also has an interesting metaphorical use here: it literally means 'to bear a shield beside', so 'to fight beside' or 'to stand by'. Therefore, it underlines the agency of the weapons, which fight beside the hero, rather than being simply manipulated by him. Moreover, the root of this compound verb, the noun ἀσπίς, 'the shield', suggests that the bow and arrows had perhaps essentially a defensive action, protecting the sides of the hero, rather than attacking the enemy. This is a strikingly new vision of this weapon, infused with affective value, which contrasts with the Homeric one.

In *Trojan Women*, Euripides expresses the symbiotic relationship between Hector and his shield in a similar way: the object that pathetically kept the imprint of the hero's body, protected his arm (the verb σῴζειν reappears with the participle σῴζουσ', 1195), while being at the same time protected by his guardian (φύλακ').

The 'prosthetic' weapon in tragedy: an extension of the self or an independent other?

In this last point, I will discuss the ways in which weapons seem to acquire another status, more independent than that of self-extensions. The prosthetic metaphor reaches perhaps its limits; in the end, objects are like 'detachable prostheses' and tragic playwrights seem to have experimented with this dramatic opportunity, too. When it occurs, the separation from well-loved weapons is staged as a physical and emotional moment of crisis where the heroes are losing not only a part of themselves, but also the only *philoi* that they had:

> Beloved bow, out of my loving hands you were forced! You look with
> pity, I think, if you have a mind, upon the unhappy friend of Heracles
> who shall never use you anymore, but, in the grasp of a cunning man
> you are plied instead, looking on his shameful deceptions and on the
> loathsome enemy, who, against me, contrived innumerable evils from
> shameful deeds![66]

In this formal apostrophe to the bow, Philoctetes addresses his bow as his
friend (φιλός), his only companion on his desert island. His words anthropo-
morphise the object to the point of attributing it eyes to see (ὁρᾷς) and a
conscious mind (φρένας τινας), capable of empathy for his misfortunes (ἐλεινὸν).
Even out of his hands, the object continues to live on and exist as an
autonomous self, capable of observing and judging people. It therefore seems
to acquire a proper identity, separate from that of Philoctetes.

In the case of Heracles' bow and arrows, objects seem to be doubly identified
as parts of the hero's extended body but also surrogates for his lost kin (φιλοί).
In a comparable lyric apostrophe to the weapons, loving words used first to
qualify filial love between relatives (κοινωνίαι, 'embrace') are then transposed
to the relationship between the hero and his weapons.

> O painful pleasure of kissing you, painful embraces of these weapons![67]

Just as Megara and her children were united in death in a 'dire embrace'
(κοινωνίαν δύστηνον, 1363), Heracles and his weapons are companions of
infortune (λυγραί τε τῶνδ' ὅπλων κοινωνίαι) until death do they part. In spite
of his qualms, the hero will not discard his weapons after the killing but hold
them again in his arms (ὠλέναις) or let them dangle against his sides, just like
his children did hang onto his clothes or to his knees – the same verb
προσπίπτω is suggestively used by Euripides for the children and the weapons.[68]
A *philos* in Greek, e.g., a friend or a kinsman, may be perceived as another
self.[69] Yet, in the case of Heracles and Philoctetes, an evolution from a
'prosthetic relation' towards an affective companionship with an object conceived as a separate entity, differentiated from the self, is perceptible.

This evolution might be related to the generic nature of tragedy: as an
essentially dialogical and material art form, theatre needs to build situations of
exchange between two visible entities, be they human or non-human. The
over-determination of form may have encouraged this experimentation of the
detachment of 'prosthetic weapon' from their possessors. The objects can then
be used as interlocutors in their own right. They are physically present and,
at the same time, suggest the absence of any human being that could bring
assistance to the distressed hero. The object's autonomy can therefore be seen
as a dramatic device used to stage the solitude of the tragic hero in a more
powerful way.

Conclusion

In the beginning of this chapter, I acknowledged the methodological and ethical issues aroused by a too-extensive and disordered use of the prosthetic metaphor. A wide gap has opened up between the real experience of prosthetic wearers and the imaginary reconstruction of prosthesis as a body-incorporation, which does reiterate the same body as before or even enhance it. This awareness may be even more necessary when one thinks about the experience of prosthetics in antiquity: Martha Rose reminds us that:

> it is difficult to believe that any prosthetic device would have been practical as well as cosmetic. Even today, with advanced understanding of pre-prosthetic preparation and a wide array of prosthetic choices, prosthetic devices are often discarded because of the great energy expenditure that it takes to use them.[70]

However, my point was to show that the 'prosthetic imagination' is not necessarily a modern deformation, deriving from science fiction or our current fascination with high-tech advances. The dream of a perfect replacement, restoring a body's integrity, may go back to the first extant literary depiction of a prosthesis in Pindar's *Olympian* 1. I also argued that Pindar's elaboration of Pelops' ivory shoulder is a creative response to the Homeric man–weapon symbiotic relationship. Concomitantly, Greek dramatists elaborated their own responses to it on the tragic stage, deepening the reciprocal and affective relationship between heroes and weapons, perhaps to the point of invalidating the 'prosthetic metaphor' to some extent. The transfer of living qualities onto the objects may go as far as granting some of them the status of *philoi* endowed with a separate identity.

This historical and literary investigation into 'prosthetic imagination' should then maybe lead to the acceptation of the independence and licence of the imaginative thinking, however unsettling it can be, in respect of our rational and societal need for an authentic and scientific account of this experience of disability. The 'prosthetic literary imagination' does not speak directly of daily experience in our world. Ancient Greek literature makes this explicit: Pelops, Heracles, Ajax, Philoctetes or Achilles are not normal human beings but 'larger-than-life' heroes, sometimes demi-gods that possess superhuman abilities.[71] They enjoy an idealised and magnifying relationship with objects that extend their human agency and make them match perfectly the description of the 'prosthetic gods' of Freud:

> With every tool man is perfecting his own organs, whether motor or sensory, or is removing the limits to their functioning. . . . Man has, as it were, become a prosthetic god. When he puts on all his auxiliary organs he is truly magnificent: but those organs have not grown on him and they still give him much trouble at times.[72]

Simple human beings may only wish their 'trouble' and pain to be soothed and live normally, without being constantly concerned with their prostheses.[73] Traditional myths and stories that convey a dream of symbiosis between humans and objects nevertheless deserve to be considered as part of the prosthetic experience, in so far as imagination and fantasy are a part of reality and contribute to shape it.

Notes

1 I would like to warmly thank Jane Draycott for her support and for having read my paper at the 'Prostheses in Antiquity' conference, in which I was unable to take part physically. Her helpful comments were greatly appreciated. I am also grateful to Professor Nagy and the staff of Harvard's Center for Hellenic Studies for having provided me with ideal conditions to write this chapter.

2 Jain, 1999, p. 52.

3 Sobchack, 2009, p. 280.

4 Sobchack, 2009, p. 279.

5 Jain, 1999, p. 33.

6 Serlin, 2006, p. 51.

7 Serlin, 2006, p. 51.

8 Adams, this volume; Knappett, 2005, p. 169; Malafouris-Clark, 2008, pp. 222–232; Malafouris, 2008.

9 Sobchack, 2009, pp. 190–192.

10 Pindar, *Olympian Ode* 1.23–28 (trans. W. H. Race, modified): Λάμπει δέ οἱ κλέος ἐν εὐάνορι Λυδοῦ Πέλοπος ἀποικίᾳ· τοῦ μεγασθενὴς ἐράσσατο Γαιάοχος Ποσειδᾶν, ἐπεί νιν καθαροῦ λέβητος ἔξελε Κλωθώ, ἐλέφαντι φαίδιμον ὦμον κεκαδμένον.

11 Nagy, 1986; Drew Griffith, 2000; Patten, 2009; Krummen, 2014, pp. 196–214; Morgan, 2015, pp. 234–240.

12 For other mentions of prostheses in Greek and Latin literature, see Bliquez, 1996; Rose, 2003, p. 26. On prosthetic toes, see Finch, this volume. On prosthetic legs, see Eitler and Binder, this volume.

13 Lorimer, 1936.

14 Sophocles, fr. 453 (Odysseus wounded by the spine).

15 Vernant, 1991, p. 37.

16 Krummen, 2014, p. 204.

17 'Pure cauldron' or 'purifying cauldron', a new presentation of the cauldron that was probably meant to contrast with the soiled cauldron in which Tantalus had boiled his children. See Krummen, 2014, pp. 205–209: her interpretation of Pindar's reworking of Pelops' myth as a new explanation of 'the traditional structure and materials of the ancient myth's restoration scene' seems very convincing to me. At Lycophron, *Alexandra* 156 Pelops is said to be a youth twice.

18 Patten, 2009, p. 137.

19 See also Apollodorus, *Epitome* 2.3: Pelops is even more beautiful (ὡραιότερος) after his return to life (ἐν τῇ ἀναζωώσει). Patten, 2009, p. 137; Morgan, 2015, p. 234, and note 48.

20 Pindar, *Olympian Ode* 1.23–28 (trans. G. Nagy).

21 Nagy, 1986, pp. 87–88.

22 Drew Griffith, 2000, p. 22.

23 Pausanias, *Description of Greece* 5.13.4–5.

24 Drew Griffith, 2000, p. 31; Patten, 2009, p. 138.

25 Nagy, 1986, p. 88.

26 For instance *Iliad* 4.135, 7.252 = 11.436, etc.; see Frontisi-Ducroux, 1975, p. 65; Longo, 1996; Lissarrague, 2008; Purves, 2015.

27 *Iliad* 22.134–136; Frontisi-Ducroux, 1975, p. 67.

28 See the comment of Eustathius on *Iliad* 4.126: the passion of the feeling person is transferred onto the weapon. *Iliad* 13.444 = 16.613 = 17.529; the participle μαιμώων, 'quivering with eagerness', is also applied to weapons (4.126; 5.661; 14.542), see Kokolakis, 1980, p. 90.

29 Longo, 1996, pp. 25–26 notes that such a supernatural being existed in near Eastern civilisation (Nart Batradz).

30 Longo, 1996, p. 28.

31 *Iliad* 14.376 sq., 381 sq.: ἐσθλὰ μὲν ἐσθλὸς ἔδυνε, χέρεια δὲ χείρονι δόσκον, 'good armor did the good warrior put on, and the worse they gave to the worse'.

32 For instance, *Iliad* 11.18; 16.132; 19.370: κνημῖδας καλὰς ἀργυρέοισιν ἐπισφυρίοις ἀραρυίας, 'beautiful greaves fitted with silver ankle-pieces'. Bliquez, 1996, pp. 2667–2673 builds on the archaeological evidence of *cnemides*, to imagine what an ancient peg leg could look like.

33 See the pair of greaves, from Vergina, Royal Tomb II. Museum of the Royal Tombs of Aigai, Vergina, Macedonia, Greece, BM 2587.

34 On the historical burial of warriors with their weapons in the Iron Age see Whitley, 2002; Lloyd, 2015.

35 Longo, 1996, p. 29; Griffin, 1980, p. 39: 'homeric weapons sympathize with the warrior who wields them in force'.

36 *Iliad* 20.399; 15.542; Griffin, 1980, pp. 34–36.

37 *Iliad* 18.317 and 24.478–479.

38 Vernant, 1991, p. 37.

39 Drew Griffith, 1998, pp. 230–256.

40 For a discussion raising the question of whether a stick or crutches may be considered as prostheses, see Sobchack, 2009, p. 289. On human aids, see van Schaik, this volume.

41 Worman, 2000; Rose, 2003, p. 19; Miller, 1944 refers to a fragment from Aeschylus' lost *Philoctetes*, which also contains medical terminology. On the Hoby Cup, a first century CE Roman silver skyphos (National Museum of Copenhagen) Philoctetes is shown being treated by his comrades immediately after the snake bite, and as a crippled recluse sometime later (thanks to Jane Draycott for having pointed this cup out to me).

42 Grassi *et al.*, 1999.

43 Rose, 2003, p. 21.

44 Rose, 2003, p. 19. On the use of a prosthetic leg in conjunction with a crutch, see Eitler and Binder, this volume.

45 Sophocles, *Philoctetes* 1437.

46 We do not have any visual representations of a walking Philoctetes. In those extant, Philoctetes appears seated on a rock, with his bow lying on the ground next to him. See *LIMC*, s.v. 'Philoctetes'; for example, Philoctetes on Lemnos, red-figure squat lekythos, 450–400 BCE, New York, Metropolitan Museum: 56.171.58.

47 Mueller, 2016, p. 222, n. 4; see also pp. 135, 147.

48 Notably, Ajax is named αἴθωνα λέοντα, 'blazing lion' at Homer *Iliad* 11.548.

49 Thanatos questions the presence of the bow, which draws the attention of the spectators on this weapon; see Monbrun, 2007; Noel, 2014.

50 See Harsh, 1960; Musurillo, 1967, p. 121; Lada-Richards, 1997; Taplin, 1971 and 1978, pp. 77–100; Segal 1980–1, pp. 125–142; Gill, 1980; Mueller, 2016, pp. 38–39.

51 *Iliad* 4.122, 4.125, 15.463 and 15.469; Monbrun, 2007, pp. 48, 161.

52 Monbrun, 2007, pp. 160–165.

53 *Iliad* 6.116–118; 7.238–239.

54 Brillet-Dubois, 2010.
55 For example, Boston Pelike, Museum of Fine Arts Inv. 1920.187, Tafel 4 in Rabe, 2008; Lonis, 1979, p. 129; see Figure 3 in Jackson, 1991, p. 234. In his 1971 film version of Euripides' *Trojan Women*, Michael Cacoyannis also reproduced this visual arrangement of weapons (original production by Kino Lorber Edu).
56 The same pleonastic insistance appears when Electra holds the urn supposedly containing the ashes of her dead brother (Sophocles, *Electra* 1129–1216).
57 Sophocles, *Philoctetes* 1004–1005 (trans. H. Lloyd-Jones, modified): ὦ χεῖρες, οἷα πάσχετ' ἐν χρείᾳ φίλης. νευρᾶς, ὑπ' ἀνδρὸς τοῦδε συνθηρώμεναι.
58 Sophocles, *Philoctetes* 1128–1129 (trans. H. Lloyd-Jones, modified): ὦ τόξον φίλον, ὦ φίλων χειρῶν ἐκβεβιασμένον.
59 For instance, the French Hellenist Mazon translates by 'épaule' (shoulder) (CUF, Belles Lettres); so do Berguin and Duclos ('épaules', GF, 1966); Kovacs 'on my arm' (Loeb).
60 Euripides, *Trojan Women* 762, 1142; *Phoenician Women* 300, 306.
61 Euripides, *Trojan Women* 1194–1199 (trans. D. Kovacs, modified): Ὦ καλλίπηχυν Ἕκτορος βραχίονα σῴζουσ', ἄριστον φύλακ' ἀπώλεσας σέθεν. Ὡς ἡδὺς ἐν πόρπακι σὸς κεῖται τύπος ἴτυός τ' ἐν εὐτόρνοισι περιδρόμοις ἱδρώς, ὃν ἐκ μετώπου πολλάκις πόνους ἔχων ἔσταζεν Ἕκτωρ προστιθεὶς γενειάδι.
62 For an illuminating parallel, see Aeschylus, *Seven against Thebes* 488, 521 (τύπος means imprint on blazons).
63 Griffin, 1980, p. 39 'homeric weapons sympathize with the warrior who wields them in force, but the poet does not allow them to act simply by themselves'.
64 See Monbrun, 2007, p. 160.
65 Euripides, *Heracles* 1098–1100 (trans. D. Kovacs): πτερωτά τ' ἔγχη τόξα τ' ἔσπαρται πέδῳ, ἃ πρὶν παρασπίζοντ' ἐμοῖς βραχίοσιν. ἔσῳζε πλευρὰς ἐξ ἐμοῦ τ' ἐσῴζετο.
66 Sophocles, *Philoctetes* 1128–1131) (trans. H. Lloyd-Jones, modified): ὦ τόξον φίλον, ὦ φίλων χειρῶν ἐκβεβιασμένον, ἦ που ἐλεινὸν ὁρᾷς, φρένας εἴ τινας ἔχεις, τὸν Ἡράκλειον ἄθλιον ὧδέ σοι οὐκέτι χρησόμενον τὸ μεθύστερον, ἄλλου δ' ἐν μεταλλαγᾷ πολυμηχάνου ἀνδρὸς ἐρέσσῃ, ὁρῶν μὲν αἰσχρὰς ἀπάτας, στυγνὸν δὲ φῶτ' ἐχθοδοπόν, μυρί', ἀπ' αἰσχρῶν νατέλλονθ', ὃς ἐφ' ἡμῖν κάκ' ἐμήσατ'.
67 Euripides, *Heracles* 1376–1377 (trans. D. Kovacs): Ὦ λυγραὶ φιλημάτων. τέρψεις, λυγραί τε τῶνδ' ὅπλων κοινωνίαι.
68 προσπίτνοντ': Euripides, *Heracles* 1379 and προσπεσὼν: 986; see also for the same action, 79; *Alcestis* 948; *Trachiniai* 762, *cf.* Bond, comm. *ad loc.*
69 Aristotle, *Eudemian Ethics* 1245a29–30; *Nicomachean Ethics* 1166a 31–32; *Great Ethics* 1213a11–13; *Rhetoric* 1385b28–29; Belfiore, 2000, p. 101.
70 Rose, 2003, p. 26.
71 Nagy, 2013, p. 107.
72 Freud, 1962 (1930), p. 42.
73 Sobchack, 2009, p. 294.

Bibliography

Belfiore, E. S. (2000) *Murder among Friends: Violation of Philia in Greek Tragedy*. Oxford and New York, NY: Oxford University Press.
Bennett, J. (2010) *Vibrant Matter: A Political Ecology of Things*. Durham, NC: Duke University Press.
Bliquez, L. J. (1996) 'Prosthetics in Classical Antiquity: Greek, Etruscan, and Roman Prosthetics', *ANRW* II 37.3, pp. 2640–2676.
Bond, G. W. (1981) *Euripides' Heracles*. Oxford and New York, NY: Clarendon Press.

Brillet-Dubois, P. (2010) 'Astyanax et les orphelins de guerre athéniens. Critique de l'idéologie de la cité dans *Les Troyennes* d'Euripide', *REG* 123, pp. 29–49.

Clark A. (2008). *Supersizing the Mind: Embodiment, Action and Cognitive Extension.* Oxford: Oxford University Press.

Coole, D. and Frost, S. (2011) *New Materialisms: Ontology, Agency, and Politics.* Durham, NC: Duke University Press.

Drew Griffith, R. (1998) 'Corporality in the Ancient Greek Theatre', *Phoenix* 52.3/4 (Autumn–Winter), pp. 230–256.

Drew Griffith, R. (2000) 'Pelops and the Speal-bone (Pindar "Olympian" 1.27)', *Hermathena* 168, pp. 21–24.

Freud, S. (1962, first German edition 1930) *Civilization and its Discontents.* Edited by J. Strachey. New York, NY: Norton.

Frontisi-Ducroux, F. (1975) *Dédale, Mythologie de l'artisan en Grèce ancienne.* Paris: F. Maspero.

Gell, A. (1991) *Art and Agency: An Anthropological Theory.* Oxford and New York, NY: Clarendon Press.

Gildersleeve, B. L. (1885) *The Olympian and Pythian Odes.* New York, NY: Harper & Brothers.

Gill, C. (1980) 'Bow, Oracle and Epiphany in Sophocles' *Philoctetes*', *G&R* 27.2, pp. 137–146.

Grassi, G., Farina, A. and Cervini, C. (1999) 'The Foot of Philoctetes', *The Lancet* 354.9196, pp. 2156–2157.

Griffin, J. (1980) *Homer on Life and Death.* Oxford: Clarendon Press.

Fennell, C. A. M. (1879) *Pindar: The Olympian and Pythian Odes.* Cambridge: University Press.

Harsh, P. W. (1960) 'The Role of the Bow in the *Philoctetes* of Sophocles', *AJP* 81.4 (Oct.), pp. 408–414.

Hodder, I. (2012) *Entangled: An Archaeology of the Relationships between Humans and Things.* Malden, MA: Wiley-Blackwell.

Jackson, A. H. (1991) 'Hoplites and the Gods: The Dedication of Captured Arms and Armour', in Hanson, V. D. (ed.) *Hoplites: The Classical Greek Battle Experience.* London and New York, NY: Routledge.

Jain, S. (1999) 'The Prosthetic Imagination: Enabling and Disabling the Prosthesis Trope', *Science, Technology and Human Values* 24.1, pp. 31–54.

Knappett, C. (2005) *Thinking Through Material Culture: An Interdisciplinary Perspective.* Philadelphia, PA: University of Pennsylvania Press.

Knappett, C. and Malafouris, L. (edd.) (2008). *Material Agency: Towards a Non-Anthropocentric Approach.* New York, NY: Springer.

Kokolakis, M. (1980) 'Homeric Animism', *Museum Philologicum Londiniense* IV, pp. 89–113.

Krummen, E. (2014) *Cult, Myth, and Occasion in Pindar's Victory Odes: A Study of Isthmian 4, Pythian 5, Olympian 1, and Olympian 3* (English translation by J. G. Howie). Prenton, UK: Francis Cairns Publications, ARCA.

Lada-Richards, I. (1997) 'Neoptolemus and the Bow: Ritual *thea* and Theatrical Vision in Sophocles' *Philoctetes*', *JHS* 117, pp. 179–183.

Lissarrague, F. (2006) 'De l'image au signe: objets en représentation dans l'imagerie grecque', *CCRH* 38, pp. 11–24.

Lissarrague, F. (2008) 'Corps et armes: figures grecques du guerrier', in Dasen, V. and Wilgaux, J. (edd.) *Langages et métaphores du corps dans le monde antique.* Rennes: Presses universitaires de Rennes, pp. 15–27.

Lloyd, M. (2015) 'Death of a Swordsman, Death of a Sword: The Killing of Swords in the Early Iron Age Aegean (ca. 1050 to ca. 690 B.C.E.)', in Lee, G., Whittaker, H. and Wrightson, G. (edd.) *Ancient Warfare: Introducing Current Research* Volume I. Newcastle-upon-Tyne: Cambridge Scholars Publishing, pp. 14–31.

Longo, O. (1996) 'Le héros, l'armure, le corps', *Dialogues d'histoire ancienne* 22.2, pp. 25–51.

Lonis, R. (1979) *Guerre et Religion en Grèce à l'époque Classique*. Paris: Les Belles Lettres.

Lorimer, H. L. (1936) 'Gold and Ivory in Greek Mythology', in *Greek Poetry and Life = Festschrift Gilbert Murray*. Oxford: Clarendon Press, pp. 14–33.

Malafouris, L. (2008) 'Is it "Me" or is it "Mine"? The Mycenaean Sword as a Body-part', in Borić, D. and Robb, J. (edd.) *Past Bodies: Body-Centered Research in Archaeology*. Oxford: Oxbow Books, pp. 115–123.

Miller, H. W. (1944) 'Medical Terminology in Greek Tragedy', *TAPA* 75, pp. 156–167.

Monbrun, P. (2007) *Les voix d'Apollon: l'arc, la lyre et les oracles*. Rennes: Presses universitaires de Rennes.

Morgan, K. A. (2015) *Pindar and the Construction of Syracusan Monarchy in the Fifth Century B.C.* Oxford and New York, NY: Oxford University Press.

Mueller, M. (2016) *Objects as Actors: Props and the Poetics of Performance in Greek Tragedy*. Chicago, IL and London: University of Chicago Press.

Musurillo, H. A. (1967) *The Light and the Darkness: Studies in the Dramatic Poetry of Sophocles*. Leiden: Brill.

Nagy, G. (1986) 'Pindar's *Olympian* 1 and the Aetiology of the Olympic Games', *TAPA* 116, pp. 71–88.

Noel, A.-S. (2014) 'L'arc, la lyre et le laurier d'Apollon: de l'attribut emblématique à l'objet théâtral', *Gaia: revue interdisciplinaire sur la Grèce archaïque* 17, pp. 105–128.

Patten, G. (2009) *Pindar's Metaphors: A Study in Rhetoric and Meaning*. Heidelberg: Winter.

Puech, A. (1958) *Pindare* 1. Paris, Soc. d'éd. 'Les belles lettres'.

Purves, A. (2015). 'Ajax and Other Objects: Homer's Vibrant Materialism', *Ramus* 44.1–2, pp. 75–94.

Rabe, B. (2008) *Tropaia: tropē und skola: Entstehung, Funktion und Bedeutung des griechischen Tropaions*, Rahden/Westf: M. Leidorf.

Rose, M. L. (2003) *The Staff of Oedipus: Transforming Disability in Ancient Greece*. Ann Arbor, MI: University of Michigan.

Segal, C. (1980) 'Visual Symbolism and Visual Effects in Sophocles', *CW* 74.2, pp. 125–142.

Serlin, D. (2006) 'The Other Arms Race', in Davis, L. J. (ed.) *The Disability Studies Reader: Second Edition*. New York, NY and London: Routledge, pp. 49–65.

Snodgrass, A. M. (1967) *Arms and Armour of the Greeks*. London: Thames and Hudson.

Sobchack, V. (2009) 'A Leg to Stand on: Prosthetics, Metaphor, and Materiality', in Candlin, F. and Guins, R. (edd.) *The Object Reader*. London and New York, NY: Routledge, pp. 17–41.

Taplin, O. (1971) 'Significant Actions in Sophocles' *Philoctetes*', *GRBS* 12.1, pp. 25–45.

Taplin, O. (1979) *Greek Tragedy in Action*. Berkeley, CA: University of California Press.

Vernant, J.-P. (1991) 'Corps obscurs, corps éclatants' = 'The Body of the Divine', translated into English by Wilson, A. and revised by Zeitlin, F. (1991) *Mortals and Immortals: Collected Essays*. Princeton, NJ: University Press, pp. 27–49.

Von Wees, H. (1998) 'Greeks Bearing Arms: The State, the Leisure Class, and the Display of Weapons in Archaic Greece', in Fisher N. and Von Wees, H. (edd.) *Archaic Greece: New Approaches and New Evidence*. London: Duckworth, pp. 333–378.

Whitley, J. (2002) 'Objects with Attitude: Biographical Facts and Fallacies in the Study of Late Bronze Age and Early Iron Age Warrior Graves', *CAJ* 12, pp. 217–232.

Worman, N. B. (2000) 'Infection in the Sentence: The Discourse of Disease in Sophocles' *Philoctetes*', *Arethusa* 33.1, pp. 1–36.

8 The psychology of prostheses: substitution strategies and notions of normality

Ellen Adams

Introduction

The standard definition of a prosthesis – an artificial aid that replaces a missing body part or function – is straightforward on the surface. However, the clinical use of such devices has major implications for our notions of personhood, normality and identity. The central aim of this chapter is to explore the range of responses to prostheses, with a consideration of disability studies, psycho-prosthetics and sign language. After briefly considering limb prostheses, it turns to modern auditory aids and the Deaf community, which has experienced a particularly fraught relationship with technological developments and medical professionals. The tension between the clinical approach to fixing the body (the 'medical model') and cultural adaptations (particularly sign language: see the 'social model') has at its core different attitudes to substitution strategies and normality. This chapter argues that, despite a shortfall in evidence about disabled people from the ancient world, we can benefit from an engagement with disability studies regarding a variety of issues, including prosthetic solutions. The chapter concludes with suggestions about how the alternative mode of communication of sign language may inform our understanding of the ancient world, particularly with reference to oratory, pantomime, and art history.

Prostheses: definitions, evidence and identity politics

This chapter grapples with the challenge of assessing whether the wealth of modern evidence can and should be applied to antiquity. The term 'prosthesis' was coined in the mid-sixteenth century to describe a syllable added to the beginning of the word; later, at the beginning of the eighteenth century, it took on a medical meaning.[1] Nowadays, dictionaries define a prosthesis as an artificial body part, such as an arm, foot or tooth, that replaces a missing part.[2] In practice, modern prostheses may replace bodily functions rather than parts (for example, a hearing aid attempts to substitute the hearing, not the ear), and, as technology advances, prostheses may also *enhance* functions.

In some areas of the Humanities and Social Sciences, prostheses are defined very broadly – even to refer to 'any machine or technology that intervenes in human subjectivity', which can extend to a telephone or computer, or even the virtual world via the internet.[3] It has been claimed that 'we may even go so far as to class objects as bodily and cognitive prosthetics', or that human culture is '*by definition* of the order of prosthetic extensions'.[4] De Preester and Tsakiris refer to Plato's *Phaedrus* in support of the idea that writing, as external memory, is also a prosthetic extension (this reference indicates how the ancient world influences modern psychological or cognitive studies in perhaps unexpected ways).[5] Furthermore, the adjective 'prosthetic' has been used as a metaphor that loses sight of the aid itself, such as 'prosthetic aesthetic' and 'prosthetic territories'.[6] A rather more focused definition is taken here, whereby a prosthesis is a replacement aid and/or strategy for a body part and/or function.[7]

There is considerable evidence for dental prostheses in the ancient world, but much less for limb substitutions.[8] A replacement right leg was found in Capua, made of wood with bronze sheeting and dating to around 300 BCE. Bliquez concludes that this device did not have a foot attached, and could not have performed particularly well as a replacement leg (people probably had peg legs).[9] There are literary sources, such as Herodotus' reference to a wooden foot that Hegesistratus had made, following a self-amputation (*Histories* 9.37). However, there is no mention of prosthetic devices in the Hippocratic corpus.[10] Undoubtedly war wounds and other accidents occurred in the ancient world, although the lack of anaesthetics and antiseptic would have rendered death more likely than today, reducing the need for prostheses.

Prosthetic devices developed for soldiers in the two World Wars irrevocably changed ideas of replacement, compensation and rehabilitation. It has even been argued that 'today's special-education programs are direct descendants of the medical discourse of rehabilitation from the two World Wars'.[11] Wheelchairs and prosthetic limbs support those with mobility problems, implants mend those with chronic illnesses or cosmetic disfigurements, and even living things, such as guide dogs, can help those with sensory disabilities.[12] Lack of space prevents consideration of the related phenomenon of phantom limbs, but mind and body do not always agree on issues of bodily 'absence'.[13] The considerable differences between the technologies of the ancient and modern worlds render comparisons highly problematic.

Any human attempt at fixing the body, including the use of aids, aims to render it normal again. This chapter argues, however, that this 'normality' is a highly contested notion that lies at the heart of disability identity politics. For example, deafness is a communication disability in addition to a hearing impairment. Sign language, which overcomes any communication barrier, has been categorised as a kind of 'primitive prosthesis'.[14] In sharp contrast, audists have argued that a strict oral education (with signing banned) offers the 'prosthetic device that would make people who were lacking a part of their human body whole'.[15] This disagreement arises from different substitution strategies, resulting in turn from conflicting notions of normality.

Disability studies can shed light on the potential range of personal responses, and has the advantage of engaging with the actual *users* of prostheses. The same aid can be viewed very differently – for example, is a wheelchair an enabler or a restrictor? If ancient evidence for prosthetic devices is sparse, then indications concerning how individuals responded to such aids is virtually non-existent. While we cannot project back modern experiences, they can offer vital insights – at least highlighting the variability of human responses to such tools.

I have compared Alison Lapper's and Oscar Pistorius' comments regarding their prosthetic devices elsewhere.[16] Pistorius – perhaps protesting too much – stated that he would not necessarily desire 'normal' legs if they could be magically applied.[17] Recalling childhood memories with his brother, he stated: 'every morning while Carl put on his shoes, I would slip on my prostheses; it was all the same to me'.[18] His supreme achievements in normalising led to a denial of being disabled, and this in itself can become a considerable mental strain. On 14 February, 2013, he killed his girlfriend, Reeva Steenkamp. Pistorius illustrates how people tend to categorise disabled people at polar opposites: superhero or supervillain, or, in his case, both.[19] Oscar Pistorius' relationship with his impairment and his replacement (arguably enhancing) prostheses is not universally experienced.

Alison Lapper recalls her childhood fittings for prostheses as an enforced necessity: 'they wanted to normalize us. I can see that from an able-bodied person's point of view that is the logical thing to do'.[20] Lapper's negative experience of prostheses is not unique, as Diane DeVries demonstrates.[21] The double leg amputee Aimee Mullins represents a third response. As a Paralympic sprinter and model, cheetah legs boosted the former achievement (they are modelled on the hind legs of a cheetah), while Barbie-inspired 'pretty legs' supported the latter.[22] At one point, Cinderella glass (or clear polyethylene) slippers/legs were made for her. Aesthetics and technology combined to enable certain (fantasy) roles to be enacted, with the permission and indeed encouragement of the human actor.

This range of experiences denotes that we should be wary of generalizing about how people engage with prosthetic devices, and it is also the case that people change their mind over time. For example, the initial response to an amputation is often a desire to be viewed as before, as 'normal'. But then the strain of pretending and passing as 'normal' often gives way to the acceptance and even celebration of the new body in a revised framework of identity politics, and the imitation prosthetic devices are rejected.[23] This time delay, often of years, indicates how responses to prostheses are not static or universal.

These accounts do not match the common clinical assumption that prostheses are universally desired because they 'complete' and 'normalise' a body.[24] In some cases, the prosthesis 'may become psychologically invested into the self'.[25] It is true that users may feel a reliance on them, feeling bereft if there is a technical fault. Furthermore, it has been suggested that, even when not actually attached to the individual, a prosthesis 'may continue to embody a person's sense of identity and sense of ability or disability'.[26] However, the tendency to label such users as 'posthuman', for example, has been rightly critiqued and criticised, notably by a prosthesis user.[27]

It is important to inject a more emotionally aware approach to the traditional pathogenic or deficit model of disability.[28] Only relatively recently has it been recognised that people require psychological support when adapting to prostheses, and that a level of trauma can accompany a medical 'cure'.[29] 'Psychoprosthetics' has become a specific field of interest, which highlights the range of responses to such aids, focusing on limb loss and prosthetic devices.[30] Unfortunately, scholars in the Humanities and Social Sciences, who are interested in the relationship between people and things, have not taken up this research.

This chapter demonstrates that the relationship between people, practices and things is highly complex when considered through the experience of prosthetic use. We are frustrated by the lack of evidence from the ancient world regarding such aids, but an awareness of the subject from the point of view of disability studies will highlight the range of responses people have to prostheses and substitution strategies, and caution us against leaping to firm assumptions based on slight evidence.

Human–object relationships – and cyborgs

Archaeology, by the nature of its evidence, considers very closely the relationship between humans and things.[31] At times, material culture becomes embodied, and *vice versa*. Olson states: 'embodiment becomes a process of materialization whereby selfhood, gender, cosmological entities, and so on are imbued in matter'.[32] Furthermore, the deceased body becomes material culture, particularly in the manner that it is discovered and studied archaeologically.[33] But what of the agency of objects?[34] The active nature of objects and symbols has long been recognised, in that humans use them, and they have an impact on people's lives.[35] Objects, clothing, adornment and gadgets are indispensable in everyday life. A sword, for example, is said to be 'alive', 'having the role of a dynamic attractor that draws out of the Mycenaean body a novel predisposition for action not previously available'.[36] However, to state that an object has a cultural biography does not mean that it lived a life as such, and overemphasising the agency of objects may result in the dehumanisation of a person – particularly when the objects involved are prostheses.[37] As they are made for 'broken' bodies, this is a particularly sensitive area. There is a two-way dynamic between humans and objects, but things do not have the primary agency of human consciousness. If archaeologists engaged with disability studies and research into modern prostheses, then certain pitfalls would be avoided. Instead, it has drawn from fields such as philosophy.

Ancient philosophers offer insights into attitudes towards health and disease; indeed, there was a close relationship between philosophy and practitioners or physicians.[38] They have often been consulted regarding the senses, and the body's engagement with the world.[39] In modern terms, it is notable that it was a philosopher who was given responsibility for producing the UK's 1978 Warnock Report on special educational needs. Explorations of the mind may serve the body and its failings. This dialogue between antiquity and modernity, archaeology (and Classics) and philosophy is healthy, but it has also resulted in some troubling developments.

For example, in support of the argument that the body is not confined by the boundary of the skin, archaeologists and social scientists often cite Merleau-Ponty's interpretation of a blind man with a cane;[40] these numerous references mean that this blind man certainly gets about.[41] The scholarly consensus is that Merleau-Ponty 'grounded perception in the experienced and experiencing body', but the point seems to be rather undermined if one actually ignores the voice and perspective of the blind man – which we are not given in this account.[42] Stated rather more bluntly: 'academics who want to make comments about the impact of impairment, might do well to base their analysis on empirical evidence about how disabled people feel about their embodiment'.[43] In psychoprosthetics, it is considered useful to contrast the empirical approach, which clinically treats the patient as an object of study, with the phenomeno-logical method, which deploys testimonials and questionnaires as research tools, drawing from the user's lived experience.[44] Ironically, one of the leading protagonists of phenomenology here applies the former approach; the blind man is an object of study, and we do not hear from him himself.[45] Accounts of the blind experience from an experiential 'view' are far rarer.[46]

A Greek epigram describes an old lame (not blind) woman who went to the Nymphs' spring of Etna; her prayers were answered and she no longer needed her staff (*Greek Anthology* 6.203).[47] As thanks to the nymphs, she left it as a votive offering. The stick was a disposable tool or aid, not absorbed into the body. Hamilakis describes extensions like this stick as 'sensorial prostheses'; however, a staff is not always considered to be a prosthetic device, in the sense that a prosthetic limb is.[48] In fact, a staff may symbolise age and therefore wisdom, rather than denoting weakness.[49] Elsewhere, I have argued that anatomical votives should be considered as ritual prostheses, in that they aim to achieve wholeness through the ritual sphere.[50] A key part of the argument of this current chapter is that such experiences will vary immensely, so philosophical musings that lead to so-called universal truths can be very misleading – and this situation is bewildering when there are sources of emic evidence available, as there are in modern times.

Some authors have been so keen to break down any barriers between people and things that terms such as 'cyborg' and 'hybrid' are deployed.[51] 'Cyborg' may simply mean 'the extension of human abilities by mechanical components inserted in the body'.[52] However, it is not clear that (internal) cochlear implants would render a person a 'cyborg' more than (external) hearing aids, for example; it is also unclear whether it matters if the instrument is electromechanical or not. The cyborg-creature has been popularised in cinema, novels and TV series. Such objectification of the impaired body leads quickly to negative portrayals – as Garland Thomson notes, 'literary texts necessarily make disabled characters into freaks, stripped of normalizing contexts and engulfed by a single stigmatic trait'.[53] These cultural representations have highly influenced such discussions of cyborgs, which do not bother the users of such aids and prostheses for accounts of their experiences.[54]

When prostheses-users are presented as cyborgs, they are dehumanised.[55] This is rather ironic, as it is our profound engagement with tools that is often presented as definitional to humanity.[56] Such dehumanising language justified the slaughter of disabled people in Nazi Germany, and less extreme oppression is still current today. They have also been de-bodied by scholars such as Gray and Mentor: 'speaking of "the" body, "my" body, is in some ways a strange thing for a cyborg to say'.[57] Donna Haraway's work has highly influenced cyborg studies, and it has been argued that she has been oversimplified to produce a crude idea of human–machine hybridity.[58] Haraway in fact viewed all humans as cyborgs, 'theorized and fabricated hybrids of machine and organism'.[59] To single out aid-users is unnecessary and problematic, and it also ignores very clear alternative identities and engagements with prostheses.

It is worthwhile exploring an example of cyborg-prosthesis in more detail. Cochlear implants involve an invasive procedure into the head. Users have been viewed as objects of curiosity, and useful examples to deploy when thinking about bodies and things. The users themselves are not necessarily consulted.[60] These implants do not have agency. They may be able to tune into certain frequencies, but they are programmed to do so – they are not decision-making entities.[61] Nothing is clear-cut in this debate, however, as some prostheses-users have chosen to 'own' the term cyborg. Michael Chorost's account of childhood deafness is standard – his hearing parents viewed sign language as a last resort, only to be tried if integration into 'normal' life failed.[62] He received cochlear implants as an adult, and, very shortly after (when the eagerness to normalise is generally at its strongest), wrote *Rebuilt: How Becoming Part Computer Made Me More Human*. He rejected the negative feedback on his use of the word 'cyborg' from longer-term wearers – as explored above, values associated with prostheses can change over time.[63] It is clear from his later book that the implants by no means render him hearing, and at this point he had started to learn sign language.[64]

I could have focused on limb prostheses (as several other chapters in this volume do), especially as such bodily aesthetics have appealed so much to classical art historians.[65] Furthermore, modern artists, such as Marc Quinn and Mary Duffy, have provided much food for thought regarding fragmentary bodies and their (non)restoration.[66] However, the invisible disability of deafness and modern auditory prostheses offer particular insights and challenges to the replacement of a function (hearing) rather than a bodily part (in addition to the advantage that I am a life-long user of them). The technology in this area has improved at the same pace as limb prostheses,[67] but the procedures that have been developed are considerably more diverse. Hearing is crucial to oral communication – and the level of sophistication that humans have achieved in this area is often argued to be what separates us from other animals. So what happens when this goes wrong? Are those who cannot talk less than human?

There is a further complexity. In parallel with – and defiance of – the clinical aim to 'fix' the impaired individual, the Deaf community has developed sign language as an alternative solution, which renders a physical prosthesis unnecessary. Indeed, the recent development of this auditory technology coincides with the recognition of sign as a real language. There is considerable tension between advocates of these different types of coping mechanisms, which are framed around different ideas of normality and identity. Auditory prostheses therefore open up a range of responses and debates not seen in other areas, and serve to demonstrate just how problematic it is to generalise about the relationship between people and things.

Deafness, communication and sign language

Evidence regarding deaf people in antiquity will be explored elsewhere.[68] Suffice to say, this evidence is sparse, but literary and philosophical accounts are mostly concerned with the muteness or communicative aspect than the individual's lack of hearing. The issue here is not the lack of hearing, but the absence of communication skills, that resulted in being 'dumb' in both the modern senses. There do not seem to have been auditory prostheses of any kind, including ear trumpets.[69] Clay representations of ears were given as votive offerings, and, as deafness and muteness were considered together, models of mouths might also represent deafness.[70] It has been argued elsewhere that such votives served as a kind of ritual prosthesis in the healing process.[71] We do not know whether the gestures used by the speechless mentioned in Plato's *Cratylus* was full sign language (see also Xenophon *Anabasis* 4.5.33). It is unlikely, however, that there was a large enough concentration of deaf people to produce it, and there is no proof of the presence (or absence) of full sign language in the ancient world.[72]

Given that it is highly unlikely that a deaf person could have become literate and communicated using writing, this would mean that all communication would be on the level of gesture.[73] There are various elements of sign that are considerably more natural, iconic or innate than spoken language, hence the deployment today of non-language, gestural communication programmes such as Makaton.[74] Sufficient communication can be expressed in gesture for deaf people to perform basic manual tasks in an agricultural setting, so it may have been more of a problem for roles expected of the elite.[75] Over-all, our understanding of the lives and treatment of deaf individuals is rather weak, despite the best efforts of scholars to consider this group in antiquity. I want, therefore, to focus on modern responses to deafness and its range of prostheses, in order to demonstrate how medical and social interventions can reveal diverse and even contradictory values in terms of bodily norms and ideals.

Before turning to this group, it is worth outlining some of the key topics in disability studies that help to shed light on the startlingly different attitudes held towards auditory prostheses (as explored above with limb prostheses). Modern medicine provides treatments and cures that those in the ancient world would not have dreamt of. The doctor treats the patient using surgery, aids and drugs, with increasing authority – to an almost godlike extent. This process of clinically fixing the body is known as the medical model. The social model argues that disabled people are such because of the prejudicial beliefs and actions of the majority, which results in environmental constraints.[76] The modern focus of disability studies is an assessment of a *disabling society*.[77] The term 'disability' is therefore distinguished from 'impairment', the physiological and biological missing part or defective element of various kinds, such as mobility, learning, sensory, communication and mental difficulties, cosmetic disfigurements and chronic illness. The ancient world had words and labels for various impairments, but does not appear to have had a single one for 'disability'; the implications of this are reviewed elsewhere.[78] Elements of both the medical and social model may be detected in the ancient world, alongside a third one: the ritual, or moral, model. Here, one 'deserves' good health by keeping on the right side of the gods, and, where the cause of a disease was unclear, divine or demonic, agency could be blamed.[79] The extensive use of sanctuaries for Asclepius and the dedication of anatomical votives demonstrate this practice.[80]

The above models take very different approaches to normality. Since the early nineteenth century, the word normal 'has been used to describe how things are, as well as to prescribe how they ought to be – often both at once': modern medical practice takes a statistical approach towards establishing the typical body.[81] Furthermore, prostheses have contributed to the stereotype of the disabled as superhuman or subhuman at the extremes of normality. It is a further step to decide whose responsibility it is to 'normalise' an impairment. The medical model attempts to render the individual as able-bodied as possible and to fix them, so that they can have a 'normal' life. The aim is to use technology to allow spoken language to be developed. The social model argues that it is normal for any given society to have 15 per cent disabled people (as calculated by the 2011 WHO Report), so it should adapt to accommodate these requirements – supporting, for example, sign language use. A middle ground between the two positions may be found;[82] both individual and society seek to contribute towards integration by various means.

Different attitudes to normality are distinguished in the d/Deaf contrast. The lower case 'deaf' are those with a physiological hearing loss, either congenitally or from later on in life, who may well use an auditory prosthesis in order to get by, or 'pass' as hearing. The Deaf, however, view themselves as a cultural group or linguistic minority, based on their sign language (e.g. BSL, British Sign Language). Since 1960, signed languages have been fully recognised as such (a fully formed language). They had previously been caught in a catch-22 cycle: investigations had not yet demonstrated that they possessed a formal grammar and syntax, and were therefore worthy of linguistic research. Viewing sign language as the key positive attribute to being Deaf is a particularly sensitive matter as BSL was only officially recognised as a language in Britain in 2003 (although it does not yet have legal protection as a formal minority language). This recognition was vital in terms of practical access and rights, but it also served a subtler benefit. The acknowledgment that this mode of communication was equal to spoken language *changed the parameters of normality*. Deaf people had a proper language, as is 'normal' for humans, and were not restricted to animal gesture. The debate over whether sign language should be tolerated, celebrated or completely banned has at its heart the cultural concept of normality: if communication separates humans from animals, and the civilised from the primitive, then this is no superficial debate.[83]

Today in Britain, it is still possible to meet people who experienced an inappropriately orally based education, which involved having their arms bound in order to prevent them from signing. On the whole, the history of deaf education (and therefore lives) is bleak, consisting of a series of experiments made by hearing professionals, with the prime aim to achieve speech – the 'medicalization of cultural deafness'.[84] Medical approaches develop prostheses in order to rehabilitate the patient into the hearing world.[85] It is notable that standard clinical surveys of hearing loss and their appropriate prosthetic devices do not include sections on sign language as a compensation strategy.[86] Some state that it is language – specifically spoken language – that distinguishes humans from animals.[87] Many clinical works give 'lip service' to sign language, and then ignore it.[88]

In contrast, others, in the mould of the social model, have argued that sign language must be supported as a human right to language.[89] A further 'alternative normality' can be seen in the area of Martha's Vineyard where the entire community grew to be bilingual in both English and sign language.[90] This was due to the unusually high proportion of deaf births, due in turn to the restricted genetic pool. The hearing members of the community picked up that strand of sign language as a matter of course, and it was 'normal' for hearing people to sign among themselves. This ended when children began to be sent to deaf school at some distance, and met future partners, which mixed up the gene pool. Martha's Vineyard is an excellent example of social adaptation that resets the terms of the norms (the social model). It is this tension that makes auditory prostheses such a rich area to review, although, as stated above, it is unclear whether sign language as a replacement strategy should count as a prosthesis.

A further relevant issue is whether such profound differences in communication may affect one's cognitive norms. 'Deaf Students are not hearing students who cannot hear' – the difference is more fundamental, in terms of categories and concepts constructed by the brain.[91] There are fundamental differences between spoken and sign languages, and the cognitive impact of learning them. Iconic and/or indexic representation is easier in sign language.[92] Saussure's ideas on the dualism between the signifier and the signified have a very different relevance for sign languages. For example, Saussure's 'sign' system is not iconic – there is no physical relationship between the word 'chair' (the signifier) and the signified concept.[93] The sign(s) for chair is/are iconic in sign language, however. Sign deploys cinematic elements of panning, close-up and slow-motion, and there is nothing comparable in spoken language.[94] There is some evidence that deaf and hearing signers are faster in generating mental images, and that level, not age of sign acquisition, is important in gaining advantage in mental rotation task.[95] However, in sequential tests, deaf people performed worse, which may be due to the linear nature of spoken English.[96]

To conclude: a remarkable parallel (but apparently contradictory) pair of developments has occurred over the last couple of decades: sign language is now flourishing, partly thanks to its formal recognition. The Deaf argue that there is no problem that needs to be medically fixed by technological developments: in fact, technological advances such as video messaging (e.g. FaceTime) facilitate long-distance signed communication (which cannot be written down). It seems perverse from the outsiders' point of view to focus on the management of a condition rather than finding a cure, but this movement in the Deaf community is mirrored in others, such as autistic people.[97] Silberman's work is a fascinating exploration of the modern West's attempt to deal with a condition that medicine cannot cure – and raises the vital question: should we try? Hans Asperger's thesis (submitted to the University of Vienna in 1943) referred to the 'monstrous idea of human perfectibility' – brave thoughts for that time and place.[98]

This section is a further reminder not to generalise about strategies for dealing with impairments and the varying reactions to them, associated with different ideas of norms and completeness. The case of deafness is rather more subtle than physical completeness, and this discussion is only applicable to modern values, which cannot be projected onto the past. However, this chapter aims to highlight the range of human responses to dealing with human bodies, even if the debates about these prostheses are anachronistic regarding the classical world. We now turn to auditory prosthetics, as they have been termed, and the range of responses to them by users and professional bodies.[99]

Modern aids for the deaf

Evolving from ear trumpets, modern hearing aids have improved dramatically over time.[100] Once a constraining box hung around the neck, behind-the-ear analogue hearing aids impeded mobility much less. The introduction of digital hearing aids in 1996 greatly improved the quality of the sound. Cochlea damage reduces frequency selectivity, or the ability of the ear to focus on desired frequencies (mainly the higher ones for voices) and reduce background noise. So it is not just that people hear less, but also that they hear of lesser quality, and with an impaired ability to select the desired sounds. The solution of making everything louder can have painful consequences when wearing auditory prostheses. They are therefore an aid, not a cure, and it is insightful to compare the attitude of two key British institutions in response to them, the hearing-led Action on Hearing Loss (AHL), and the Deaf-led British Deaf Association (BDA). 'Hearing loss' defines people by what they lack (the medical model), whereas the BDA campaigns on many social issues on behalf of the Deaf community (the social model).

On the British National Health Service website, an audiology specialist from AHL makes reassuring noises about the small and discrete design of modern digital hearing aids in order to tackle the stigma many feel (one private company is called 'Hidden Hearing'). This fear is not unrealised: deaf children may be called 'aliens' due to their prosthetics.[101] Louise Hart states: 'We need a new attitude to hearing aids. Wearing them should be as unremarkable as wearing glasses.'[102] She is suggesting that users will be able to 'pass' as normal or hearing, or, as Mitchell and Snyder state, 'prosthetic devices, mainstreaming, and overcompensation techniques, all provide means for people with disabilities to 'fit in' or to 'de-emphasize' their differences'.[103] Such is the perceived power of technology to 'normalise' and 'cure'.[104] This medical fixing approach can have significant psychological implications. Ironically, being told that an aid *should* make you complete can make you feel even more inadequate when it fails to do so.[105] In contrast, the BDA promotes the use of BSL and the acceptance of Deaf culture. These institutions take very different stances, stemming from very different views of normality.

One might expect the promotion of hearing aids to be an uncontroversial issue. The Starkey Foundation, for example, is keen to promote its charitable work in providing hearing aids for those unable to purchase them, with considerable support from dignitaries such as Bill Clinton and George W. Bush. The Daily Moth (a Deaf-based group) has asked: 'how much impact does Starkey have on framing how our disability and community is perceived?'[106] The deaf are presented as problems to be fixed, for whom there is no chance of education, training or work unless they are incorporated into the hearing sphere. The California Association of the Deaf (CAD) posted an open letter to the Starkey Foundation on 14 February 2016, requesting that the issue be presented differently: 'Hearing aids will not end language deprivation. American Sign Language can.' Complaints also concerned the evangelical nature of the event. To film and publish the 'switch-on' moment is a peculiar staging of a clinical procedure,[107] and this glorification of technological aids has been branded 'inspiration porn'. This is far removed from the support required for a successful adaptation to such prostheses.[108] Elsewhere I have made a distinction between the modern and ancient world, arguing that a ritual/moral model is relevant for antiquity.[109] However, an emotive element is also present in this performance, as a kind of modern ritual prosthesis.

Hearing aids are worn on the body, whereas cochlear implants require invasive surgery, which destroys any residual hearing. Twelve to twenty-two electrodes are implanted in the cochlea, essentially replacing the work of thousands of minute hair cells, with varied results; any level of success is only possible due to the plasticity of the human brain.[110] While the technology is improving, they are no cure: their adoption renders users partially deaf or hard of hearing, and the finer nuances of language (such as intonation and stress) will be lost.[111] The type of sound cochlear implants provide is very different from that experienced by a hearing person. To put this in an everyday context, music is poorly (or 'differently') perceived because of the weak information about pitch.[112] This is obviously a problem for tonal languages, such as Mandarin.[113] They are not, therefore, a panacea – 'in common with other prostheses, they are a tool for living, one among many, appropriate for some and not others'.[114] An awareness of such varied experiences is vital when thinking about how people engage with objects and prostheses, as noted above.

The medical approach is keen to implant or use 'appropriate intervention' as early as possible, 'to minimize disruption to language development'.[115] In America, it was only hearing people – including a representative from the cochlear implant industry – who sat on the committee that decided that it would be appropriate to install them on children from age two.[116] In contrast, Nittrouer points out that the same argument is made for learning sign language as young as possible.[117] A survey of studies of people with cochlear implants suggests that they were not necessarily caught between two worlds, but assumed 'more of a bicultural stance or comfort in shifting identities'.[118] Most users of all kinds of auditory prosthetics are grateful for the opportunities they create.[119] But Jo Milne also notes that, after she received cochlear implants, she is still lip-reading, that she tires easily and that there was a great pleasure in escaping to silence.[120] Over-heightened expectations of the technology can cause problems later.[121] Rehabilitation is now acknowledged to play a major role in the success of all prostheses; in the case of auditory ones the brain needs to be retrained to process this new information, and a programme of speech therapy needs to be embarked upon. An immediate 'switch-on' moment is unlikely to be fully successful in cases of significant hearing loss.

Furthermore, the presence of a prosthetic can lead to the assumption that the patient is then 'cured' and now hearing, reducing the obligation on others to adapt their behaviour. Many coping strategies are not reliant on technology, but involve lip-reading, body language-reading and great feats of guesswork. This involves great focus and concentration on the part of the deaf, quite often with little or no adaptation on the part of the hearing people present. Parents welcome the benefits that auditory prosthetics can bring, stating that being able to chat with their children when not being able to see each other's face was important, thereby displaying a striking lack of deaf awareness, and without apparently grasping the considerable effort required on the (still non-'hearing') child.[122] In this case, who does the prosthesis serve? Part of a full rehabilitation programme should include role-play in issues such as 'requesting changes in the environment'.[123] Lack of space has necessitated a focus on just prosthetic devices for deafness, but it is clear from this example alone that 'replacing' parts of the body is extremely controversial. Aside from the important observation that prostheses do not necessarily offer a cure-all, there are more positive lessons to be learned from the development of substitution strategies, particularly sign language. These can, in perhaps unexpected ways, be applied to the ancient world.

Sign language and traditional areas of Classics

While the visible nature of limb prostheses may appear to have more obvious relevance to our understanding of the ancient world, there are several subtle insights that may be drawn from the modern experience of being deaf. There are clear limitations to this exercise – disability awareness, technological advances and substitution strategies are incomparable between the ancient and modern worlds. However, it is incumbent upon me to indicate how and why a serious engagement with disability studies may benefit Classics and cognate disciplines, even beyond the study of disabled people themselves. Bragg takes the view that classicists should not necessarily be interested in sign language, as it is highly unlikely that one existed in the ancient world.[124] However, it is here tentatively presented as a form of prosthesis. This hesitation arises because the suggestion that it is a second-best replacement for spoken language fails to acknowledge the potential fresh insights it can bring into areas such as oratory, drama/pantomime and classical art.

It might be asked whether a substitution strategy should be seen as an imperfect prosthesis. We are set in a fixed and overwhelmingly negative view of disability, which, while probably shared by most in antiquity, is not the only way to face impairments, and can unnecessarily shut out avenues of exploration (and is again an unfortunate consequence of the ableism that steeps through the Humanities). Deaf pride, identity and culture do not simply allow the individual to make the most of a bad lot; they also flip the status of 'hearing loss' to 'deafness gained'.[125] From the perspective of the able-bodied, impairments equal loss; from that of the affected individual, they can mean simply difference. Indeed, the argument has been made that the impairment results in compensatory skills that can have a high value in themselves, such as deaf police officers monitoring security cameras due to enhanced visual concentration.[126] These 'alternative realities' may be preferable to the attempt to pass as 'normal', and in celebrating a heightened visual awareness, 'we are not making the case that hearing individuals should intentionally become deaf; but we do call into question the reverse notion, that deaf individuals should intentionally become hearing'.[127] We may begin with a consideration of the role of gesture in communication, oratory and even rhetoric.

Kahne's book focuses on twelve necessary consequences of dealing with deafness that can actually serve as useful tips in all modes of communication.[128] Consultants stress the importance of body language in success in life and work; sign language sweeps gestures, eye contact and gaze, facial expressions and all kinds of visual signaling into a coherent syntax. As part of the widening of psycholinguistic approaches, co-speech gestures are being debated, and 'investigators of language are moving away from our ancient written language bias'.[129] In this case, classicists may welcome the attention to non-verbal communication, and begin to apply it back onto the ancient world.

The importance of non-verbal communication has been recognised for a long time in the modern age. John Bulwer produced five works on bodily communication in the seventeenth century, which shed light on the influence of Classics in our modern ideas of communication, explored the role of gestural communication, and emphasised the distinction between gesture and posture. In *Chirologia and Chironomia*, he builds upon Aristotle's studies of the body by considering gesture, 'of great use and advantage, as being no small part of civill prudence'.[130] A section near the end on 'Certain cautionary notions extracted out of the Ancient and Modern rhetoricians, for the compleating of this art of manuall rhetorique, and the better regulating the important gestures of the hand and finger' illustrates the close engagement with classical sources. By including references to Plato, Seneca, Virgil, Livy and Plutarch, he carries the implication that gestures are universal, but he was also frustrated by the lack of evidence for ancient gesture, and recognised that those of his day would differ in some ways.[131] Furthermore, he challenged ancient sources when he felt it was appropriate to do so, such as questioning Aristotle's assertion that deafness was an impairment only humans experienced.[132] 'Cephalelogia', or the language of the head and facial expression, receives less attention in this work; this is provided later.[133]

Bulwer's *Philocophus* is the first English work on deaf communication forms, including lipreading and the first publication of finger-spelling.[134] He stressed the relation between communication and movement; for the 'Deafe and Dumbe', hearing is 'nothing else but the due perception of motion'.[135] As speech 'is a voluntary Action, and therefore perform'd by Motion', all communication is some form of movement, breaking down any divide between speech and sign.[136] Bulwer's *Pathomyotomia* (1649) explores motion and the 'muscles of the affections', or how internal emotions are exposed to the world from the body via the muscles. Again, this book is the first substantial work in English on the topic.[137] Unfortunately, unlike antiquity's continuing influence, he was little regarded by later authors. The eighteenth-century elocutionary movement drew heavily from Demosthenes and his emphasis on delivery, including gesture and action. One of the group, Reverend Gilbert Austin, used the title of *Chironomia* for his 1806 work. Austin berates the lack of attention to delivery and action by previous scholars – while failing to refer to John Bulwer.[138] With just two references to the deaf in his work (but many to ancient sources), Austin also failed to acknowledge that this group of people could offer insights into visual communication. This has set a trend that is followed still today, with little reference to the 'prosthetic' of sign language, including works that advocate interdisciplinary approaches.[139]

Rarely has the history of deaf communication and other visual-kinetic communication systems, such as Roman pantomime, been considered together.[140] It has been well noted that the eighteenth century witnessed much interest in pantomimic acting in England and France.[141] In 1709, Richard Steele referred to the opera singer Nicolini Grimaldi, whose 'every Limb and every Finger contributes to the Part he acts, insomuch as a deaf Man might go along with him in the Sense of it'.[142] The pantomime of compositions such as Ovid's *Metamorphoses* is a growing area of scholarship.[143] The *Metamorphoses* 'prove hospitable to pantomime-inflected readings', and, if Roman pantomime was mainstream, then certain conventions could build over time into something much more sophisticated than may be assumed.[144] Can a visual language give us insights into how ancient pantomime might have been performed?

The performance of narrative in sign language relies on role shift, or referential shift, where the account is presented from the point of view of a particular participant. 'Role shift is signaled in three ways: *shifted expressive elements, shifted gaze and/or posture* and *shifted reference*'.[145] The signals that the signer uses to 'shift' between characters can be extremely subtle, and one would expect a more exaggerated version in pantomime. Lada-Richards discusses the possible pantomime version of the story of Apollo and Daphne, involving the rather more cumbersome exit and entry of different characters.[146] But with role shift, this would not be necessary, and the mourning sisters can also be seamlessly depicted. While there is no documentation for practice such as role shift in the ancient world, the thought experiment of linking Ovid to pantomime might extend to a consideration of the incorporation of these modern techniques.[147]

Unfortunately, the potential similarity with this grammatical aspect of sign language falls down with the realisation that Roman pantomime actors would be masked – anathema for the practice of role shift.[148] However, this comparison has merits. 'Pantomime was the only ancient performative genre where identity/role-changes were effected primarily by means of the body, that is to say, with changes of gait, posture, gestures, attitude, range and types of movement': add facial expression, and you have role shift.[149] Change of role could be indicated by a different mask – or even without this physical adjustment. Indeed, Libanius (*Oration* 64.66) refers to gestures 'such as the meaningful tilting of the head or torso or a codified leap or spin to signal the moment of character change'.[150] Conventionalised leaping is easy to imagine; we know from role shift in sign language that a mere change in eye gaze can signal the same effect. The central issue here is the performance of narrative, and much can be learned from the 'substitution strategy' of sign language about this.

As stated, Bulwer was keen to distinguish between the movement of gesture as communication and the stillness of posture; this has relevance in art history. Work on gesture is generally found to be problematic and lacking in methodological rigour by critics familiar with the sophistication of sign language.[151] A recent work on Hellenistic body language draws from twentieth-century works on body language, non-verbal communication and anthropology; sign language is briefly referred to, but the main focus is on how the body supports (or indeed undermines) communication.[152] Masséglia sets out a fascinating series of postures, and makes a convincing case that this kind of framing warrants close analysis. But the study of pose and posture is not necessarily the same as gesture as movement (although certain art forms, such as Emma Hamilton's *Attitudes*, may switch between the two).[153] Kinaesthetic activity may be represented in art, but it is crucially frozen.[154] Classical art is essentially the two-dimensional and three-dimensional motionless representation of life experience, and therefore shares certain qualities with sign language dictionaries. These are ultimately unsatisfactory and even more problematic: not only do they freeze the action, but they also fail to register facial expression and mouth shapes.

In terms of approaches to art history, communicating about it in a visual language opens up many opportunities. Several works have approached classical (or specifically Roman) art as though it were a grammatical language or system of communication.[155] It remains the case, however, that few approaches to ancient art enter the emic sphere of understanding.[156] Recent discussions of ekphrasis – the vivid description of the visual – has explored intermediality, or the rhetoric of visual–verbal relations.[157] Some even argue that all art history is ekphrasis, and Simonides' dictum: 'a picture is a silent poem and a poem is a speaking picture' is a cornerstone for intermedial approaches.[158] It is notable that these pictures are normally still, rather than moving, but spoken and written language is also extremely limited in its linear form. Pich and Squire also consider 'bringing about seeing through hearing', but the question raised here is whether we may take this further, and explore intermodiality – different *modes* of communication as the basis of these relations.[159]

British Sign Language includes visual iconicity and cinematographic elements such as zooming.[160] It is performed in four dimensions – whereas speech is argued to be delivered in just one (time), and written language in two.[161] The implications of this in terms of understanding, studying and communicating about art will be explored in a future project, but it remains to state here that art historians are more constrained by the mode of interaction than is realised – 'the medium is not just the channel of the message but a co-constructor of its content, too'.[162] It is also the case that artists are often obsessed with the language of the body, and certain compensatory strategies, or behavioural prostheses, may affect this. For example, Goya was only 46 years old when he became deaf, and it has been argued that this forced him to evaluate the role of gesture with more consideration and insight than most.[163] He wrote of using sign language, and his 1812 work on *A Study of Gestural Language* appears to demonstrate fingerspelling.[164]

We return to Plato's discussion of observed communication via gesture by deaf people – unlikely to be a sign language, but relevant nonetheless. We need to consider the possibility that gestures could be conventionalised beyond the iconicity of mime in the ancient world, and to adjust our assumptions accordingly. The irony of this argument is that sensory studies have long tried to suppress the predominant role of the visual in most, if not nearly all, media. This approach, however, suggests that the visual has been under-represented in studies about human communication, due to the emphasis on oral and written modes in traditional areas of study such as oratory, pantomime and art history.

Conclusion

This chapter has drawn from disability studies, psychoprosthetics and sign language studies in order to highlight the complexities of this volume's topic. The definition of 'prosthesis' is important: the metaphorical use of the term can be somewhat confusing, and detracts from the fact that the implications of using such a device is impossible to generalise about: we have seen this with both limb and auditory prostheses. In particular, we can detect much tension between the clinical approach (represented by Action for Hearing Loss and the Starkey Foundation) and the cultural one (represented by the British Deaf Association and the California Association of the Deaf). This has been recognised in disability studies as the medical and social models. The use of prostheses is set against the development of sign language, a very different form of substitution strategy, and both reveal very different ideas of 'normality'. One hopes for integration into the normal hearing world, the other adapts the social norms themselves, as in the case of Martha's Vineyard. Perhaps unexpectedly, disability studies offer a fresh way at looking at how cultural norms are defined.

The range of modern prosthetic devices would have been unimaginable in the ancient world. Insights from disability studies are unlikely to have direct relevance for our understanding of ancient Greece and Rome, but other fields, such as gender studies, have paved the way in demonstrating how Classics may incorporate modern thinking into old material.[165] While the application of modern psychoprostheses may be considered invalid, this should at least serve as a warning not to generalise too much about early prostheses, while demonstrating that the use of such tools is deeply intertwined with notions of normality and identity. It is notable that this chapter has repeatedly called attention to how ancient authors have been referenced in modern times regarding the disabled and deaf body: the role of Classics in the ableism inherent in the modern West is one that deserves further study.

The use of aids by people with impairments is an important area for archaeologists and classicists to consider, for the light it sheds on the wider issue of the role objects have in shaping personhood. The ancient disabled body is too often studied in a clinical, etic manner, as representations in art, literature or mythology. An understanding of disability studies allows for the experienced, emic voice to be heard, and for a rather more positive approach to be taken than is often the case when dealing with the impaired. Notably, an understanding of the nature of sign language may be transferred to diverse areas of traditional study, such as oratory, pantomime and art history. The strategies people develop, whether technological or linguistic, are a testament not merely to the failure of the human body, but also to the adaptability and originality of the human mind.

Notes

1 Jain, 1999.
2 I would like to thank Jane Draycott for organising such a fascinating and timely conference. I am very grateful to Dan Orrells and Michael Squire for reading a very early draft of this chapter.
3 Serlin, 2006, p. 51.
4 Knappett, 2005, p. 169; de Preester and Tsakiris, 2009, p. 308, italics in original; see also Lury, 1998.
5 De Preester and Tsakiris, 2009.
6 See Sobchack, 2006 for an overview of these uses. See also Jain, 1999, p. 41 who has explored this term in general literature and the 'oddly constructed – or perhaps underconstructed and overobjectified – disabled body standing in for questions about bodies, selves, agency and technology'.
7 See for example Scully, 2009.
8 On dental prostheses, see Becker and Turfa, this volume, Draycott, this volume, and Lehmhaus, this volume; on extremity prostheses, see Finch, this volume, Eitler and Binder, this volume.
9 Bliquez, 1996, p. 2670.
10 Rose, 2003, p. 26.
11 Quayson, 2007, p. 10.
12 An issue raised in Trentin, 2013, p. 110 is the availability of slaves in the ancient world in order to assist the disabled, in this case the blind. Given the low status of slaves, they may have been perceived along the lines of modern aids.
13 See for example Crawford, 2014; the 'phantom limbs' that pervade classical art in terms of the absent limbs of sculptures are barely discussed in the scholarship; this is a subject for future development and comparison.
14 Davis, 2013, p. 78; Lane, 2006, p. 89.
15 Davis, 2008, p. 315.
16 Adams, 2017.
17 Pistorius, 2012, p. 119.
18 Pistorius, 2012, pp. 22–23.
19 Harvey, 2015.
20 Lapper, 2015, p. 32.
21 Murray, 2008, pp. 125–126.
22 Sobchack, 2006.
23 Crawford, 2015.
24 See for example de Preester and Tsakiris, 2009.
25 MacLachlan, 2004, p. 129.
26 Gallagher, Desmond and MacLachlan, 2008, p. 7.
27 Sobchack, 2006, p. 22.
28 Gallager, Desmond and MacLachlan, 2008, p. 2; 2002.
29 See for example Pedley, Giles and Hogan, 2005; Murray, 2008.
30 See for example Murray, 2008; Pray, 1996.
31 See for example Miller, 1987; Olsen, 2010; Hodder, 2012.
32 Olson, 2010, p. 35.
33 See for example Sofaer, 2006.
34 See for example Knappett, 2005; Knappett and Malafouris, 2008; see also Gell, 1998; Dobres and Robb, 2000.
35 See for example Hodder, 1982.
36 Malafouris, 2008a, p. 118.
37 Appadurai, 1986; Kurzman, 2001; Sobchack, 2006.
38 Macfarlane, 2010; Holmes, 2010, pp. 93–96.
39 See for example Hamilakis, 2013, pp. 25–26; Squire, 2016.

40 Merleau-Ponty, 2002, pp. 165–166.
41 See for example, Knappett, 2005, p. 24; Scully, 2009, p. 66; de Preester and Tsakiris, 2009; Malafouris, 2008b; 2009, p. 96; Mills, 2013.
42 Paterson, 2012, p. 165.
43 Shakespeare, 2014, p. 67.
44 Mills, 2013.
45 Mills, 2013, p. 789.
46 See for example Saerberg, 2010; see also Rodaway, 1994, p. 53.
47 Lacon or Philippus of Thessalonica. Thanks to Jessica Hughes and Alexia Petsalis-Diomidis for this reference. This epigram is followed by those referring to craftsmen dedicating their tools upon leaving their profession, a different type of association between people and things.
48 Hamilakis, 2013, pp. 67–69, p. 113, p. 197.
49 Masséglia, 2015, p. 87.
50 Adams, 2017.
51 See for example Knappett, 2005 *passim*.
52 Leigh, 2009, p. 146.
53 Garland Thomson, 1997, p. 11.
54 See for example Featherstone and Burrows, 1995; Ott, 2002, p. 3.
55 Kurzman, 2001; Sobchack, 2006, p. 17.
56 For example Black, 2014, p. 34.
57 Gray and Mentor, 1995, p. 230.
58 Kurzman, 2001, pp. 381–382.
59 Haraway, 2004, p. 8.
60 See for example Knappett 2005, p. 25; insights by users are available from, for example, Snell, 2015.
61 *pace* Chorost, 1995, p. 40.
62 Chorost, 1995, p. 28.
63 Chorost, 1995, p. 98.
64 Chorost, 2011. Communication disabilities such as deafness have two relevant issues: the relation between individual humans and objects/aids (prostheses), and the role that objects have in maintaining communications between humans, see Adams, in preparation a.
65 See for example Squire, 2011; more generally: Smith and Morra, 2006; Gallagher, Desmond and MacLachlan, 2006.
66 Quinn, 2004.
67 Recent reports in the media have explored the development of a sense of touch for such devices: for example, http://www.independent.co.uk/news/science/prosthetic-limbs-could-soon-feel-after-scientists-develop-skin-that-can-sense-touch-a6695786.html (accessed 18 February 2016).
68 Adams, in preparation a; see also Laes, 2011; Rose, 2003; 2006.
69 These were not invented before the second half of the seventeenth century: Jütte, 2005, p. 115.
70 Rose, 2006, p. 19.
71 Adams, 2017.
72 Rose, 2003, p. 75; Rose, 2006, p. 21.
73 There have been several recent studies of ancient gesture, for example Cairns, 2005; Fögen, 2009; Masséglia, 2015.
74 Stokoe, 2001. See also Armstrong and Wilcox, 2007, which begins with a discussion of Plato's *Cratylus*.
75 Laes, 2011, p. 46. A slightly different example is Battos the Lame of Cyrene, who lost political sovereignty because of his disability, Cosi, 1987, pp. 134–135; after Herodotus *Histories* 4.161.
76 Anderson and Carden-Coyne, 2007; Thomas, 2007; Schillmeier, 2010.

77 Swain, French and Cameron, 2003, p. 1.
78 Adams, in preparation b.
79 Holmes, 2010, p. 86; Oliver and Barnes, 2012.
80 Adams, 2017.
81 Baynton, 1996, p. 141; Davis, 1995; Crawford, 2014; Adams, 2017; Adams, in preparation b.
82 See also Shakespeare, 2006, p. 43.
83 Baynton, 1996.
84 Lane, 1992, p. 120.
85 See for example Hull, 2010.
86 See for example Sataloff and Sataloff, 2005.
87 Nittrouer, 2010, pp. 43–44; sign language is mentioned throughout (for example pp. 2–3, p. 51), for example in terms of how manual signs can be used to support the learning of English (Total Communication, or Sign Supported English). This is telling as the author, in the preface, claims to enjoy interacting with the Deaf community, and later acknowledges ASL as a 'true' language (p. 8); but the stance is undeniably audist.
88 See for example Baguley and Graham, 2009, p. 5; see also the evasive comment in Marriage, 2007, p. 142.
89 See for example Siegel, 2008.
90 Groce, 1985; see de Vos, 2011 for a contemporary example in Bali; Kusters, 2014.
91 Marschark *et al.*, 2010, p. 129.
92 Armstrong and Wilcox, 2007; Mathur and Rathmann, 2014.
93 Example given in Knappett, 2005, pp. 88–89.
94 Bauman, 2006.
95 Marschark and Spencer, 2010; Leigh, 2010.
96 Marschark and Spencer, 2010.
97 Silberman, 2015.
98 Silbermann, 2015, p. 108.
99 See for example Zeng, Popper and Fay, 2012.
100 Hersh and Johnson, 2003; Frost, 2009.
101 Archbold and Wheeler, 2010, p. 235.
102 www.nhs.uk/Livewell/hearing-problems/Pages/hearing-aids.aspx (accessed 22 April 2016).
103 Mitchell and Snyder, 2000, p. 3.
104 Leigh, 2010, p. 204; Crawford, 2014, p. 14.
105 See the patient case studies of 'Jack' and 'Rick' in Hogan, 2005, pp. 2–3.
106 https://www.facebook.com/TheDailyMoth/videos/487858631416042/ (accessed 23 February 2016).
107 https://www.starkeyhearingfoundation.org/ (accessed 7 March 2016).
108 That deaf people have a significantly greater tendency to encounter mental health issues than hearing people is now acknowledged: Du Feu and Chovaz, 2014; Austen, 2009; McKenna and O'Sullivan, 2009.
109 Adams, 2017.
110 Cooper, 2009; Nittrouer, 2010, p. 21; Fu and Galvin III, 2012, p. 257.
111 NHS Commissioning Board, 2013, p. 3; Marshark *et al.*, 2010, pp. 129–130.
112 See for example Plack, 2014, p. 253.
113 Zeng, 2012, p. 1.
114 Lane, 1992, p. 135.
115 Plack, 2014, pp. 248–249; see also Archbold and Wheeler, 2010, p. 227; Shapiro, 1993, p. 224; Marshark *et al.*, 2010, p. 133 argue that it is not necessarily the case that the earlier the cochlear implant is installed, the better. Concerns have also been raised concerning the medical profession possibly misleading parents about the results of such surgery, Lane, 1992.

116　Lane, 1992, p. 204. See also a YouTube compilation of switching on cochlear implants for the first time, including an apparently distressed child: https://www.youtube.com/watch?v=mbe7x8GP2Ds (accessed 7 March 2016).
117　Nittrouer, 2010, p. 14.
118　Leigh, 2009, p. 158.
119　For example, Milne, 2015, pp. 10, 183, 213.
120　Milne, 2015, pp. 221, 245.
121　Pedley and Giles, 2005, p. 30.
122　Archbold and Wheeler, 2010, p. 230; see also Baynton, 1996, pp. 80–81.
123　Lind and Dyer, 2005, p. 160.
124　Bragg, 1997, p. 2.
125　Bauman and Murray, 2014, p. xv.
126　Bauman and Murray, 2014, p. xxv.
127　Bauman and Murray, 2014, p. xxvii.
128　Kahne, 2013; see also Hauser and Kartheiser, 2014.
129　Slobin, 2008, p. 115.
130　Bulwer, 1644, no pagination.
131　Bulwer, 1644, pp. 131–132.
132　Bulwer, 1648, p. 88.
133　Bulwer, 1649.
134　Bulwer, 1648, p. 181; Bulwer's work is enhanced by his engagement with deaf people, although it is notable that this work is focused mainly on the lack of speech (or the implications for it, such as the nasalisation common for deaf people and need to lipread) than the adoption of sign. This work was produced some years before Dr John Wallis demonstrated a form of signing in front of the Royal Society in 1662, Geen and Tassinary, 2002, p. 276.
135　Bulwer, 1648, no pagination.
136　Bulwer, 1648, p. 16.
137　Greenblatt, 1995; Geen and Tassinary, 2002.
138　Goring, 2014.
139　See for example Poulakos, 2007.
140　But see Baynton, 1996, pp. 86–87; Bragg, 1997.
141　Lada-Richards, 2010, p. 22, with reference to a work by John Weaver on ancient pantomime from 1712.
142　*The Tattler* 115, 3 January 1709, quoted in Lada-Richards, 2010, pp. 32–33.
143　See Lada-Richards, 2016 and references.
144　Lada-Richards, 2016, p. 133.
145　Johnston and Schembri, 2007, p. 273, italics in original.
146　Lada-Richards, 2016, p. 146.
147　See also Slaney, 2017.
148　It is also worth stressing that most signers are quick to disassociate their language from the art form of mime, mainly due to the historical fight to obtain language recognition.
149　Lada-Richards, 2013, p. 122; see also Lada-Richards, 2016, p. 146 on Manilius *Astronomica* 5.480b, 483.
150　Lada-Richards, 2016, p. 148; little evidence remains for the texts for pantomimes, with one possible libretto: Hall, 2008.
151　See for example Bremmer and Roodenburg, 1992; Bragg, 1997, p. 7.
152　Masséglia, 2015.
153　Lada-Richards, 2003.
154　See for example Masséglia, 2015, p. 62.
155　See for example Zanker, 1988; Hölscher, 2004.
156　Elsner, 2014, p. 1.
157　See for example Squire, 2015.

158 Elsner, 2010; Pich and Squire, 2016.
159 Pich and Squire, 2016.
160 See for example Russo, 2004.
161 Sacks, 2012, p. 71, citing a paper delivered by William Skotoe at the New York Academy of Sciences in 1979. Note that Bulwer's insistence that speech requires movement, and therefore represents four dimensions, takes a slightly different perspective here.
162 Young and Temple, 2014, p. 176.
163 Tal, 2010; see also Mirzoeff, 1995, p. 106.
164 Tal, 2010, p. 116. Lack of space does not allow a more detailed exploration of artists and their engagement with the deaf (for example da Vinci: Mirzoeff, 1995, p. 13) or deaf artists (for example Reynolds: Mirzoeff, 1995, pp. 27–28), or indeed the engagement of neoclassical artists and deafness (for example David's students: Mirzoeff, 1995, p. 70).
165 Adams, in preparation b.

Bibliography

Adams, E. (2017) 'Fragmentation and the Body's Boundaries: Reassessing the Body in Parts', in Draycott, J. and Graham, E.-J. (edd.) *Bodies of Evidence: Ancient Anatomical Votives Past, Present and Future.* Abingdon: Routledge, pp. 193–213.

Adams, E. (in preparation a) 'Deafness', in Laes, C. (ed.) *A Cultural History of Disability in Antiquity.* London: Bloomsbury.

Adams, E. (in preparation b) 'The Forgotten 'Other': Disability Studies and the Classical Body'.

Anderson, J. and Carden-Coyne, A. (2007) 'Enabling the Past: New Perspectives in the History of Disability', *European Review of History* 14, pp. 447–457.

Appadurai, A. (ed.) (1986) *The Social Life of Things: Commodities in Cultural Perspective.* Cambridge: Cambridge University Press.

Archbold, S. and Wheeler, A. (2010) 'Cochlear Implants: Family and Young People's Perspectives', in Marschark, M. and Spencer, P. E. (edd.) *Oxford Handbook of Deaf Studies, Language, and Education. Volume 2.* Oxford: Oxford University Press, pp. 226–240.

Armstrong, D. and Wilcox, S. (2007) *The Gestural Origin of Language.* Oxford: Oxford University Press.

Austen, S. (2009) 'Mental Health and Pre-lingual Deafness', in Graham, J. and Baguley, D. (edd.) *Ballantyne's Deafness: Seventh Edition.* Chichester: Wiley-Blackwell, pp. 202–212.

Austin, Rev. G. (1806) *Chironomia: Treatise on Rhetorical Delivery.* London: Bulmer and Co.

Baguley, D. and Graham, J. (2009) 'Introduction', in Graham, J. and Baguley, D. (edd.) *Ballantyne's Deafness: Seventh Edition.* Chichester: Wiley-Blackwell, pp. 1–5.

Bauman, H.-D. L. (2006) 'Towards a Poetics of Vision, Space and the Body: Sign Language and Literary Theory', in Davis, L. J. (ed.) *The Disability Studies Reader: Second Edition.* London: Routledge, pp. 355–366.

Bauman, H.-D. L. and Murray, J. (2014) 'Deaf Gain: an Introduction', in Bauman, H.-D. L. and Murray, J. (edd.) *Deaf Gain: Raising the Stakes for Human Diversity.* Minneapolis, MN and London: University of Minnesota Press, pp. xv–xlii.

Baynton, D. C. (1996) *Forbidden Signs: American Culture and the Campaign against Sign Language.* Chicago, IL and London: University of Chicago Press.

Black, D. (2014) 'Where Bodies End and Artefacts Begin: Tools, Machines and Interfaces', *Body and Society* 20, pp. 31–60.

Bliquez, L. (1996) 'Prosthetics in Classical Antiquity: Greek, Etruscan and Roman Prosthetics', in *ANRW* II 37.3, pp. 2640–2676.

Bragg, L. (1997) 'Visual-kinetic Communication in Europe before 1600: A Survey of Sign Lexicons and Finger Alphabets Prior to the Rise of Deaf Education', *Journal of Deaf Studies and Deaf Education* 2, pp. 1–25.

Bulwer, J. (1644) *Chirologia: or the Naturall Language of the Hand. Composed of the Speaking Motions, and Discoursing Gestures thereof. Whereunto is added Chironomia: or, the Art of Manuall Rhetoricke. Consisting of the Naturall Expressions, Digested by Art in the Hand, as the Chiefest Instrument of Eloquence.* London: Thomas Harper.

Bulwer, J. (1648) *Philocopus, or the deaf and dumbe mans friend.* London: Humphrey and Moseley.

Bulwer, J. (1649) *Pathomyotomia, or A dissection of the significative muscles of the affections of the minde.* London: Humphrey Moseley.

Cairns, D. (ed.) (2005) *Body Language in the Greek and Roman Worlds.* Swansea: Classical Press of Wales.

Chorost, M. (2005) *Rebuilt: How Becoming Part Computer Made Me More Human.* London: Souvenir Press.

Chorost, M. (2011) *World Wide Mind: The Coming Integration of Humanity, Machines and the Internet.* New York, NY, London, Toronto and Sydney: Free Press.

Cooper, H. (2009) 'Cochlear Implants', in Graham, J. and Baguley, D. (edd.) *Ballantyne's Deafness: Seventh Edition.* Chichester: Wiley-Blackwell, pp. 229–241.

Cosi, D. M. (1987) 'Jammed Communication: Battos, the Founder of Cyrene, Stammering and Castrated', in Ciani, M. G. (ed.) *The Regions of Silence: Studies on the Difficulty of Communicating.* Amsterdam: J. C. Gieben, pp. 115–144.

Crawford, C. (2014) *Phantom Limb: Amputation, Embodiment, and Prosthetic Technology.* New York, NY and London: New York University Press.

Crawford, C. (2015) 'Body Image, Prostheses, Phantom Limbs', *Body and Society* 21, pp. 221–244.

Davis, L. (1995) *Enforcing Normalcy: Disability, Deafness and the Body.* London: Verso.

Davis, L. (2008) 'Postdeafness', in Bauman, H.-D. L. (ed.) *Open Your Eyes: Deaf Studies Talking.* Minneapolis, MN and London: University of Minnesota Press, pp. 314–325.

Davis, L. (2013) *The End of Normal. Identity in a Biocultural Era.* Ann Arbor, MI: University of Michigan Press.

De Preester, H. and Tsakiris, M. (2009) 'Body-extension Versus Body-incorporation: is There a Need for a Body-model?', *Phenomenology and the Cognitive Sciences* 8, pp. 307–319.

De Vos, C. (2011) 'Kata Kolok Color Terms and the Emergence of Lexical Signs in Rural Signing Communities', *The Senses and Society* 6, pp. 68–76.

Dobres, M.-A. and Robb, J. (edd.) (2000) *Agency in Archaeology.* London: Routledge.

Du Feu, M. and Chovaz, C. (2014) *Mental Health and Deafness.* Oxford: Oxford University Press.

Elsner, J. (2010) 'Art History as Ekphrasis', *Art History* 33, pp. 10–27.

Elsner, J. (2014) 'Introduction', in Elsner, J. and Meyer, M. (edd.) *Art and Rhetoric in Roman Culture.* Cambridge: Cambridge University Press, pp. 1–35.

Featherstone, M. and Burrows, R. (1995) 'Cultures of Technological Embodiment: An Introduction', *Body and Society* 1, pp. 1–19.

Fögen, T. (2009) '*Sermo corporis*: Ancient Reflections on *gestus, vultus* and *vox*', in Fögen, T. and Lee, M. (edd.) *Bodies and Boundaries in Graeco-Roman Antiquity*. Berlin and New York, NY: Walter de Gruyter, pp. 15–43.

Frost, G. (2009) 'Hearing Aids', in Graham, J. and Baguley, D. (edd.) *Ballantyne's Deafness: Seventh Edition*. Chichester: Wiley-Blackwell, pp. 213–228.

Fu, Q.-J. and Galvin III, J. J. (2012) 'Auditory Training for Cochlear Implant Patients', in Zeng, F.-G., Popper, A. N. and Fay, R. R. (edd.) *Auditory Prostheses: New Horizons*. Springer Handbook of Auditory Research 39. New York, NY: Springer-Verlag, pp. 257–278.

Gallagher, P., Desmond, D. and MacLachlan, M. (2008) 'Psychoprosthetics: An Introduction', in Gallagher, P., Desmond, D. and MacLachlan, M. (edd.) *Psychoprosthetics*. London: Springer, pp. 1–10.

Garland-Thomson, R. (1997) *Extraordinary Bodies: Figuring Physical Disability in American Culture and Literature*. New York, NY: Columbia University Press.

Geen, T. R. and Tassinary, L. G. (2002) 'The Mechanization of Emotional Expression in John Bulwer's "Pathomyotomia" (1649)', *American Journal of Psychology* 115, pp. 275–299.

Gell, A. (1998) *Art and Agency: An Anthropological Theory*. Oxford: Oxford University Press.

Goring, P. (2014) 'The Elocutionary Movement in Britain', in MacDonald, M. (ed.) *The Oxford Handbook of Rhetorical Studies*. Oxford: Oxford University Press: online.

Gray, C. H. and Mentor, S. (1995) 'The Cyborg Body Politic and the New World Order', in Brahm Jr, G. and Driscoll, M. (edd.) *Prosthetic Territories: Politics and Hypertechnologies*. Boulder, CO, San Francisco, CA and Oxford: Westview Press, pp. 219–247.

Greenblatt, S. (1995) 'Toward a Universal Language of Motion: reflections on a Seventeenth-Century Muscle Man', in Foster, S. L. (ed.) *Choreographing History*. Bloomington, IN: Indiana University Press, pp. 25–31.

Groce, N. E. (1985) *Everyone Here Spoke Sign Language: Hereditary Deafness on Martha's Vineyard*. Cambridge, MA: Harvard University Press.

Hall, E. (2008) 'Is the "Barcelona *Alcestis*" a Latin Pantomime Libretto?', in Hall, E. and Wyles, R. (edd.) *New Directions in Ancient Pantomime*. Oxford: Oxford University Press, pp. 258–282.

Hamilakis, Y. (2013) *Archaeology and the Senses: Human Experience, Memory and Affect*. Cambridge: Cambridge University Press.

Haraway, D. (2004) *The Haraway Reader*. New York, NY and London: Routledge.

Harvey, C. (2015) 'What's Disability Got to Do with it? Changing Constructions of Oscar Pistorius before and after the Death of Reeva Steenkamp', *Disability and Society* 30, pp. 299–304.

Hauser, P. and Kartheiser, G. (2014) 'Advantages of Learning a Signed Language', in Bauman, H.-D. L. and Murray, J. (edd.) *Deaf Gain: Raising the Stakes for Human Diversity*. Minneapolis, MN and London: University of Minnesota Press, pp. 133–145.

Hersh, M. and Johnson, M. (2003) *Assistive Technology for the Hearing-impaired, Deaf and Deafblind*. London: Springer.

Hodder, I. (1982) *Symbols in Action: Ethnoarchaeological Studies of Material Culture*. Cambridge: Cambridge University Press.

Hodder, I. (2012) *Entangled: An Archaeology of the Relationships between Humans and Things*. Chichester: Wiley-Blackwell.

Hogan, A. (2005) 'Introduction: towards a more Holistic and Transdisciplinary Model of Rehabilitation', in Pedley, K., Giles, E. and Hogan, A. (edd.) *Adult Cochlear Implant Rehabilitation*. London and Philadelphia, PA: Whurr Publishers, pp. 1–7.

Holmes, B. (2010) 'Medical Knowledge and Technology', in Garrison, D. (ed.) *A Cultural History of the Human Body in Antiquity*. Oxford and New York, NY: Berg, pp. 83–105.

Hölscher, T. (2004) *The Language of Images in Roman Art*. Cambridge: Cambridge University Press.

Hull, R. (ed.) (2010) *Introduction to Aural Rehabilitation*. San Diego, CA, Oxford and Brisbane: Plural Publishing.

Jain, S. (1999) 'The Prosthetic Imagination: Enabling and Disabling the Prosthesis Trope', *Science, Technology and Human Values* 24, pp. 31–54.

Johnston, T. and Schembri, A. (2007) *Australian Sign Language (Auslan): An Introduction to Sign Language Linguistics*. Cambridge: Cambridge University Press.

Jütte, R. (2005) *A History of the Senses: From Antiquity to Cyberspace*. Cambridge: Polity.

Kahne, B. (2013) *Deaf Tips: Twelve Lessons from the Deaf World to Improve Your Communication in Your Personal, Social, and Professional Life*. CreateSpace Independent Publishing Platform.

Knappett, C. (2005) *Thinking Through Material Culture: An Interdisciplinary Perspective*. Philadelphia, PA: University of Pennsylvania Press.

Knappett, C. and Malafouris, L. (edd.) (2008) *Material Agency: Towards a Non-Anthropocentric Approach*. London: Springer.

Kurzman, S. (2001) 'Presence and Prosthesis: A Response to Nelson and Wright', *Cultural Anthropology* 16, pp. 374–387.

Kusters, A. (2014) 'Deaf Gain and Shared Signing Communities,' in Bauman, H-D. L. and Murray, J. (edd.) *Deaf Gain: Raising the Stakes for Human Diversity*. Minneapolis, MN and London: University of Minnesota Press, pp. 285–305.

Lada-Richards, I. (2003) ' "Mobile Statuary": Refractions of Pantomime Dancing from Callistratus to Emma Hamilton and Andrew Ducrow', *International Journal of the Classical Tradition* 10, pp. 3–37.

Lada-Richards, I. (2010) 'Dead but not Extinct: on Reinventing Pantomime Dancing in Eighteenth-century England and France', in Macintosh, F. (ed.) *The Ancient Dancer in the Modern World Responses to Greek and Roman Dance*. Oxford: Oxford University Press, pp. 19–38.

Lada-Richards, I. (2013) '*Mutata corpora*: Ovid's Changing Forms and the Metamorphic Bodies of Pantomime Dancing', *TAPA* 143, pp. 105–152.

Lada-Richards, I. (2016) 'Dancing Trees: Ovid's *Metamorphoses* and the Imprint of Pantomime Dancing', *AJP* 137, pp. 131–169.

Laes, C. (2011) 'Silent Witnesses: Deaf-mutes in Graeco-Roman Antiquity', *CW* 104, pp. 451–473.

Lane, H. (1992) *The Mask of Benevolence: Disabling the Deaf Community*. New York, NY: Knopf.

Lane, H. (2006) 'Construction of Deafness', in Davis, L. J. (ed.) *The Disability Studies Reader: Second Edition*. London: Routledge, pp. 79–92.

Lapper, A. (2005) *My Life in my Hands*. London: Pocket.

Leigh, I. (2009) *A Lens on Deaf Identities*. Oxford: Oxford University Press.

Leigh, I. (2010) 'Reflections on Identity', in Marschark, M. and Spencer, P. E. (edd.) *Oxford Handbook of Deaf Studies, Language, and Education. Vol. 2*. Oxford: Oxford University Press, pp. 195–209.

Lind, C. and Dyer, L. (2005) 'Social-interactional Elements of Communication Therapy for Adult Cochlear Implant Recipients', in Pedley, K., Giles, E. and Hogan, A. (edd.) *Adult Cochlear Implant Rehabilitation*. London and Philadelphia, PA: Whurr Publishers, pp. 148–163.

Lury, C. (1998) *Prosthetic Culture: Photography, Memory and Identity*. London and New York, NY: Routledge.

Macfarlane, P. (2010) 'Health and Disease', in Garrison, D. (ed.) *A Cultural History of the Human Body in Antiquity*. Oxford and New York, NY: Berg, pp. 45–66.

MacLachlan, M. (2004) *Embodiment: Clinical, Critical and Cultural Perspectives on Health and Illness*. Maidenhead: Open University Press.

Malafouris, L. (2008a) 'Is it "Me" or is it "Mine"? The Mycenaean Sword as a Body-part', in Borić, D. and Robb, J. (edd.) *Past Bodies: Body-Centered Research in Archaeology*. Oxford: Oxbow, pp. 115–123.

Malafouris, L. (2008b) 'Beads for a Plastic Mind: the "Blind Man's Stick" (BMS) Hypothesis and the Active Nature of Material Culture', *CAJ* 18, pp. 401–414.

Malafouris, L. (2009) 'Between Brains, Bodies and Things: *Tectonoetic* Awareness and the Extended Self', in Renfrew, C., Frith, C. and Malafouris, L. (ed.) *The Sapient Mind: Archaeology Meets Neuroscience*. Oxford: Oxford University Press, pp. 89–104.

Marriage, J. (2007) 'Habilitation of Children with Permanent Hearing Impairment', in Graham, J. and Baguley, D. (edd.) *Ballantyne's Deafness: Seventh Edition*. Chichester: Wiley-Blackwell, pp. 139–150.

Marschark, M., Sarchet, T., Rhoten, C. and Zupan, M. (2010) 'Will Cochlear Implants Close the Reading Achievement Gap for Deaf Students?', in Marschark, M. and Spencer, P. E. (edd.) *Oxford Handbook of Deaf Studies, Language, and Education*. Vol. 2. Oxford: Oxford University Press, pp. 127–143.

Marschark, M. and Spencer, P. E. (2010) 'The Promises (?) of Deaf Education: from Research to Practice and Back Again', in Marschark, M. and Spencer, P. E. (edd.) *Oxford Handbook of Deaf Studies, Language, and Education*. Vol. 2. Oxford: Oxford University Press, pp. 1–14.

Masséglia, J. (2015) *Body Language in Hellenistic Art and Society*. Oxford: Oxford University Press.

Mathur, G. and Rathmann, C. (2014) 'The Structure of Sign Language', in Goldrick, M., Ferreira, V. and Miozzo, M. (edd.) *The Oxford Handbook of Language Production*. Oxford: Oxford University Press, pp. 379–392.

McKenna, L. and O'Sullivan, A. (2009) 'Psychological Aspects of Acquired Hearing Loss', in Graham, J. and Baguley, D. (edd.) *Ballantyne's Deafness: Seventh Edition*. Chichester: Wiley-Blackwell, pp. 189–201.

Merleau-Ponty, M. [Trans. C. Smith] (2002) *Phenomenology of Perception*. London and New York, NY: Routledge.

Miller, D. (1987) *Material Culture and Mass Consumption*. Oxford: Blackwell.

Mills, F. B. (2013) 'A Phenomenological Approach to Psychoprosthetics', *Disability and Rehabilitation* 35, pp. 785–791.

Milne, J. (2015) *Breaking the Silence*. London: Coronet.

Mirzoeff, N. (1995) *Silent Poetry: Deafness, Sign and Visual Culture in Modern France*. Princeton, NJ: Princeton University Press.

Mitchell, D. T. and Snyder, S. L. (2000) *Narrative Prosthesis: Disability and the Dependencies of Discourse*. Ann Arbor, MI: University of Michigan Press.

Murray, C. (2008) 'Embodiment and Prosthetics', in Gallagher, P., Desmond, D. and MacLachlan, M. (edd.) *Psychoprosthetics*. London: Springer, pp. 119–130.

NHS Commissioning Board 2013: *NHS D09/S/A. NHS Standard contract for cochlear implants.* NHS England. www.england.nhs.uk/commissioning/wp.../d09-ear-surg-coch-0414.pdf. Downloaded 12 June 2015.

Nittrouer, S. (2010) *Early Development of Children with Hearing Loss.* San Diego, CA, Oxford and Brisbane: Plural Publishing.

Oliver, M. and Barnes, C. (2012) *The New Politics of Disablement.* Basingstoke: Houndsmills.

Olsen, B. (2010) *In Defense of Things: Archaeology and the Ontology of Objects.* Lanham, New York, NY, Toronto and Plymouth: Altamira Press.

Ott, K. (2002) 'The Sum of its Parts: an Introduction to Modern Histories of Prosthetics', in Ott, K., Serlin, D. and Mihm, S. (edd.) *Artificial Parts, Practical Lives: Modern Histories of Prosthetics.* New York, NY and London: New York University Press, pp. 1–42.

Paterson, K. (2012) 'It's about Time! Understanding the Experience of Speech Impairment', in Watson, N., Roulstone, A. and Thomas, C. (edd.) *Routledge Handbook of Disability Studies.* London: Routledge, pp. 165–177.

Pedley, K. and Giles, E. (2005) 'The Assessment of Adult Cochlear Implant Candidates', in Pedley, K., Giles, E. and Hogan, A. (edd.) *Adult Cochlear Implant Rehabilitation.* London and Philadelphia, PA: Whurr Publishers, pp. 8–49.

Pedley, K., Giles, E. and Hogan, A. (edd.) (2005) *Adult Cochlear Implant Rehabilitation.* London and Philadelphia, PA: Whurr Publishers.

Pich, F. and Squire, M. (2016) 'Reading as Seeing: A Conversation on Ancient and Modern Intermedialities', *Arabeschi* 8, pp. 44–76.

Pistorius, O. (2012) *Blade Runner.* London: Virgin.

Plack, C. J. (2014) *The Sense of Hearing: Second Edition.* London: Psychology Press.

Poulakos, R. (2007) 'Modern Interpretations of Classical Greek Rhetoric', in Worthington, I. (ed.) *A Companion to Greek Rhetoric.* Oxford: Blackwell Publishing, pp. 16–24.

Pray, J. L. (1996) 'Psychosocial Aspects of Adult Aural Rehabilitation', in Mosely, M. and Bally, S. (edd.) *Communication Therapy: An Integrated Approach to Aural Rehabilitation with Deaf and Hard of Hearing Adolescents and Adults.* Washington, DC: Gallaudet University Press, pp. 128–148.

Quayson, A. (2007) *Aesthetic Nervousness: Disability and the Crisis of Representation.* New York, NY: Columbia University Press.

Quinn, M. (2004) *Marc Quinn: The Complete Marbles.* New York, NY: Mary Boone Gallery.

Rodaway, P. (1994) *Sensuous Geographies: Body, Sense and Place.* London and New York, NY: Routledge.

Rose, M. L. (2003) *The Staff of Oedipus: Transforming Disability in Ancient Greece.* Ann Arbor, MI: University of Michigan Press.

Rose, M. L. (2006) 'Deaf and Dumb in Ancient Greece', in Davis, L. J. (ed.) *The Disability Studies Reader: Second Edition.* London: Routledge, pp. 17–31.

Russo, T. (2004) 'Iconicity and Productivity in Sign Language Discourse: An Analysis of Three LIS Discourse Registers', *Sign Language Studies* 4, pp. 164–197.

Sacks, O. (2012) *Seeing Voices: A Journey into the World of the Deaf.* London: Picador.

Saerberg, S. (2010) 'Just Go Straight Ahead', *The Senses and Society* 5, pp. 364–381.

Sataloff, R. T. and Sataloff, J. (edd.) (2005) *Hearing Loss: Fourth Edition.* New York, NY and London: Taylor and Francis.

Schillmeier, M. (2010) *Rethinking Disability: Bodies, Senses and Things.* New York, NY and London: Routledge.

Scully, J. L. (2009) 'Disability and the Thinking Body', in Kristiansen, K., Vehmas, S. and Shakespeare, T. (edd.) *Arguing About Disability: Philosophical Perspectives.* London: Routledge, pp. 57–73.

Serlin, D. (2006) 'The Other Arms Race', in Davis, L. J. (ed.) *The Disability Studies Reader: Second Edition.* London: Routledge, pp. 49–65.

Shakespeare, T. (2006) *Disability Rights and Wrongs.* London: Routledge.

Shakespeare, T. (2014) *Disability Rights and Wrongs Revisited.* Routledge.

Shapiro, J. (1993) *No Pity: People with Disabilities Forging a New Civil Rights Movement.* New York, NY: Three Rivers Press.

Siegel, L. M. (2008) *The Human Right to Language: Communication Access for Deaf Children.* Washington, DC: Gallaudet University Press.

Silberman, S. 2015. *Neurotribes: The Legacy of Autism and How to Think Smarter about People who Think Differently.* Crows Nest: Allen and Unwin.

Slaney, H. (2017) 'Motion Sensors: Perceiving Movement in Roman Pantomime', in Betts, E. (ed.) *Senses of the Empire: Multisensory Approaches to Roman Culture.* Abingdon and New York, NY: Routledge, pp. 159–175.

Slobin, D. I. (2008) 'Breaking the Molds: Signed Languages and the Nature of Human Language', *Sign Language Studies* 8, pp. 114–130.

Smith, M. and Morra, J. (edd.) (2006) *The Prosthetic Impulse: from a Posthuman Present to a Biocultural Future.* Cambridge, MA and London: MIT.

Snell, L. (2015) 'Documenting the Lived Experiences of Young Adult Cochlear Implant Users: "Feeling" Sound, Fluidity and Blurring Boundaries', *Disability and Society* 30, pp. 340–352.

Sobchack, V. (2006) 'A Leg to Stand on: Prosthetics, Metaphor, and Materiality', in Smith, M. and Morra, J. (edd.) *The Prosthetic Impulse: from a Posthuman Present to a Biocultural Future.* Cambridge, MA and London: MIT Press, pp. 17–41.

Sofaer, J. R. (2006) *The Body as Material Culture: A Theoretical Osteoarchaeology.* Cambridge: Cambridge University Press.

Squire, M. (2011) *The Art of the Body: Antiquity and its Legacy.* London: I. B. Tauris.

Squire, M. (2015) 'Ecphrasis: Visual and Verbal Interactions in Ancient Greek and Latin Literature', Oxford Handbooks Online: 10.1093/oxfordhb/9780199935390.013.58.

Squire, M. (ed.) (2016) *Sight and the Ancient Senses.* London and New York, NY: Routledge.

Stokoe, W. C. (2001) *Language in Hand: Why Sign Came Before Speech.* Washington, DC: Gallaudet University Press.

Swain, J., French, S. and Cameron, C. (2003) 'Introduction: Enabling Questions', in Swain, J., French, S. and Cameron, C. (edd.) *Controversial Issues in a Disabling Society.* Oxford: Oxford University Press, pp. 1–7.

Tal, G. (2010) 'The Gestural Language in Francisco Goya's Sleep of Reason Produces Monsters', *Word and Image* 26, pp. 115–127.

Thomas, C. (2007) *Sociologies of Disability and Illness: Contested Ideas in Disability Studies and Medical Sociology.* Basingstoke and New York, NY: Palgrave Macmillan.

Trentin, L. (2013) 'Exploring Visual Impairment in Ancient Rome', in Laes, C., Goodey, C. F. and Rose, M. L. (edd.) *Disabilities in Roman Antiquity: Disparate Bodies A Capite ad Calcem.* Leiden: Brill, pp. 89–114.

The Warnock Report (1978) *Special Educational Needs. Report of the Committee of Enquiry into the Education of Handicapped Children and Young People.* London.

The WHO Report (2011) *World Health Organization Report on Disability.* World Health Organization.

Young, A. and Temple, B. (2014) *Approaches to Social Research: The Case of Deaf Studies.* Oxford: Oxford University Press.

Zanker, P. (1988) *The Power of Images in the Age of Augustus.* Ann Arbor, MI: University of Michigan Press.

Zeng, F.-G. (2012) 'Advances in Auditory Prostheses', in Zeng, F.-G., Popper, A. N. and Fay, R. R. (edd.) *Auditory Prostheses: New Horizons.* Springer Handbook of Auditory Research 39. New York, NY: Springer-Verlag, pp. 1–12.

Zeng, F.-G., Popper, A. N. and Fay, R. R. (edd.) (2012) *Auditory Prostheses: New Horizons.* Springer Handbook of Auditory Research 39. New York, NY: Springer-Verlag.

Index

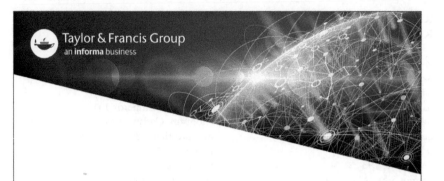

Milton Keynes UK
Ingram Content Group UK Ltd.
UKHW040102071024
449327UK00019B/744

9 780367 733605